MEDICAL EDUCATION
AT ST BARTHOLOMEW'S HOSPITAL
1123–1995

TO JENNY

MEDICAL EDUCATION AT ST BARTHOLOMEW'S HOSPITAL 1123–1995

Keir Waddington

THE BOYDELL PRESS

First published 2003

Published by The Boydell Press
An imprint of Boydell & Brewer Ltd
PO Box 9, Woodbridge, Suffolk IP12 3DF, UK
and of Boydell & Brewer Inc.
PO Box 41026, Rochester, NY 14604–4126, USA
website: www.boydell.co.uk

ISBN 0 85115 919 2

A catalogue record for this book is available from the British Library

Library of Congress Cataloging-in-Publication Data
Waddington, Keir, 1970–
Medical education at St. Bartholomew's Hospital, 1123–1995 /
Keir Waddington.
p. cm.
Includes bibliographical references.
1. St. Bartholomew's Hospital (London, England)–History. 2. Teaching
hospitals–Great Britain–London–History. I. Title.
RA988.L8 S323 2003
362.1'094212–dc21
2002012483

Typeset by Keystroke, Jacaranda Lodge, Wolverhampton
Printed in Great Britain by
St Edmundsbury Press Ltd, Bury St Edmunds, Suffolk

Contents

CONTENTS

Illustrations

Figures

Plates

Tables

Acknowledgements

In writing this book, my main debt lies with Marion Rae and Sally Gilbert in the Archive at St Bartholomew's. Without their help, support and company I doubt this book would have appeared in the way that it has. The archivists at the Wellcome Library have been invaluable in aiding me reconstruct the broader picture of London medical education. I also want to thank the librarians at Guildhall Library, and the archivists at the University of London for their patient assistance. In addition, Murray Milgate and Brian Callingham provided valuable assistance, unearthing information about the wartime experiences of students from St Bartholomew's at Queens' College, Cambridge. At the Rockefeller Archive Centre, gratitude is owed to Michelle Powers for information about the time spent in the USA by Walter Fletcher, Francis Fraser and Wilmot Parker Herringham. I would also like to thank the staff at the Public Record Office for their aid. I am grateful to the staff of the London Metropolitan Archive and to those at the British Library, Royal College of Physicians, Royal College of Surgeons, Institute of Education Library, Cardiff Arts and Social Sciences Library, and the Wellcome Library for their invaluable help.

At St Bartholomew's, a debt is owed to Peter McCrorie, Adam Feather and Anne Musker, and to the rest of the staff in the Centre for Medical and Dental Education, for giving me a desk and providing support. I would also like to thank the Archives Committee for their encouragement, along with Jackie Roe at the Guild of Nurses. In the medical school, considerable support was provided not only by all those who were kind enough to agree to be interviewed, but in particular by Julian Axe, Michael Besser, Michael Farthing, Cedric Gilson and David Lowe.

I am grateful to the Archives and Museum of St Bartholomew's Hospital for permission to reproduce the plates in the book.

Considerable assistance has also been provided by numerous colleagues and friends. A considerable debt is owed to Anne Hardy and Bill Jones whose careful reading and many useful comments have been invaluable. I am grateful to Bill Bynum, Roger Cooter, Elsbeth Heaman, Chris Lawrence, Roy Porter, Carole Rawcliffe, Harriet Richardson, Julia Shepherd, John Warner and Susan Williams who read parts of this book during the writing process and offered many useful insights and comments. I am also indebted to Kaye Bagshaw, Martin Daunton, Sue Gold, Lesley Hall, John Henderson, Pat Hudson, Caroline Overy, Sally Sheard and Trevor Turner for their suggestions and support. I would also like to thank Peter Sowden at Boydell for making this book possible and for his support throughout the publication process. As usual, a considerable debt is owed to Jennifer Haynes for her enthusiasm, questioning and willingness to help me. Any mistakes are of course my own.

Without the generous support of the Special Trustees of St Bartholomew's Hospital and the assistance of John Dennis this book would not have been possible.

Keir Waddington
Cardiff University, February 2002

Abbreviations

AHA	Area Health Authority
BECC	British Empire Cancer Campaign
BHM	*Bulletin of the History of Medicine*
BLQ	Bartholomew's, London and Queen Mary's
BMA	British Medical Association
BMJ	*British Medical Journal*
BMS	basic medical science
CELC	City and East London Confederation
CVCP	Committee of Vice-chancellors and Principals
DHSS	Department of Health and Social Security
EcHR	*Economic History Review*
EHR	*English Historical Review*
EMS	Emergency Medical Service
EMIS	Educational and Medical Illustration Services
FRCS	Fellow of the Royal College of Surgeons
GMC	General Medical Council
HEFCE	Higher Education Funding Council for England
ICRF	Imperial Cancer Research Fund
JMERG	Joint Medical Education Research Group
LCC	London County Council
LGB	Local Government Board
LMA	London Metropolitan Archive
LRCP	Licentiate of the Royal College of Physicians
LSA	Licentiate of the Society of Apothecaries
LSMW	London School of Medicine for Women
MAB	Metropolitan Asylums Board
MCQ	multiple choice question
MOH	Medical Officer of Health
MRC	Medical Research Council
MRCP	Member of the Royal College of Physicians
MRCS	Member of the Royal College of Surgeons
MTC	Merchant Taylors' Company
NEMRHA	North East Metropolitan Regional Health Authority
NETRHA	North East Thames Regional Health Authority
NHS	National Health Service
OSCE	objective structure clinical examination
PBL	problem-based learning
PRO	Public Record Office

QMC	Queen Mary College
QMW	Queen Mary and Westfield College
RAWP	Resource Allocation Working Party
RC	Royal Commission
RHA	Regional Health Authority
SC	Select Committee
SDL	self-directed learning
SHM	*Social History of Medicine*
SIFT	Service Increment for Teaching
SSM	special study modules
SU	Students' Union
TES	*Times Education Supplement*
THES	*Times Higher Education Supplement*
UFC	University Funding Council
UGC	University Grants Committee
ULL	University of London Library

Introduction

> The presence of an undergraduate medical school in a hospital gives rise to two groups of requirements, which are not existent in a hospital concerned only with the care of patients. First, there must be the physical space needed by the medical school wholly for its teachers and students. Secondly, the construction of the wards, outpatient departments, operating theatres, pathology departments of a teaching hospital must be on a larger scale and more elaborate than would be needed for patients alone, in order that effective teaching may take place.[1]

So said the governors of St Bartholomew's Hospital after a dispute with the lecturers in the Medical College in 1965. Although the subsequent agreement over teaching and clinical space recognised the role St Bartholomew's had as a teaching hospital, when teaching started is less certain. While the hospital and priory were established in 1123, provision for the training of doctors took longer to emerge. Several versions of how clinical instruction started at the hospital have been put forward, although few have explained why a school was relatively slow to evolve. Some have claimed that effective instruction commenced in 1765 when Percival Pott delivered his lectures on surgery. Other evidence suggests that apprentices had at least been present since the mid-seventeenth century. Although no formal charter or foundation existed until 1921, the presence of a medical school at St Bartholomew's had been referred to since the 1800s. For many, the College went on to symbolise tradition, fierce institutional loyalty and a particular style of academic medicine. However, little is known about how the institution worked and developed, or about its culture.[2]

The same might be said for the history of medical education. It has customarily been ancillary to larger themes in medical history, forming what

---

[1] Memorandum from the governors, 1965, HA 41. Unless otherwise stated, all archival sources are held at the St Bartholomew's Hospital archives, West Smithfield, London.

[2] Victor Medvei and John Thornton, *The Royal Hospital of Saint Bartholomew's, 1123–1973* (London, 1974); Susan C. Lawrence, *Charitable Knowledge: Hospital Pupils and Practitioner in Eighteenth-Century London* (Cambridge, 1996), while her '"Desirous of Improvement in Medicine": Pupils and Practitioners in the Medical Societies at Guy's and St Bartholomew's Hospitals, 1795–1815' (*BHM* lix (1985), pp. 89–104) looks at the hospital's medical society. Other historians, including Thomas N. Bonner (*Becoming a Physician: Medical Education in Britain, France, Germany, and the United States, 1750–1945* (New York, 1995)) refer to the College but only as part of the larger story.

Vivian Nutton and Roy Porter have described as a 'peaceful backwater'.[3] Medical schools have frequently been seen as the locus for change rather than an object for study. Investigations have been biased towards London and Edinburgh, with the evolution of private and hospital schools in the eighteenth and nineteenth centuries attracting most attention. Although Bonner has sought to produce a comparative study that seeks to analyse training in national terms,[4] far less research has been undertaken on the twentieth century; and little on the postwar period.[5] All too often students have appeared as passive participants. In institutional histories, the hospital's teaching function has been subsumed as part of its general history, or only the dramatic and pioneering included. General histories have focused on the role of book learning and the position of universities in the medieval period; on the institutionalisation of training in the eighteenth century; or on debates over the value of science to training.[6] Where studies have looked beyond 1900, it is to analyse the development of laboratory medicine or science.

Research in the 1980s began to break out of this mould. It started to analyse how medieval practitioners were educated, or the type of training gained at Oxford or Cambridge rather than just what was happening at the more famous European universities.[7] The eighteenth century received renewed critical attention. In her study *Charitable Knowledge*, Susan Lawrence set out to articulate a new vision of the institutionalisation of training that integrated culture, the clinic and the notion of a profession. Her work has analysed the production and role of knowledge in the construction of medical education and professional identities.[8] Other studies have put forward a critical assessment of the role of the Hunters and the impact of Paris

[3] 'Introduction', *The History of Medical Education in Britain*, ed. Vivian Nutton and Roy Porter (Amsterdam, 1995), p. 2.

[4] Bonner, *Becoming a Physician*.

[5] See W. F. Bynum, 'Sir George Newman and the American Way', in *Medical Education*, ed. Nutton and Porter, pp. 37–56; George Graham, 'The Formation of the Medical and Surgical Professorial Units in the London Teaching Hospitals', *Annals of Science* xxvi (1970), pp. 1–22; Jack Morrell, *Science at Oxford, 1914–1939: Transforming an Arts University* (Oxford, 1997); Steve Sturdy, 'The Political Economy of Scientific Medicine: Science, Education and the Transformation of Medical Practice in Sheffield, 1890–1922', *Medical History* xxxiv (1992), pp. 125–99; Mark Weatherall, *Gentlemen, Scientists, and Doctors: Medicine at Cambridge, 1800–1940* (Woodbridge, 2000).

[6] See Andrew Cunningham, 'Aspects of Medical Education in the Seventeenth and Early Eighteenth Centuries' (unpublished Ph.D. diss., London, 1974); Charles Newman, *Evolution of Medical Education in the Nineteenth Century* (London, 1957).

[7] Faye Getz, 'Charity, Translation, and the Language of Medical Learning in Medieval England', *BHM* lxiv (1990), pp. 1–17; Margaret Pelling, 'Knowledge Common and Acquired: The Education of Unlicensed Medical Practitioners in Early-Modern London', in *Medical Education*, ed. Nutton and Porter, pp. 250–79; Peter Murray Jones, 'Reading Medicine in Tudor Cambridge', ibid., pp. 153–83.

[8] Lawrence, *Charitable Knowledge*.

on how doctors were trained.[9] Rosner and Jones have gone some way to redress the anonymity of students. They have suggested that students played an important role in shaping provision; that they were far from passive in the educational process.[10] Studies by Butler, Sturdy and Jacyna on Victorian provincial schools have given valuable insights into how science was integrated into teaching and how medicine was merged into civic universities.[11] However, notwithstanding calls by Brieger to see medical education as 'part of the history of education', few studies have placed medical education in Britain within the historiography of higher education.[12]

Despite the growing historical interest in how doctors were trained, it is the contribution of medical education to the creation of a professional identity and the tensions surrounding the role of science in training that have attracted historians. For Lawrence, the history of modern Western medical education has been 'intimately connected with the history of the medical profession'.[13] Sociological and historical interest in professionalisation in the 1970s, and moves by historians in the 1980s to re-evaluate the range of practitioners in the eighteenth century, firmly linked professionalisation and occupational closure to training.[14] Medical education and the construction of practitioners' professional identity were it seemed intimately connected. The same association may be detected between the orthodox 'knowledge' students were instructed in and the debates surrounding how that knowledge should be constructed.[15] London's medical schools were a locus for these ideas and debates. These same institutions have also been perceived as central to the

---

[9] W. F. Bynum and Roy Porter, ed., *William Hunter and the Eighteenth-Century Medical World* (Cambridge, 1985).

[10] Lisa Rosner, *Medical Education in the Age of Enlightenment: Edinburgh Students and Apprentices, 1760–1826* (Edinburgh, 1991); Colin Jones, 'Montpellier Medical Students and the Medicalisation of Eighteenth-Century France', in *Problems and Methods in the History of Medicine*, ed. Roy Porter and Andrew Wear (London, 1987), pp. 57–80.

[11] Stella V. F. Butler, 'A Transformation in Training: The Formation of University Medical Faculties in Manchester, Leeds and Liverpool, 1870–84', *Medical History* xxx (1986), pp. 115–32; Stella V. F. Butler, 'Centres and Peripheries: The Development of British Physiology, 1870–1914', *Journal of the History of Biology* xxi (1988), pp. 473–500; Sturdy, 'The Political Economy of Scientific Medicine', pp. 125–99.

[12] Gert H. Brieger, '"Fit to Study Medicine"', *BHM* lvii (1983), p. 6.

[13] Susan C. Lawrence, 'Medical Education', in *Companion Encyclopaedia of the History of Medicine*, ed. W. F. Bynum and Roy Porter, 2 vols (London, 1993), Vol. 2, pp. 1151–3.

[14] See Noel and Parry Jones, *The Rise of the Medical Profession: A Study of Collective Social Mobility* (London, 1976); M. Jeanne Peterson, *The Medical Profession in Mid-Victorian London* (Berkeley, 1978). For recent studies see Irvine Loudon, *Medical Care and the General Practitioner, 1750–1850* (Oxford, 1986); Margaret Pelling, 'Medical Practice: Trade or Profession?', *The Professions in Early Modern England*, ed. W. Prest (London, 1987), pp. 90–128.

[15] See Michel Foucault, *The Birth of the Clinic: An Archaeology of Medical Perceptions*, trans. A. M. Sheridan (London, 1972); Toby Gelfand, *Professionalising Modern Medicine:*

controversies surrounding the value of the laboratory to clinical practice that underlay debates on the nature of medicine in the late nineteenth century. Hospital schools formed one part of an arena with the medical press and the General Medical Council (GMC) in which tensions between experimental science, the laboratory and a liberal education were negotiated.[16]

What can a study of medical education at St Bartholomew's contribute to this historiography? While Bonner has stressed the importance of discontinuities and change based around 'creative individuals or powerful centres of innovation', *Medical Education at St Bartholomew's Hospital* suggests a different story – one of continuity and discontinuity, of institutional cultures, students, and individuals. It is not one of steady or heroic progress. The history of the College spans the period in which training was institutionalised in the eighteenth century, formalised in the nineteenth, and moulded into the university sector and National Health Service (NHS) in the twentieth. A product of the growing market for medicine and medical knowledge in the eighteenth century and of individual initiatives, St Bartholomew's became an important part of the metropolitan educational community, a bastion of the medical establishment. By the 1890s, it had emerged as the largest school in London. In looking at the College, the experiences of the pupils and staff and the forces that shaped institutional development are explored to investigate the interaction between knowledge, education and the institution. A study of this kind helps redress the *terra incognita* of the medical school to rescue it from those who have endeavoured to ensure that 'no breath of scandal, no imputation of incompetence, no scrap of human error, should ever be associated with their beloved institution'.[17] It can tell us much about how medical knowledge was created and transmitted; about the social environment of medical schools; and about the circular debates that shaped the organisation of learning.

Throughout its history, St Bartholomew's has been a number of institutions that coexisted simultaneously. It has been branded as backward looking, resistant to change – an image that has damaged its position on several occasions. While the College saw value in tradition, an alternative institution may be seen. St Bartholomew's was also pioneering, with

---

Paris Surgeons and Medicine Science and Institutions in the Eighteenth Century (Westport, Conn., 1980); Erwin H. Ackerknecht, *Medicine at the Paris Hospital, 1794–1848* (Baltimore, 1967). Caroline Hannaway and Ann La Berge (ed., *Constructing Paris Medicine* (Amsterdam, 1998)) offer a revisionist assessment of the Paris school.

[16] See Stella V. F. Butler, 'Science and the Education of Doctors during the Nineteenth Century' (unpublished Ph.D. diss., UMIST, 1982); Gerald L. Geison, *Michael Foster and the Cambridge School of Physiology: The Scientific Enterprise in Late Victorian Society* (Princeton, 1978); Christopher Lawrence, 'Incommunicable Knowledge: Science, Technology and Clinical Art in Britain, 1850–1914', *Journal of Contemporary History* xx (1985), pp. 503–20.

[17] 'Introduction', *Medical Education*, ed. Porter and Nutton, p. 2.

innovation motivated by concerns about competition, by new technology and key individuals, and by efforts to redress perceived deficiencies. Like many of its contemporary institutions, the College was both conservative and ground breaking, a situation that frequently resulted in tension.

Medical schools, for all their internalism, could not be self-contained worlds. Those in London formed part of a quartet with their associated hospital, with the University of London and with the state. At a basic level, hospital and college at St Bartholomew's were hard to separate. After the creation of the NHS, the boundaries between the two became more blurred. However, the relationship was not always easy. Just as the College was linked to the hospital, so it was also intimately connected to what was happening at a metropolitan and national level. Lecturers were often closely involved in the politics of medical education. Anxiety about competition and the need for lecturers to deliver courses that matched the requirements of the examining bodies had a considerable impact on the organisation of teaching. After St Bartholomew's became a constituent college of the University of London in the 1840s, lecturers looked increasingly to the University as the College internalised an academic ethos.

The remaining part of the quartet was the state. After 1858, the College came under the indirect influence of the state through the GMC, University Grants Committee (UGC) and Medical Research Council (MRC), although it was not until after 1918 that these bodies started to play a more assertive role. Guidelines from the GMC and grants from the UGC helped direct the structure of learning. In the second half of the twentieth century, both bodies had a marked effect on the organisation of the College, with the 1980s witnessing open conflict with the UGC. The state had a further impact. The formation of the NHS placed London's teaching hospitals in a privileged position but included them in a service in which education, patient care and funding exerted contrary pressures on teaching. NHS reforms required regular rethinking of the curriculum, while pressure on the hospital and a rise in student numbers forced the College to develop links with other institutions. After the publication of the Todd Report in 1968, which attempted to balance changes in higher education and healthcare, the College became embroiled in protracted and at times bitter negotiations over merging with The London and Queen Mary College. The College's stance called into question the authority of the University and UGC. Although a compromise was reached and a confederation formed, further attempts to reform healthcare in London in the 1990s forced the final merger of the three institutions in 1995.

The history of medical education at St Bartholomew's is therefore the story of an institution and the history of that institution's interaction with other bodies. It is also the history of medical education in London.

Several themes have emerged in the course of the College's development. The first is the nature of institutional medical education. Changing concepts of how disease should be understood and an expanding market for medicine sustained the rise of medical schools in the eighteenth century. Medical education moved outside the library and on to the wards. New ways of delivering knowledge through demonstrations and clinical lectures emerged, often slowly and in the face of opposition. Tensions developed between staff and subjects as new institutional arrangements for teaching were fitfully expanded. Student demand, licensing requirements, individual lecturers, medical knowledge and worries about institutional inadequacies all combined to shape teaching. How the institution affected the socialisation of students and the development of a collegiate culture raises further questions.

The second theme may be defined as the use of science. The shift in medical gaze between the 1790s and 1830s underpinned the hospital as an educational environment and confirmed the importance of the bedside to teaching. In the teaching hospital, a new technical language of the body helped differentiate the orthodox practitioner. Science and craft were combined, but new ways of looking at disease and the growth of the experimental sciences in the mid-Victorian period merged with anxieties about the value of a liberal education to introduce discord. Beneath the self-confident exterior projected by St Bartholomew's, there were tensions over what type of medicine should be taught. Divisions in the College reflected anxieties about the role of the laboratory that was part of transatlantic debates surrounding attempts to make medicine into an experimental science. In the College, the experimental sciences were initially included through the pre-clinical subjects under pressure from the licensing bodies. The integration came later in the clinical subjects, and relied less on external pressure than on the practical application of pathology and bacteriology. However, old practices continued. Many of the discoveries hailed as symbolising a new form of medicine were initially opposed, and it was only in the 1890s that the empiricism that had dominated the College was challenged.

The 1880s and 1890s were a period of adaptation; one that left St Bartholomew's less confident. As disquiet mounted about the position of the London teaching hospitals, reformers outside the College began to argue that teaching, science and research should be fused through the University. Interest focused on the need to develop clinical academic units as a way of merging the bench and the bedside. These ideas received powerful support from the Haldane Commission established in 1909 to reform the University of London. Influential staff at St Bartholomew's shared this enthusiasm and advocated a professorial system. Rather than being part of a Flexnerian agenda, interest was based on a desire to develop academic medicine. War interrupted planning and it was not until 1918 that St Bartholomew's founded the first professorial clinical units in Britain. Experience differed from the ideal and the units were often marginalised. In the interwar period, the academic style of medicine advocated by Haldane and embodied in the units vied with a view that upheld traditional notions, highlighting the different approaches on how medical knowledge was constructed. By the

1950s, the need to orientate medical schools around a university system had been accepted. The gap between science and the bedside had been bridged, but debate continued over the nature of academic medicine. If science had been accepted as an integral part of a doctor's training, old divisions between clinical and pre-clinical study were challenged as uncertainly grew about the location and content of training. Concerns about science and vocational training, so familiar to the Victorians, had been relabelled and redefined.

The third theme is curriculum reform. Throughout the history of medical education those involved in the process of 'producing' doctors have appeared to be constantly worried about the nature of training. For Porter and Nutton, modifications to how and what medicine has been taught have coexisted 'with periodic episodes of soul searching'.[18] As medical knowledge expanded, pressure on the curriculum grew so that it became 'more and more compressed and indigestible'.[19] Concerns about overcrowding, science, assessment and the role of lectures repeatedly resurfaced. How and where new subjects should be added was balanced against a desire for a liberal education. By the late Victorian period, uncertainty about the role of science had refocused debate. Outside London, medical schools moved closer to universities, stimulating metropolitan fears about competition. However, medical education was not a sterile, reactive field in which new ways of acquiring knowledge were grafted on to an already overburdened curriculum. The demands placed on teaching hospitals by students, and the need to integrate new disciplines into learning, ensured that medical education had a direct impact on clinical care. Here training was central to the introduction of new specialties in the face of clinical resistance. A similar cross-fertilisation occurred through the laboratory, with teaching interests shaping the development of laboratory accommodation.

The twentieth century presented new challenges. Greater stress was placed on the importance of a university education as a way of integrating science and research into clinical teaching. The pre-clinical sciences were reinvigorated but how to merge medicine and the university proved allusive. As ideas changed on how doctors should be educated, the curriculum was repeatedly reformed. Although the GMC and the University of London shaped development, medical schools were also encouraged to experiment. Emphasis shifted from the need to produce safe general practitioners to a desire to provide a basic training as a platform for further study. Assessment and mechanisms of learning were questioned as the primacy of the teaching hospital was challenged. Greater attention focused on the role of the community, reflecting changes in the NHS and budgetary pressure on healthcare and higher education. By the 1990s, a revolution in attitudes to medical education was felt to be underway. The College both followed these

---

[18] Ibid., p. 13.
[19] AGM, 15 January 1969, MS 27/4.

developments and led the way, helping pioneer a curriculum with The London that was felt to provide the model for the GMC's *Tomorrow's Doctors*.

The final theme is the development of a research culture. St Bartholomew's was not just about the transmission of knowledge; it was also about its production. Until the late nineteenth century, research was a marginal pursuit in the College, confined to converted cupboards and dedicated individuals. Here the demands of the classroom and the expansion of specialisation shaped development. The introduction of experimental physiology pushed the creation of a makeshift physiological research laboratory in the 1870s, but it was in bacteriology and pathology that the first institutional investment was made. As the laboratory rose in status as a source of knowledge, work in pathology and bacteriology between the 1890s and the 1920s, and in radiology from the 1920s, stimulated clinical research. The formation of the MRC in 1912 and support from such bodies as the Rockefeller Foundation acted as a further spur. Determined not to fall behind, greater encouragement was given to research – especially clinical research – throughout the 1920s and 1930s and new laboratories were added. Although the College became one of main recipients of MRC funding as part of its policy to stimulate academic medicine, it was unable to match the profile of University College or assume the same leadership in shaping national research policy. By the late 1930s, a research ideology had penetrated the establishment at St Bartholomew's. However, this was not always compatible with the teaching, clinical work or private practice. Tensions remained, and although research had a pedagogic function, it was often considered marginal.

While the professorial units and individual departments provided a focus, a number of informal research 'schools' emerged. From the start, these were more than small groups of scientists pursuing a reasonably coherent programme of research in the same institutional context.[20] Tensions between clinical and pre-clinical staff, and the diversity of work carried out in the College and hospital, ensured that St Bartholomew's was never able to become a single research school. However, it did provide a framework for a shifting number of research 'schools' grouped around particular areas, forms of technology and often charismatic staff, linked, as Morrell has suggested, to 'intellectual, institutional, technical . . . and financial circumstances'.[21] Radiology and oncology were the first such 'school' in the College. In the postwar period, similar developments were seen in gastroenterology, in radioimmunoassay and in endocrinology. External support was sought and internal funding made available through a Research Committee, which after its inception in 1948 aimed to stimulate research at St Bartholomew's. The

[20] Gerald L. Geison, 'Scientific Change, Emerging Specialties, and Research Schools', *History of Science* ix (1981), p. 23.
[21] Jack Morrell, 'The Chemist Breeders: The Research Schools of Liebig and Thomson', *Ambix* xix (1972), pp. 1–46.

1960s saw a further drive to develop the research culture. Once more concerns about status and inadequate facilities played their part. External funding rose dramatically throughout the 1980s and a number of initiatives were begun to extend research facilities throughout the College.

Medical Education at St Bartholomew's Hospital brings together these strands to investigate how teaching started and evolved at St Bartholomew's. The intention is not to provide an institutional history of one medical school but to explore wider themes in the development of medical education through the history of the College. Although St Bartholomew's became closely linked with a number of institutions, a strong tradition remained that at times was both an asset and a hindrance.

Part I

Foundations 1123–1880

1

A slow evolution

Institutionalising education

Until the nineteenth century, medical education was generally informal and unregulated, seldom rigidly confined within an institution. Training traditionally embraced 'any means by which a person absorbs the knowledge and skills that a community recognises to produce a healer'.[1] An institutional focus in a hospital setting evolved in England only during the late eighteenth century. The systematisation of informal arrangements between practitioner and student and the old practice of walking the wards encouraged this transition, while a growing demand for doctors added a stimulus to expand educational provision. Development was haphazard, often accidental; and it was not until the nineteenth century that a concerted effort was made to exclude the untrained and the unorthodox. Because the way doctors learned is 'bound up with *what* they learned', how medical education developed at St Bartholomew's needs to be explained in relation to these developments.[2]

Medicine and learning, c.1000–c.1600

Medicine at the time of the foundation of St Bartholomew's in 1123 comprised a number of overlapping interpretations. In medieval hospitals care was equated with Christian doctrines based on 'medicine for the soul', with cure attributed to prayer, miracles or relics, not any system of treatment. Most early hospitals offered little more than rest, good diet and spiritual comfort until the fifteenth century.[3] Outside the hospital, illness was explained by a complex set of ideas that merged religion, magic and folklore. These overlapping systems needed little in the way of formal training. Learned medicine, or that practised by a small group of elite physicians, was different. It formed a corpus of knowledge that was transmitted through text-based medicine and a philosophical interpretation of Graeco-Roman views of

---

[1] Susan C. Lawrence, 'Medical Education', in *Companion Encyclopaedia of the History of Medicine*, ed. W. F. Bynum and Roy Porter, 2 vols (London, 1994), Vol. 2, p. 1151.
[2] Ibid., p. 1153.
[3] Carole Rawcliffe, 'Hospitals of Later Medieval London', *Medical History* xxviii (1984), pp. 1–3.

the body. Classical authors gave medicine a philosophical rationale, but in essence practice was centred on the regulation of lifestyle (or regimen) and based on the system of the four humors: blood, yellow bile, black bile and phlegm. Illness was related to an imbalance of one of these humors. This was medicine for the literate.

How was this knowledge transmitted? In early modern medicine, medical learning was acquired in a number of ways. Families handed down medical knowledge and remedies. Monastic libraries built up medical holdings for monk-apothecaries and writers interested in human physical nature. A vernacular medical tradition provided an important source of information for those unschooled in learned medicine and supplemented knowledge for those who were. With the audience for physic expanding in the early modern period and medicine becoming a significant, stratified occupation, a large number of medical tracts and compendia were produced.[4] Practical in nature, they drew heavily on classical authorities. Staff from St Bartholomew's contributed to this wealth of vernacular medical literature. The earliest and most famous of these texts was the *Breviarium Barthlomei* (Breviary of Bartholomew's) written between 1380 and 1395 by John of Mirfield. Mirfield was a contemporary of Chaucer who lived within the Priory at St Bartholomew's and was closely connected to the hospital where Faye Getz has suggested the *Breviarium* was used as a medical encyclopaedia. Although some have dismissed it as the product of a medical amateur, the *Breviarium* covered every aspect of medicine to aid those who did not have access to many books, or who needed a summary. It is one of the first examples of a hospital producing a medical text, suggesting that St Bartholomew's played a limited educational role but one that extended outside the hospital into the medical and lay community. The *Breviarium* represented a hospital library in miniature, extolling doctors to use treatments whose actions had been approved by ancient authorities.[5] Later surgeons at the hospital also published important textbooks. The boundary between popular and learned medicine was frequently blurred, with many of these books combining classical and popular learning.

Physicians, as the self-conscious elite of learned practitioners, made claims to learning that lay outside this vernacular tradition. Few in number, physicians were concentrated in towns where the population had enough money to pay for their services. It was believed that the best physician was not necessarily the most experienced, but the one who devoted the most time

[4] Faye Getz, 'Charity, Translation and the Language of Medical Learning in Medieval England', *BHM* lxiv (1990), pp. 1–17; Nancy G. Siraisi, *Medieval and Early Renaissance Medicine: An Introduction to Knowledge and Practice* (Chicago, 1990), pp. 52–4.
[5] Faye Getz, 'John Mirfield and the *Breviarium Bartholomei*: The Medical Writings of a Clerk at St Bartholomew's Hospital in the Later Fourteenth Century', *Bulletin (Society for the Social History of Medicine)* xxxvii (1985), pp. 24–6.

to classical texts, logic, natural philosophy and astronomy.[6] It was around this philosophical and classical training that an institutional form of medical education first developed. With four to seven years of study after passing an Arts degree required for an orthodox practitioner, training as a physician was suited to a university environment. Universities across Europe set up faculties of medicine to provide a framework for these subjects, encouraged by religious and political authorities who used them as a source of reliable practitioners. The effect was to reinforce the authority of book learning and systematise its transmission.

A style of medical training based on book learning pioneered at Salerno in the tenth century became the basis of learned medicine. Its model of lectures and discourse stressed medicine's philosophical roots and drew heavily upon scholastic methods used in the study of theology. As Salerno's reputation declined in the thirteenth century, other schools in northern Europe acquired a leading position in the training of physicians. Until the Renaissance, differences between institutions were reflected in their size, reputation and position, not in the teaching they offered. However, in England medical teaching was slow to emerge. Oxford and Cambridge borrowed their curriculum from Paris, where medicine was initially a minor subject, and could not match the facilities and reputations of the major European schools. This discouraged students from taking a medical degree in England. More successful and less conservative university schools were established in Scotland. Even after instruction in medicine had started at Oxbridge in the fourteenth century, ambitious English students still opted in growing numbers to travel to Scotland or Europe for part of their training.[7]

A university education represented an ideal, not a comprehensive or universal education for all branches of medicine. It was not necessary for practice and leading practitioners were able to attract pupils who wanted to learn their skills outside a university framework. For those who did attend, many left after they had acquired what they believed was an adequate knowledge.[8] Surgeons were excluded from this commonwealth of learning after the Fourth Lateran Council in 1215 insisted that priests in higher orders, who formed the body of those studying medicine, could not shed blood. Under this ruling, surgery was marginalised in university education and became a largely lay province, although this did not mean that surgeons were not learned and latinate. Divisions between 'internal' medicine and 'external' manipulation were upheld at an intellectual and practical level. Although anatomy was seen as an important part of rational university

---

[6] Margaret Pelling, 'Medical Practice in Early Modern England: Trade or Profession?', in *The Professions in Early Modern England*, ed. Wilfred Prest (London, 1987), pp. 90–128.

[7] Siraisi, *Medieval and Early Renaissance Medicine*, pp. 48–9, 55–65.

[8] Margaret Pelling and Charles Webster, 'Medical Practitioners', in *Health, Medicine and Mortality in the Sixteenth Century*, ed. Charles Webster (Cambridge, 1979), pp. 165–235.

medicine, with doctors using it to show that the body was intelligible, surgery occupied a precarious position as an academic discipline.[9] For the most part, training remained practical and largely guild based. In London it was centred on the elite Fellowship of Surgeons and the larger Company of Barber-Surgeons, chartered in 1376. Like other medieval guilds, these bodies worked to protect the public from the poorly trained or unscrupulous, combining religious and social duties with mutual aid. To promote training the surgical guilds adopted an apprenticeship system. Apprenticeship was part of a highly decentralised, locally based system of education that was both haphazard and unsystematic but managed to survive into the mid-nineteenth century. The two companies (forcibly merged under Henry VIII in 1540) required a minimum of seven years' service to a master before a licence to practice was granted. Based on one-to-one learning, it was a less expensive form of education. With the master in *loco parentis*, apprentices were not just taught the secrets of the trade but were also 'encouraged to learn and to display the rights and duties of good citizenship'. In 1563, apprenticeship was made a legal requirement for all trades and crafts. Even before this, it had conferred on surgeons a legal right to practice and a status that was essential for a practitioner's livelihood. Much depended on the master, however. Those attached to a London surgeon, who were often extremely learned biblio-philes, had better opportunities for learning and practice afterwards.[10]

War and the invention of gunpowder greatly extended the realm of surgery. It led to the emergence of a new class of surgeon who based his practice on anatomy and dissection. In England, the formation of the United Company of Barbers and Surgeons out of the two existing guilds created a more active organisation and a move to regulate training. It continued the system of apprenticeship, but with the help of an annual grant of four executed criminals, a course of instruction and dissection was added.[11] Dissection had been used as an aid to teaching in the Italian universities since the early twelfth century, although it was not widely accepted until the fourteenth century. It was only with the formation of the United Company that a similar move was made in England to organise a course of dissection. The College of Physicians (founded in 1518 to licence physicians in London) followed with an annual dissection after 1566. However, interest in medical

[9] Roger French, 'The Anatomical Tradition', in *Companion Encyclopaedia*, ed. Bynum and Porter, Vol. 1, pp. 82–3.

[10] Joan Lane, 'Role of Apprenticeship in Eighteenth-Century Medical Education in England', in *William Hunter and the Eighteenth Century Medical World*, ed. W. F. Bynum and Roy Porter (Cambridge, 1985), p. 57; Juanita Burnby, 'An Examined and Free Apothecary', *The History of Medical Education in Britain*, ed. Vivian Nutton and Roy Porter (Amsterdam, 1995), p. 17.

[11] The Company was part of a European move to control and license medical activity that most expressed itself at a civic rather than a national level: Pelling, 'Medical Practice', p. 92.

education in the two medical guilds remained limited. College and Company combined a sense of responsibility to the public with a need for minimum standards, but their courses were intended for those already practising. Dissections were largely intended to support classical theories rather than expand knowledge of the body. Obligatory anatomical lectures were introduced in 1569 by the College of Physicians, and fellows were expected to read Galen's *De Simplici Medicine* and *De Usu Partium* within a year of joining, but no other requirements were enforced. Neither did the United Company outline a basic curriculum while attendance at its lectures was not required for a licence.[12] Surgeons saw lectures as a supplement to apprenticeship rather than a necessary part of training and it was often difficult for students to see any dissections before they started to practise.

'Younge doctors': early teaching at St Bartholomew's

Text-based medical studies and apprenticeship did not rule out using medieval and early modern hospitals to gain clinical experience. Although neither St Bartholomew's nor any other medieval English hospital acquired a contemporary reputation as a 'school', most of those trying to become physicians or surgeons did spend some time at a hospital, either paying one of the staff to walk the wards or to be his pupil.[13] The College of Physicians encouraged the newly qualified to gain practical experience in a hospital. Cambridge's statutes also required candidates to have practised medicine for two years before they could become a doctor, though they did not specify that this had to be in a hospital.[14] This ensured that the different strands of medical education (apprenticeship, university education, and time spent in a hospital) ran in parallel, and students combined them according to their chosen career path, opportunities and ability to pay. It would therefore be expected that St Bartholomew's and St Thomas's, as the two largest hospitals in London after the dissolution, would be the first in England to develop an institutional form of medical education.

St Thomas's has made the claim to be the first hospital in London to take students. A statement about the presence of apprentices in the wards in 1561, twenty-one years after the formation of the United Company, has been used to support this, although at the time no systematic training was offered at St Thomas's. Surgical apprentices made their arrangements with individuals,

---

[12] Andrew Cunningham, 'Aspects of Medical Education in the Seventeenth and Early-Eighteenth Centuries' (unpublished Ph.D. diss., London, 1974), pp. 165–6.
[13] Susan C. Lawrence, *Charitable Knowledge: Hospital Pupils and Practitioner in Eighteenth-Century London* (Cambridge, 1996), p. 25.
[14] Damian Leader, *A History of the University of Cambridge*, 2 vols (Cambridge, 1988), Vol. 1, p. 203.

not the hospital. Those managing St Thomas's did not see any need to regulate the attendance of apprentices until 1691 when it was decided that all students visiting the wards had to be an apprentice of at least two years' standing. This concern was patient led; subsequent regulations were designed to support professional hierarchies.[15]

Whether St Thomas's was the first London hospital to admit apprentices must be open to doubt. Although not limited to the sick, by the fifteenth century St Bartholomew's had acquired a reputation as one of five London institutions renowned for the care it extended to the sick poor. It was also able to survive the dissolution of the Priory in 1539 with Henry VIII's break from Rome, and in 1547, after a period of intense uncertainty and protracted wrangling, was granted to the 'mayor and commonalty and citizens of London' with a small endowment.[16] Under the management of the City, St Bartholomew's acquired its first medical staff of three surgeons and a physician, although the regular services of the latter were not secured until 1567. The hospital's function in providing medical care assumed a new importance as the City worked to improve conditions. By the 1680s, St Bartholomew's was well established. It provided 'the advice and consultations of the best physicians about this town' and had some 250 patients in the wards at any one time.[17]

Given the size and contemporary importance of St Bartholomew's and the apprenticeship regulations of the United Company it is unlikely that the hospital excluded apprentices. However, historians have suggested that students first attended St Bartholomew's in 1662.[18] They base their assessment on a complaint from the almoners – who admitted and discharged patients and occasionally visited the wards – that the two physicians, Sir John Mickelthwaite and Christopher Terne, were using 'younge Doctors' to provide locum cover. Given the emphasis on traditional academic methods, it is doubtful that these 'Gentleman Practitioners' were students. With the College of Physicians encouraging newly qualified practitioners to walk the wards, it is probable that these 'younge Doctors' were using St Bartholomew's for this purpose. However, it is clear that by the mid-1660s apprentices were regularly visiting the wards. In 1664, the almoners made another complaint that reflected directly on teaching. They were worried that the 'pressing importunityes' and 'bould and sawcye carryadge' of the surgeons' apprentices was disrupting 'theire businesse'. The almoners were concerned that this conduct raised the danger that patients were being 'abused or neglected in

---

[15] E. M. McInnes, *St Thomas's Hospital* (London, 1963), pp. 74–5.

[16] Indenture of agreement between Henry VIII and the Mayor and commonality and citizens of London, 27 December 1556, HC 1/2001.

[17] Cited in Geoffrey Keynes, *Life of William Harvey* (Oxford, 1966), p. 56.

[18] Victor Medvei and John Thornton, *Royal Hospital of Saint Bartholomew's, 1123–1973* (London, 1974), p. 44.

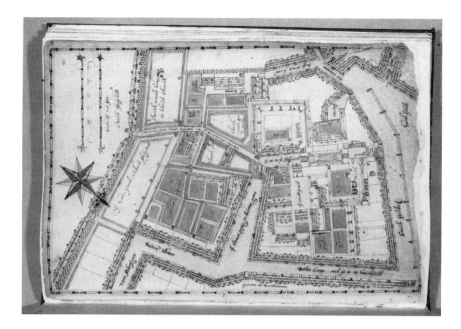

Plate 1.1 Plan of the hospital precincts, *c.*1612–17

theire severall Cures and distempers to the slander of this Hospitall'. More stringent rules were introduced: surgeons were instructed to 'dresse theire patients themselves or stand by and direct theire servants to doe the same'.[19] Apprentices were not banned, but (at least in theory) the practical experience they gained from the wards was limited.

The wording of the 1664 resolution suggests that the presence of apprentices was a common feature of life in the hospital by the mid-1660s. It is probable that apprentices visited St Bartholomew's much earlier, perhaps from the hospital's foundation in 1123, and certainly from the formation of the United Company and the re-foundation of the hospital in 1547 when a surgical staff was appointed. Norman Moore, physician and historian of the hospital, felt it was realistic to claim that 'soon after the Reformation, students used to come to the hospital chiefly from the universities', citing the example of Edward Browne who in his letters made mention of his studies at St Bartholomew's.[20] Although the attendance of students does not denote the existence of a 'medical college', it does suggest that St Bartholomew's was one of the first medical institutions in England to contribute towards the training of doctors. In addition, the role played by doctors from the hospital in generating the growing vernacular medical literature may serve as

[19] Order Book, 29 April 1662, 1 February 1664, HA 4.
[20] *RC on a University for London*, PP (1889) xxxix, p. 146.

additional evidence that St Bartholomew's indirectly contributed to text-based medicine as well as offering an opportunity for training. Teaching had started in the hospital long before any formal structure was established, but it was only when students started to obstruct its normal running that they attracted any formal recognition.

Not just the humors: anatomy, observation and learned medicine

The almoners' complaints about troublesome apprentices were made at a time when medical thought was in a period of flux. During the seventeenth century there was a revival of interest in the nature of learned medicine and whether medicine was an art or a science. Although the institutional form of medical education was outwardly stable, it was under attack from a number of sides. Critics saw traditional academic methods of learning medicine as too expensive and exclusive. Arguments for medical reform were closely linked to calls for political change; part of protests against clericalism, monopoly and what was seen as 'idle' knowledge.[21] Reformers called for medicine to be freely available in terms of knowledge and price, threatening the established role of the universities and medical guilds. At St Bartholomew's in 1621 the surgeons protested against the monopoly of the College of Physicians. The petition provoked an immediate reaction and conflict in the hospital that led to a restriction of the surgeons' authority.[22] Although the English Civil War saw a purging of the universities, change was hampered by revolution and the absence of intellectual preconditions for restructuring; and many of the reformers' hopes were dashed by the Restoration.[23]

It was not only in England that the establishment was being called into question. A gradual transformation in medical thought away from the classical principles required a shift in how and where doctors were trained. The work of the Swiss-born Paracelsus, with his semi-mystical faith in natural philosophy, scorn of traditional book learning, and the encouragement he gave to chemical remedies, struck at the foundations of classical medicine.[24] He started an attack on classical learning that stressed the study of nature and observation. New anatomical and physiological inquiries added a further dimension to the assault. A renaissance in anatomical inquiry and teaching to demonstrate the wonders of God's creation through the human body

[21] Charles Webster, 'The Medical Profession and its Radical Critics', in *Change and Continuity in Seventeenth Century England*, ed. John E. Hill (London, 1974), pp. 157–78.
[22] Keynes, *Harvey*, pp. 67–9.
[23] John Twigg, 'The Limits of "Reform"', *History of Universities* iv (1984), pp. 99–114.
[24] See Vivian Nutton, ed., *Medicine at the Courts of Europe, 1500–1837* (London, 1989); Charles Webster, *From Paracelsus to Newton: Magic and the Making of Modern Science* (Cambridge, 1982).

merged with these debates to challenge text-based medical studies as anatomists began to question classical assumptions. Although later viewed with fear and loathing, human dissection had become more acceptable to the public during this period, increasing the supply of cadavers where anatomists had previously relied on animals. It became a means through which doctors could claim a rational basis for medicine, and the public nature of dissection confirmed what was being seen, giving it added authority. A growing number of anatomists argued that faith should not be shown in everything that was written unless personal observation had proved it correct. Anatomical practice remained conservative, but the emphasis it placed on experience had a profound effect: it revealed that some of the classical ideas were wrong. The result was heated debate over the validity of classical authorities that split medical thought.[25] Doubt was strengthened by the pioneering work of William Harvey, physician to St Bartholomew's from 1609 to 1643, on the circulation of blood.[26] Contemporaries saw Harvey's ideas as revolutionary. They inspired further experimental investigations. These inquiries revealed that all was not well with traditional learned medicine.

The significance of Harvey's discoveries for physiology, linked to new anatomical structures, challenged classical medical thought at a time when Aristotelian natural philosophy and confessional religion were also being questioned. England became the centre of the 'Scientific Revolution' that was based on mechanical philosophy and faith in experimentation and observation. It was one solution to growing doubt about the validity of humanistic culture.[27] Questioning doctors strove to adopt the fashionable Newtonian framework and the mechanical theories of the body. Traditional academic methods were undermined and new certainties had to be found. Competing schools of thought were encouraged and no single doctrine was able to emerge unchallenged.

Thomas Sydenham has been given retrospective credit for the transition away from the Galenist tradition started by anatomists in the sixteenth and early seventeenth centuries. Sydenham was a Parliamentarian who wished to improve medicine for all.[28] Practising among the London poor, he was led

---

[25] See Andrew Cunningham, *The Anatomical Renaissance: The Resurrection of the Anatomical Projects of the Ancients* (Aldershot, 1997).

[26] Gweneth Whitteridge, *William Harvey and the Circulation of the Blood* (London, 1971), pp. 107–8.

[27] Lawrence Conrad *et al.*, *The Western Medical Tradition, 800 BC to AD 1800* (Cambridge, 1996), pp. 340–59; Roger French and Andrew Wear, ed., *The Medical Revolution of the Seventeenth Century* (Cambridge, 1989); Harold Cook, 'The New Philosophy and Medicine in Seventeenth Century England', in *Reappraisals of the Scientific Revolution*, ed. David Lindberg and Robert Westman (Cambridge, 1990), pp. 397–436.

[28] See K. Dewhurst, *Dr Thomas Sydenham (1624–1689): His Life and Original Writings* (London, 1966); Donald Bates, 'Thomas Sydenham: The Development of his Thought, 1666–1676' (unpublished MD, Baltimore, 1975).

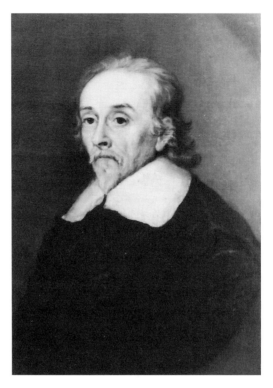

Plate 1.2 William Harvey, physician to St Bartholomew's

to a study of epidemic fevers. Although his understanding of fever differed little from classical authorities, Sydenham was influenced by Bacon and believed that to treat illness it was necessary to develop a natural history of disease to find the proper method of treatment. Sceptical of hypotheses and invisible causes, he shared anatomists' arguments that personal experience was important, arguing that observation was the key to physic. This was a revamping of Hippocratic clinical methods but a departure from the established view that limited physic to theoretical speculation. By stressing observation, Sydenham encouraged a focus on the nosology of disease and left little room for text-based medical studies, a view that extended to the Paris medical school in the late eighteenth century.[29]

Sydenham's ideas were developed at Leiden by his pupils Franciscus de la Boe Sylvius and Hermann Boerhaave. Both advocated the importance of bedside teaching and clinical instruction. In his *Institutiones Medicae*, Boerhaave outlined a view of medicine as a science where application was an art. Influenced by mechanical philosophy, he argued for a systematic approach that saw anatomy as fundamental. Students came from across

---

[29] Dewhurst, *Sydenham*, pp. 47–8, 56–9.

Europe to study under him and he encouraged them to read Sydenham's work. His methods were transmitted to Edinburgh, which became a leading centre for teaching.[30] Through the work of Sylvius and Boerhaave, Leiden became an important centre for learning where courses were organised around medical subjects, bedside teaching and dissection, not medical authors. The system had its limitations. Students were not offered raw material for independent observation, but Leiden's stress on the importance of seeing patients during study had a far-reaching impact.[31]

In England, observation and a speculative general pathology came to replace earlier ideas, forcing new explanations for existing therapies. Increasingly, medical teachers began to stress that experience was essential and the classical authorities were an obstacle to improvement. This transformation involved a shift in how students of medicine spent their time, stimulating the study of physiology and anatomy and leading to a renaissance in anatomy. However, the existing medical guilds, and Oxford and Cambridge, were slow to adapt, forcing students to depend on vernacular medical texts and private reading if they wanted to keep abreast of the new approaches. Increasingly, the system of instruction offered by Oxford, Cambridge and the medical guilds was viewed as inadequate or ancillary. Social and professional expectations of education were rising and the old monopolies were beginning to break down. Other means of delivering this new knowledge and approach had to be found.

Books and specimens

The 'bould and sawcye carryadge' of the apprentices at St Bartholomew's was seen as an affront to the smooth running of the hospital. It is significant that the almoners were complaining at the very time that some of their contemporaries were stressing the value of observation. The students' intrusion into the wards reflected the growing importance of the study of the body in a practical rather than an abstract sense. However, despite Harvey's connection with the hospital, a faith in the importance of these methods took longer to emerge at St Bartholomew's than elsewhere. In the mid-seventeenth century, the hospital was still committed to traditional academic methods based on Latin and Greek texts. Although some of the medical staff had trained at Leiden, the hospital remained conservative, fervently loyal to the Crown with a high church and Tory character.[32] This was important in

---

[30] Cunningham, 'Medical Education', pp. 134–7; Christopher Lawrence, 'Alexander Monro *Primus* and the Edinburgh Manner of Anatomy', *BHM* lxii (1988), pp. 193–214.

[31] Lawrence, 'Medical Education', p. 1162.

[32] See Craig Rose, 'Politics and the Royal London Hospitals, 1683–92', in *The Hospital in History*, ed. Lindsay Granshaw and Roy Porter (London, 1990), pp. 123–48.

defining the hospital's character in a climate where a challenge to text-based medical studies and political reform was interlinked.

In 1668, at the suggestion of Richard Mills, the treasurer, the governors voted to establish a library 'next to the Church in the Corner of the Little Cloysters'. It was an addition to the 'common library' which the Tudor chronicler, John Stow, believed existed at St Bartholomew's during the fifteenth century.[33] The decision hinted at a revised attitude to apprentices and confirmed the governors' faith in text-based medicine. Although not designed as a medical library, the governors did feel that it should be stocked with books that would interest 'university schollers'.[34] Most libraries in this period contained the Latin and Greek works of Galen and Hippocrates, along with other lesser known medical authors and anonymous medical tracts, while a growth in vernacular medical texts increased the number of medical texts in circulation.[35]

Separate libraries connected to churches became common from the fifteenth century and a large part of the precinct at St Bartholomew's was taken up by the Great Cloister and parish church. An expansion of library facilities was linked to rising literacy rates, changes in printing technology, and a move to shelve rather than chain books. Between the Reformation and the start of the eighteenth century, over 200 libraries were founded to replace what was felt to be heretical and superstitious books destroyed during the Reformation.[36] The seventeenth century also saw numerous projects for academies of learning, linked to developments in science and navigation, and dissatisfaction with existing institutions: the creation of the Royal Society in 1662 was a concrete fulfilment of these aims. Terne as one of the physicians at St Bartholomew's was one of the original fellows of the Society.[37] The new, post-Dissolution library at St Bartholomew's may be seen as part of this process.

The decision to establish a library was an optimistic one. In 1666, the Great Fire had swept across London, only stopping at the hospital gates. Although St Bartholomew's escaped destruction, much of its extensive property in the City had been destroyed, dramatically reducing income and promoting several decades of retrenchment. The creation of a library went against this trend. It is possible that the governors were merely taking advantage of an opportunity. Mills had only suggested the library because he

[33] Order book, 6 February 1668, HA 4; John Stow, *A Survey of London written in the Year 1598*, Introduction by Antonia Fraser (Stroud, 1997), p. 346.

[34] Order book, 6 February 1668, HA 4; Journal, HA 1/5.

[35] Francis Wormald and C. Wright, ed., *The English Library before 1700* (London, 1958), p. 104.

[36] Thomas Kelly, *Early Public Libraries: A History of Public Libraries in Britain before 1850* (London, 1966), pp. 38–41, 57–69.

[37] Notker Hammerstein, 'The Modern World, Sciences, Medicine and Universities', *History of Universities* viii (1989), p. 162.

had been approached by 'some persons well wishers to Learneing' willing to donate books.[38] However, other reasons, more closely connected to the hospital, may also be seen. St Bartholomew's had been seriously affected by the Great Plague in 1665. Recognisable cases of the plague were not admitted to St Bartholomew's, but the hospital quickly became infected and was not clear of cases until February 1666. Mickelthwaite and Terne, like many of their rich patients, fled from London. Despite pressure from the governors, the surgical staff and their deputies made their excuses, leaving the bulk of the work to Francis Bernard the apothecary and the matron Margaret Blagne. Although medical practice had largely returned to normal by 1668, the governors were probably eager to reassert the hospital's reputation. The plague had encouraged criticism of medicine and, reflecting efforts to found similar libraries in continental hospitals, the creation of a library might be seen as an attempt to renew confidence by showing that medicine at St Bartholomew's was a scholarly pursuit. It suggests a recognition by the mid-seventeenth century that a limited institutional structure for 'university schollers' attending St Bartholomew's was needed, and points to the governors' support of learning.

The library was an expression of faith in text-based medical study, but St Bartholomew's was not isolated from the growing importance of anatomical and pathological study. In 1722, the medical staff argued that a dissection room should be provided to aid their work. Doctors and anatomists were already offering private instruction in dissection, but it was not until 1726 that two rooms were set aside for post-mortems in the dead house at St Bartholomew's. One was for the 'more decent laying' out of patients before their burial, the other 'a Repository for anatomical or Chyrurical Preparations'.[39] This was the first museum in the hospital. Twenty years later, the governors discussed the need for a laboratory, and after an investigation of the one at St Thomas's, it was decided to go ahead with the plan.[40] With a museum and a laboratory, the hospital was developing an institutional structure that could be used for teaching and research.

Anatomy for profit

The opening of two rooms for post-mortems was an expression of the growing confidence in the value of anatomical and pathological inquiry. Outside St Bartholomew's this faith was expressed in a new type of institution, the private anatomy school. Although neither the College of Physicians, Company of Surgeons (successor to the United Company) nor the Society of

[38] Order book, 6 February 1668, HA 4.
[39] House committee, July 1722, 23 June 1726, HA 1/10.
[40] Apothecaries committee, 12 May 1747, HA 1/11.

Apothecaries expected attendance at lectures or dissections until 1815, institutional training offered subtle advantages that helped practitioners break into the highly competitive market for patients.[41]

The market for medicine had been growing since the sixteenth century; by the eighteenth century health had become firmly established as a commodity. Although the extent of rising consumption has been exaggerated, the expansion of the middle classes increased demand for doctors. Pressure was exerted on surgeon-apothecaries, as emergent general practitioners, to increase their medical knowledge and, faced with competition and a public willing to buy patent medicines, extend their traditional role from dispensing drugs. This increased demand for training beyond the established centres of learning to meet the needs of a growing body of general practitioners. As a voluntary supplement to apprenticeship, the potential rewards appeared to justify the additional expense. A rise in the numbers seeking these advantages increased demand for accessible and above all flexible teaching that neither the medical guilds nor Oxford or Cambridge was initially prepared to deliver. Medical entrepreneurs in London seized the initiative. They started to offer courses to meet demand, ensuring that London became a centre for clinical instruction and lectures.

Demand for the 'business of educating – not training – the senses' stimulated the growth of what one historian has called the 'London lecturing empire'.[42] A growing number of science lectures made London into a centre for the study of science and learning. In this environment, private anatomy teaching flourished outside the control of the medical guilds.[43] Lectures were not intended only for the doctor or amateur scientist, however. Medical learning formed part of the London spectacle and spoke to a wider audience interested in science. Medical lecturers took advantage of the broad curiosity about the natural world and fascination with experimentation. Private lecturing grew rapidly as doctors sought to advertise their clinical acumen.[44]

It was surgeons, rather than physicians, who took a leading role in these developments. The latter have been seen as passive figures in the eighteenth century, tailoring their explanation of illness and therapeutic regime to a

---

[41] See Lawrence, *Charitable Knowledge*, for her perceptive analysis of eighteenth-century teaching.

[42] Susan C. Lawrence, 'Educating the Senses: Students, Teachers and Medical Rhetoric In Eighteenth Century London', in *Medicine and the Five Senses*, ed. W. F. Bynum and Roy Porter (Cambridge, 1993), p. 155; J. N. Hays, 'The London Lecturing Empire, 1800–50', in *Metropolis and Province: Science in British Culture, 1780–1850*, ed. Ian Inkster and Jack Morrell (Philadelphia, 1983), pp. 91–119.

[43] For the development of private teaching see George C. Peachey, *Memoir of William and John Hunter* (Plymouth, 1924), 8ff.

[44] Roy Porter, 'Medical Lecturing in Georgian London', *British Journal of the History of Science* xxviii (1995), pp. 91–9; Simon Schaffer, 'Natural Philosophy and Public Spectacle in the Eighteenth Century', *History of Science* xxi (1983), pp. 1–43.

patient-dominated clinical encounter that encouraged an individualistic account of disease. The work of the surgeon, which was tied more closely to the objective experience of illness, relied less on the patient's narrative. It gave greater scope for the transmission of clinical knowledge in a climate that increasingly favoured anatomical and pathological investigation. However, knowledge was not polarised: physicians had lectured on 'internal' medicine to the United Company since the sixteenth century. This mixed approach continued, providing an education that suited the realities of practice in the growing towns and cities.[45] Neither did lecturers initially restrict themselves to anatomy, physiology or the practice of medicine and surgery. Chemistry and botany were often part of their teaching repertoire. However, it was anatomical teaching that came to dominate, reflecting London's growing reputation as a centre for surgical instruction.

The trend towards anatomico-clinical medicine, inspired by the questioning of classical authorities and shifts towards observation in the seventeenth century, stimulated teaching. Nosology was breaking down, and a view of disease based on morbid anatomy and clinical pathology was asserting itself. Although private teaching started in London, Paris, Vienna and other large European cities at about the same time, Paris has been seen by historians to symbolise these new trends. Surgeons in Paris followed the example set by teachers in Leiden and encouraged students to visit the wards.[46] Students from across Europe, attracted by the strong surgical tradition, travelled to Paris where they had previously visited Holland. Here emphasis was placed on practical instruction and the principle that each student should be allowed to dissect became standard. Fees were low and students were invited *en masse* to the wards to view a new 'type' of patient, the citizen patient who became the raw material for clinical examination and autopsy. However, research has started to suggest that the dominance and uniqueness of 'Paris medicine' represented a 'myth'.[47] The surgical emphasis on the anatomical locationisation of disease was not created or fully institutionalised in Paris and was present in London and Edinburgh. However, it was in Paris that teaching resources correlating symptoms, signs and pathological changes were combined and linked to a low fee.

Old ideas about disease and treatment persisted, but in contemporary rhetoric the 'Paris Manner' became the fashionable way to teach. By 1740, William Hewett was offering dissection 'by the Paris Method' and by 1746 so

---

[45] Lawrence, 'Educating the Senses', p. 156.
[46] See Toby Gelfand, *Professionalising Modern Medicine: Paris Surgeons and Medicine Science and Institutions in the Eighteenth Century* (Westport, Conn., 1980); Michel Foucault, *Birth of the Clinic: An Archaeology of Medical Perception*, trans. A. M. Sheridan (London, 1972); Erwin H. Ackerknecht, *Medicine at the Paris Hospital, 1794–1848* (Baltimore, 1967).
[47] See Caroline Hannaway and Ann La Berge, ed., *Constructing Paris Medicine* (Amsterdam, 1998).

was the young and energetic Scot William Hunter.[48] Hunter, aided by his brother John, established the era of the private anatomy school and helped transform the medico-scientific standing of surgery through his insistence on student dissection.[49] Private schools lacked the flexibility of individual lectures but they provided better resources for students. Spurred to be 'at the head of his profession', Hunter had arrived in London to assist James Douglas in 1741. He brought with him the new teaching methods he had experienced under Alexander Monro *primus* in Scotland, and quickly became established as an eloquent and influential teacher. Hunter's school in Great Windmill Street offered a chance to break from the narrow introduction to medicine secured through an apprenticeship or provided at an English university. Free from restrictive governors, and with a plentiful supply of cadavers and a large number of specimens, the school provided a more comprehensive course than its rivals. This, and the emphasis on student dissection, placed Hunter at an advantage in a competitive market where students could be easily lured to other teachers, or to Edinburgh or Paris. The methods adopted by Hunter were quickly adopted by other private teachers and contrasted with the practices of the Company of Surgeons where students remained spectators. Great Windmill Street provided a nursery for other private medical schools, inspiring similar projects and teaching those who would go on to found their own schools, reflecting the demand for training and stimulating a competitive market for students.[50] By transplanting the 'Paris Method' to London through private anatomy schools, the British surgical elite was able to develop its teaching resources instead of relying on Parisian initiatives. This allowed London to become a centre for medical education.[51]

Private anatomy schools remedied the perceived disadvantages of a traditional apprenticeship, offering an alternative, open cash system with no long-term obligation. Lectures gave access to materials not normally available in a framework that stressed learning rather than craft training. They reflected the needs of those with limited money to spend, and less time for study in London. With the promise of large financial rewards and freed from the medical guilds' restrictions of one student per master, ambitious instructors could teach as many as they could accommodate, and, with no regulation on the number of schools, private ventures flourished. Teaching also offered important career advantages for those unable to secure a toehold

[48] Toby Gelfand, 'The "Paris Manner" of Dissection: Student Anatomical Dissection in Early Eighteenth Century Paris', *BHM* xlvi (1972), pp. 99–130; Lawrence, 'Alexander Monro', p. 195.

[49] See Peachey, *Memoir*; Bynum and Porter, ed., *Hunter*.

[50] Roy Porter, 'William Hunter: A Surgeon and a Gentleman', in *Hunter*, ed. Bynum and Porter, pp. 13, 22–3; Robert Kirkpatrick, 'Nature's Schools: The Hunterian Revolution in London Hospital Medicine, 1780–1825' (unpublished Ph.D. diss., Cambridge, 1988).

[51] Toby Gelfand, '"Invite the Philosopher, as well as the Charitable": Hospital Teaching as Private Enterprise in Hunterian London', in *Hunter*, ed. Bynum and Porter, pp. 130–1.

in the new voluntary hospitals. Located near these hospitals but free from the regulations enforced by hospital governors not always sympathetic to teaching, such instructors provided a wider curriculum and taught all year round. Changes in the United Company further facilitated their rise, removing some of the restrictions and problems facing earlier private teachers. Until the creation of the United Company in 1746, only the Company of Surgeons was legally entitled to dissect, but this privilege was abolished with the new company, ensuring that dissection became legal in hospitals and private establishments.[52] This paved the way for anatomy classes and the entrepreneurial inclinations of leading teachers, as long as cadavers could be found.

Teaching at the London hospitals

The heyday of the private anatomy school had passed by the 1830s. The continued growth in the market for institutional teaching which they had encouraged worked against them in a period when the locus of medicine was shifting and the cost of medical education was rising. Although private schools had demonstrated that teaching was profitable, the new voluntary hospitals provided a better location for an integrated medical curriculum based on clinical instruction.

The eighteenth century saw a new form of active benevolence that aimed to help an ill-defined 'deserving' poor. This found expression in the foundation of voluntary hospitals, which evolved from an interaction of philanthropic and evangelical enthusiasm, demand for care, and the self-interest of doctors and local elites. Urbanisation and the consequent extent of disease in the nineteenth century pressurised the Victorians into further institutionalising medical services. London stood at the centre of this development, greatly increasing the clinical resources available for teaching. By 1800, hospitals were becoming an important part of regular practitioners' (and especially surgeons') professional, intellectual and financial hierarchy. Hospitals evolved into places where reputations and large practices were made and where the orthodox knowledge or 'safe' science that underpinned regular practitioners' status was constructed and disseminated.[53] Hospital experience was linked to pedagogy and knowledge, with hospital schools becoming a vehicle through which ideas were transmitted from the medical

---

[52] Ibid., p. 135.

[53] See Brian Abel-Smith, *The Hospitals 1800–1948: A Study in Social Administration in England and Wales* (London, 1964); Geoffrey Rivett, *The Development of the London Hospital System, 1832–1982* (London, 1986); John Woodward, *To Do the Sick No Harm: A Study of the British Voluntary Hospital System to 1875* (London, 1974).

elite to ordinary medical men.[54] In doing so, hospitals not only provided a forum in which professional identities were developed and confirmed but also an arena for a new type of medicine typified by observation, physical examination, statistics, anatomy and pathology. According to Woodward, changes in medical thought allied with the voluntary hospital movement to create a dramatic rise in the standard of medical education.[55] Although this view ignores the important role played by the private anatomy schools, it does reflect the dominant position hospitals had secured in the delivery of teaching by the mid-nineteenth century. This shift was part of a European trend and a gradual move towards institutionalised teaching.

The same forces that had stimulated the growth of the private anatomy schools influenced the shift of teaching into the hospital, but in the new anatomico-clinical model, London's hospitals acquired a special significance for teaching. In 1759, one commentator could argue that 'attendance at some public hospital' ought to be 'the finishing school of the clinical physician'. Others asserted that the best way for a doctor to learn was by watching a skilled practitioner in a hospital ward.[56] With the advice literature favouring a hospital education, students were attracted to London's hospitals thereby creating a large market. Provincial hospital schools were also established, but the concentration of hospitals in London ensured that by 1800 hospital training was well established in the capital with 'at least 300 students a year signed up to observe hospital practice'. Private schools were overshadowed.[57] It was not a question of the hospital replacing the lecture theatre, but a combination of the two: the theory of the lecture room was to be applied to practical observation of the wards.

London's voluntary hospitals quickly became places where experience was gained, ideas disseminated and teaching delivered, meeting the needs of clinical instruction better than their French counterparts. Surgeons who had studied in Paris brought their skills to London, helping to shift the focus of learning. Demand for new teaching facilities rose in proportion to the growing inability of the private schools, medical guilds, or Oxford and Cambridge to offer teaching resources that contemporaries saw as necessary for proper training. The situation was better in Scotland, but even Edinburgh failed to offer the resources that London's hospitals had at their disposal. Metropolitan hospitals provided ideal opportunities for teaching: they gave

---

[54] For a full discussion on how hospital medicine became central to the eighteenth-century medical world see Lawrence, *Charitable Knowledge*.

[55] Woodward, *To Do the Sick No Harm*, p. 25.

[56] Richard Davies, *General State of Education in the Universities* (Bath, 1759); James Lucas, *A Candid Inquiry into the Education, Qualifications and Offices of a Surgeon-Apothecary* (Bath, 1800); James Parkinson, *The Hospital Pupil; or, an Essay Intended to Facilitate the Study of Medicine and Surgery* (London, 1800), pp. 53–5.

[57] Hays, 'London Lecturing Empire', p. 106.

access to more patients and hence a greater variety of clinical material for demonstration and investigation. Teachers could use their patients to illustrate their lectures and the surgical theatre to demonstrate operative technique and morbid anatomy. The effect was to depersonalise the patient but attract students who were keen to watch, and were encouraged to do so by a rhetoric of observation and experience espoused in medical lectures.

For those holding hospital posts, lessons were learned from the private anatomy schools. They showed that students could provide a significant income given that most posts were unpaid, or merely honorific. A voluntary arrangement between doctors and those running the hospital fostered an entrepreneurial attitude. According to Susan Lawrence, it was precisely at those hospitals where doctors had little formal influence that schools were first able to develop.[58] Lecturing was one way of bridging the gap between qualification and a secure income. Hospital lectures offered extra knowledge to the student at a modest fee and quickly proved that hospital teaching was as lucrative as teaching in any private anatomy school.[59] The promise of high earnings lured others to start teaching. Students followed.

Students wanted to watch the leading operators and were attracted to dynamic teachers like the enigmatic and caustic John Abernethy at St Bartholomew's. To listen to these men, students at first tailored their attendance to supplement the knowledge they had acquired through apprenticeship, using a mixture of hospital schools for clinical instruction. It was only in the mid-nineteenth century that attendance at one school became the norm. For the most part, evidence suggests that many students were in London to pursue an education for general practice, overlooking professional divisions present in the medical guilds. Hospital lectures and dissections offered flexibility that was ideally suited to this, and provided a cheap form of medical education that contrasted with the expense of a university degree and cost less than an apprenticeship to a leading hospital surgeon. Those wanting to study medicine could buy tickets to hospital lecture courses, allowing them to chop and change between institutions and eminent teachers. This broke the master/apprentice relationship.

Hospital teaching became a thriving industry. A wide range of courses in the form of lectures, demonstrations, dissections and walking the wards emerged by the end of the eighteenth century, distinguishing London hospital education from other forms of science-based learning by its vocational character. The transition marked the creation of an essentially modern type of medical education, but what was established were private schools within hospitals.[60] Teaching belonged to the lecturers, not to the

---

[58] Susan C. Lawrence, 'Entrepreneurs and Private Enterprise: The Development of Medical Lecturing in London, 1775–820', *BHM* lxii (1988), p. 188.
[59] See M. Jeanne Peterson, *Medical Profession in Mid-Victorian London* (Berkeley, 1978).
[60] H. C. Cameron, *Mr Guy's Hospital, 1726–1948* (London, 1954), p. 88.

hospital. It was only when lecture fees were combined or lecturers advertised their courses together that a medical school might be said to exist, although a certain institutional framework was also needed. Often this occurred by accident rather than design and rose from an *ad hoc* need to meet rising student numbers. With most hospital governors concerned about the inconvenience to the patients, teaching was something they tolerated rather than encouraged. Boundaries could become blurred, as at Guy's where the governors played a prominent role in financing and shaping teaching.[61] The governors of Guy's and other London hospitals were persuaded that moves to create teaching facilities were a sensible investment because students represented free labour. Ironically, in most London hospitals, where governors might not have welcomed teaching, it was their financial input that invariably made it possible.

It was only at the start of the nineteenth century that recognised schools of medicine, defined at the time 'as the whole course of lectures for the improvement of pupils in chirurgical and medical knowledge ... concentrated within the verge of the respective hospitals' emerged.[62] A large staff with different interests made a broad curriculum possible, but it was the 1815 Apothecaries Act that encouraged more organised teaching. The Act confirmed the tripartite structure of medicine and built on an established system of teaching. It did not open wards to clinical instruction, as some have believed, but did build science into the curriculum in a bid to distinguish a practitioner from a quack.[63] In requiring six months' clinical work, the Act acknowledged that hospitals had a leading teaching role. It stimulated institutional teaching even if it did little to add to the content of medical education. To compete and to match the requirements of the 1815 Act, lecturers now had to offer systematic courses allowing a common core of instruction to emerge.[64] 'Everywhere the influx of students demanding to be taught and to be furnished with certificates of clinical instruction', according to the historian of Guy's, 'determined the establishment or extension of the schools'. For Negley Harte, these built on an established pattern of teaching and provided part of the impetus for the University of London.[65]

---

[61] See McInnes, *St Thomas's*, pp. 74–6, 79; Cameron, *Guy's*, pp. 89–94, 145–6.

[62] Peachey, *Memoir*, p. 300.

[63] See S. W. F. Holloway, 'The Apothecaries Act, 1815: A Reinterpretation', *Medical History* x (1966), pp. 107–29, 221–36; Susan C. Lawrence, 'Private Enterprise and Public Interest: Medical Education and the Apothecaries' Act, 1780–1825', in *British Medicine in an Age of Reform*, ed. Roger French and Andrew Wear (London, 1991), pp. 45–7; Irvine Loudon, *Medical Care and the General Practitioner, 1750–1850* (Oxford, 1986), pp. 48, 51, 129–88.

[64] Susan C. Lawrence, 'Science and Medicine at the London Hospitals: The Development of Teaching and Research, 1750–1815' (unpublished Ph.D. diss., Toronto, 1985), pp. 411–12; Lawrence, 'Private Enterprise and Public Interest', pp. 45–73.

[65] Cameron, *Guy's*, p. 82; Negley Harte, *The University of London, 1836–1986* (London, 1986), p. 52.

A college by accident

What was happening at St Bartholomew's during this time? Apprentices continued to attend the wards throughout the seventeenth and eighteenth centuries, but it was under Edward Nourse, elected assistant surgeon in 1730, that lectures were first introduced at the hospital. St Bartholomew's had risen in status since the Reformation, and Nourse was taking advantage of the growing demand for private instruction, but he was not the first member of the hospital's staff to lecture. Harvey had been Lumleian lecturer and taught anatomy at the College of Physicians in 1616, and Terne also taught medicine and anatomy at the College.[66] However, these doctors did not attempt to connect their teaching to the hospital's name. Nourse changed this practice, directly linking his teaching to his work at St Bartholomew's. He had lectured before his appointment at the United Company's theatre and at London House, Aldersgate Street, defying attempts by the United Company to control dissections.[67] In 1734, Nourse transferred his lectures to St Bartholomew's. In an advertisement in the *Evening Post* he explained that: 'desirous to have no more lectures at my own house, I think it proper to advertise that I shall begin a course of Anatomy, Chirurgical Operations and Bandages on Monday, November 11, at St Bartholomew's Hospital'.[68] These are the earliest recorded lectures delivered at a London hospital. A year later, the governors of St Bartholomew's sanctioned his activities. They resolved that 'any of the surgeons or assistant surgeons of this Hospital have leave to read Anatomical lectures in the Dissecting Room belonging to this House'. The decision was not upheld for long. In July 1735, the resolution was rescinded.[69] No indication was given as to why. They may have passed the resolution simply because Nourse had stopped teaching at St Bartholomew's and with no other staff willing to lecture there was no need for the resolution to be maintained. However, it may also reflect the fact that Nourse's lectures had disrupted the hospital, while his interest in dissection was at odds with that of the governors. The effect was to ensure that lectures by the hospital's staff had, in theory, to be given outside St Bartholomew's.

The appointment of Percival Pott as assistant surgeon in 1745 saw a concerted effort to introduce teaching at St Bartholomew's at a time when the hospital was being rebuilt. Pott served all his professional life at St Bartholomew's and improved the practice of surgery in the hospital,

---

[66] Whitteridge, *William Harvey*, pp. 82–8; Norman Moore, *The History of the Study of Medicine in the British Isles* (Oxford, 1908), pp. 73–4.

[67] Norman Moore, *The History of St Bartholomew's Hospital*, 2 vols (London, 1918), Vol. 2, p. 637; Edward Mansfield Brockbank, *The Foundation of Provincial Medical Education in England and of the Manchester School in Particular* (Manchester, 1936), p. 40.

[68] Cited in Peachey, *Memoir*, pp. 34–5.

[69] House committee, 20 November 1720, HA 1/11; general court, 31 July 1735, HA 1/11.

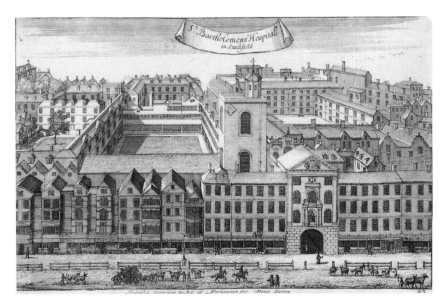

Plate 1.3 St Bartholomew's from West Smithfield, 1720. Depicts Henry VIII Gate and Smithfield frontage, with tower of St Bartholomew's-the-less and other hospital buildings behind

rendering it more humane by reducing the number of instruments and avoiding the use of cautery. Although not ahead of his time, Pott was recognised as observant and thorough, making important contributions to the treatment of fractures ("Pott's fracture"), the knowledge of tumours and occupational cancer.[70] From an educated background, Pott had been apprenticed to Nourse between 1729 and 1736, during which time he had prepared dissections for Nourse's lectures, a duty that gave Pott a solid grounding in anatomy.[71] Although he had assisted Nourse in his teaching, Pott only started lecturing on his own eight years after his appointment at St Bartholomew's. Pott may have started teaching because of the situation he found at the hospital. The year before his appointment, the governors had debated whether to discontinue paying staff gratuities on the grounds that rebuilding was sapping all the available income. In the event, the gratuities were continued, but Pott probably felt insecure and this may have encouraged him to extend his teaching.[72]

---

[70] See James Earle, *The Chirurgical Works of Percival Pott. To which are added, a short account of the life of the author* (London, 1775).

[71] D'Arcy Power, *British Masters of Medicine* (London, 1936), p. 35.

[72] General court, 5 July 1744, HA 1/11.

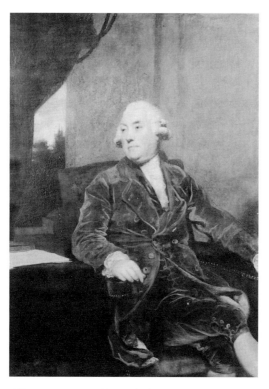

Plate 1.4 Percival Pott, surgeon to St Bartholomew's

At first, Pott's lectures were informal, designed to improve the skill of his dressers.[73] They quickly developed in to a formal course as demand rose and other lecturers established hospital-based courses. Always neat and stylish, Pott had the faculty of making his subject interesting. He was gifted with a good mode of delivery and an animated manner and, influenced by Boerhaave and Sydenham, believed in teaching by the bedside. He was one of the first lecturers in London to adopt this practice, adding to his popularity. As his reputation grew, his classes became larger and attracted students from Edinburgh.[74] By 1765, the number wanting to hear him teach persuaded Pott to transfer his lectures from his home to St Bartholomew's where he already carried out bedside teaching. Encouraged by Pott's success and the money that could be made, other doctors connected to the hospital began to offer courses. In the same year that Pott moved his lectures to St Bartholomew's, William Pitcairn, physician from 1750 to 1780 and friend of William Hunter,

[73] Peachey, *Memoir*, p. 35.
[74] Zachary Cope, 'Surgical Lectures of 150 Years Ago', in *Sidelights on the History of Medicine*, ed. Zachary Cope (London, 1957), p. 152.

started lecturing on medicine in the hospital. Following Pott's example he taught in the wards, encouraging his pupils to rely on nature.[75] Partly in recognition of Pott's work, and because of pressure from other members of the medical staff, the governors agreed in 1767 that physicians and surgeons had

> leave to make use of the Theatre for operations and also of the Room adjoining thereto in the pyle of building lately finished to read lectures in to their pupils and other purposes for the accommodation of the Physicians and Surgeons.[76]

Hospital instruction now began in earnest.

Although Pott had started systematic teaching, Abernethy provided the catalyst for a school. Frequently brusque, egotistical and capable of rudeness (especially to his patients and colleagues) Abernethy had a major impact on the early development of teaching at St Bartholomew's.[77] Before he had completed his apprenticeship with Charles Blicke, the assistant surgeon at St Bartholomew's, he was appointed assistant surgeon on Pott's retirement in 1787. With the post having few clinical responsibilities, Abernethy was attracted to teaching. In January 1788, presumably because of lack of suitable accommodation in the hospital, he advertised a course of anatomical lectures at his home in Bartholomew Close. By September, Abernethy was advertising his lectures in tandem with others teaching at St Bartholomew's. The 'usual lectures' by Pott were mentioned, along with those of William Austin, physician and a protégé of Pott's who taught chemistry and medicine, and those of Henry Krohn, physician-accoucheur at the Middlesex who taught midwifery.[78] The lectures were publicised under the heading 'St Bartholomew's Hospital', although most were delivered in Bartholomew Close.[79] Pott, Abernethy, Austin and Krohn were working together to offer a more complete course of instruction under the hospital's name. For want of better evidence, a medical school may be said to have come into existence in 1788, more as a matter of convenience than design.

Abernethy stole the limelight. At first nervous, he quickly developed a teaching style that appealed to students. They were attracted to his eccentricity, his clear and effective manner, and his style of teaching that adopted a Parisian approach. Many saw him 'as being of a superior order' and, with a large number of students attending his lectures, the governors agreed in 1791 to fund a 'Surgeons Theatre' – often referred to as the 'Medical Theatre'. The theatre was situated behind the west wing of the hospital

[75] Cited in Jane M. Oppenheimer, *New Aspects of John and William Hunter* (London, 1946), p. 117.

[76] House committee, 20 February 1767, HA 1/13.

[77] See George Macilwain, *The Memoirs of John Abernethy* (London, 1856); John Thornton, *John Abernethy: A Biography* (London, 1953).

[78] Ibid., pp. 21–2, 29.

[79] Medvei and Thornton, *St Bartholomew's*, p. 48.

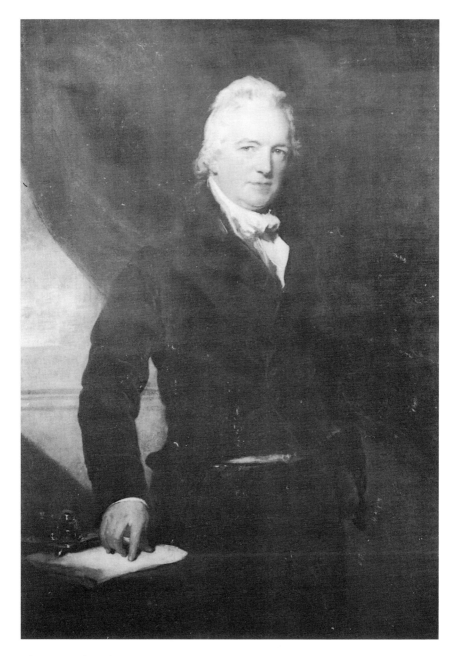

Plate 1.5 John Abernethy, surgeon to St Bartholomew's

and was fully in use when the *Morning Chronicle* advertised lectures in 'physick', anatomy, physiology, midwifery, diseases of women and children, and chemistry in 1795.[80] The opening of the new theatre was a success, helping the College to grow.

Abernethy's anatomical and surgical teaching formed the heart of the College. He provided academic guidance, and his role in founding the Medical and Philosophical Society in 1795 instituted a forum for discussion and further training. Under his encouragement, the Society established a library in 1800, although progress was slow and complaints were made in 1802 that the librarian was inclined to keep books at home. Abernethy also played a central role in attracting students, encouraging other clinicians to start teaching at St Bartholomew's. Gradually a comprehensive curriculum was developed. Lectures on anatomy, physiology and surgery were delivered by Abernethy, while others taught less prestigious courses on comparative anatomy, chemistry, physics, medicine, therapeutics, and 'the diseases of women and children'.[81] Initially many of these lecturers, such as William Osborn, lecturer on midwifery and physician at the General Lying-in Hospital, held posts at other London hospitals where opportunities for teaching were limited. These men filled gaps in experience not found in the hospital.

By 1821, so many students (numbering several hundred on the surgical side) were attending St Bartholomew's that the existing teaching accommodation was deemed inadequate. The lecturers pressed for a larger lecture theatre and the governors were asked to pay. The governors were unconvinced. They retreated behind the Henry VIII charter, in part because the first theatre had cost twice as much as planned and had been sanctioned without their approval. The charter stipulated that money could be spent only on 'the relief and cure of the sick, lame and impotent', in theory preventing funds from being spent on the College.[82] Abernethy, as the 'senior teacher', immediately presented himself to explain the benefits of the College to the hospital. Abernethy's statement was clever. The College was shown to be a utility and an asset; one that guaranteed a high standard of treatment since 'it is impossible for the Medical Officers . . . to do all that is necessary to be done for the relief of Patients' without 'recourse to the subordinate assistance of Students'. Abernethy went on to argue that the large number of students ensured that the staff were 'open to the public expression of Praise or Censure from these vigilant Observers'. It was also felt that the presence of students contributed to the development of medical science. Such assertions were part of a common rhetoric of charitable fund-raising familiar to the governors. They made underlying reference to the

---

[80] House committee, 14 April 1791, HA 1/15.
[81] *Medical and Physical Journal* vi (1801), p. 284.
[82] Special committee, 6 April 1821, HA 1/17.

powerful notion of political economy, implying that all classes of society could only benefit from the College. It was only at the end that Abernethy explained that 'the size of the Theatre is insufficient for the increased number of Students who have of late years resorted to the Hospital and the extent of the inconvenience is such as to require that this representation should be made'. To encourage the governors, Abernethy 'begged' the governors' permission to add his 'collected Specimens of various Diseases and Injuries for the instruction of Students, amounting in number of several thousands'. In addition, he volunteered that the library the surgeons had worked to establish should also be passed to the governors' control. At the very least, it was a diplomatic move that also removed the need for the College to finance the museum and library.[83]

Abernethy's statement made several important assumptions. The first was that by the early 1820s medical teaching was sufficiently advanced at St Bartholomew's for him to refer directly to a 'Medical School', even though no formal structure had been established. The second was that the origins of the College lay with the governors. This had one advantage: it gave the governors a role in teaching and implied a degree of obligation.

The governors did not make an immediate decision. They felt the matter had been 'abruptly introduced', but by April they saw no objection to using hospital funds to aid the College. The fact that there was no clause relating to medical education in the Henry VIII charter was now seen as reflecting the 'infantile state of Medical Science' at the time. Through a careful use of historical justification, the governors now argued that the hospital's founders would not have wanted to limit any improvement in medicine and therefore they felt obliged to meet the lecturers' requests. The decision, it was added, was made on the 'chief grounds of it being a measure calculated to produce the most substantial benefit and permanent good to the Hospital'.[84] The governors had accepted Abernethy's rhetoric. After an investigation of conditions at Guy's and St Thomas's, and an assessment of the practicality of extending existing accommodation, plans were drawn up for a new theatre. When the new anatomical theatre opened on 1 October 1822, 406 people attended to hear Abernethy give the first lecture.

Striving for control

By the 1820s, St Bartholomew's had established itself as the largest school in London. It had a lecturing staff under Abernethy that taught a full medical curriculum, an anatomical lecture theatre and an operating theatre, along with a museum, rudimentary library and a dead house where dissections were

---

[83] Ibid., 20 March 1822, HA 1/17.
[84] House committee, 19 April 1822, HA 1/17.

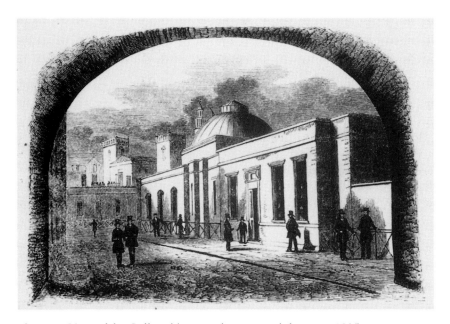

Plate 1.6 View of the College library and anatomical theatre, c.1835

undertaken. Only one major question remained to be settled: Who controlled teaching?

The issue came to a head in 1826 and continued to dominate the affairs of the hospital for a further two years. In November, the general court, the main managing body of the hospital, initiated an investigation into the conduct of the lecturers to determine if their actions had 'prejudiced' or 'injured' St Bartholomew's.[85] This was part of a general investigation of the management of the hospital established at Abernethy's insistence. It was a recognition of a growing feeling that teaching was not, as Abernethy had claimed five years earlier, beneficial to the hospital. Grievances about teaching were not new. However, Abernethy's attempts in 1825 and 1826 to resign as surgeon but continue to lecture attracted attention. He was resigning on a principle. Although appointed assistant surgeon in 1787, Abernethy had to wait until James Earle retired in 1815 before he was made a full surgeon. The frustrations he faced during this period convinced him that all staff should retire at age 60. He had petitioned the governors to enforce a retirement age, but with no action taken Abernethy decided to retire in 1825 at the age of 60. His unsuccessful resignation precipitated a crisis.

The hospital's funding of the lecture theatre in 1791 and anatomical theatre in 1821 made the governors believe they had a right to manage the

---

[85] General court, 22 November 1826, HA 1/18.

College. This attitude was revealed in 1825 when they decided 'the Medical Teachers . . . be selected from the Medical Board of the Hospital'. Existing lecturers had previously selected who taught, but the governors' resolution effectively removed their authority to control teaching and appoint staff. Unconvinced by the need to use teachers from outside the hospital, the governors insisted that the 'talents of strangers' were no longer necessary and pressed for the inclusion of teaching as part of the normal duties of the staff. Although the governors recognised 'the fostering care of Mr Abernethy', they asserted that the College had only 'arrived at a state of great reputation and usefulness through the liberality of the Governors'.[86] The resolution infuriated the lecturers. The problem had arisen because of the governors' inability to distinguish between the hospital and the College. Abernethy's persistent attempts to resign highlighted the situation. Elements within the governing body saw the posts Abernethy held as surgeon and as lecturer as synonymous, and argued that if Abernethy resigned one he should not hold the other. They were also worried that teaching was damaging care and appointed a subcommittee to investigate. There was more than Abernethy's resignation at stake. In many ways, it was a battle over who should control teaching.

In 1827, the subcommittee appointed to investigate teaching found, 'on mature deliberation', no fault with the treatment of the patients. Concerns that teaching on the wards and the rivalry this had engendered with nearby private schools (particularly the Aldersgate Street school) were acknowledged, but the subcommittee concluded that lecturing was an '*exterior*' matter, outside the purpose of the original charter, and so should be left to the lecturers. The governors did not react favourably, believing that because lectures were delivered at St Bartholomew's they were under their control. They argued that if Abernethy wanted to resign he had to do so unconditionally. The house committee, which made most of the decisions, retorted that because lectures had previously been conducted in the lecturers' homes it was a matter for the 'medical Gentlemen themselves to settle which of them should deliver lectures'. This was recognition of the private nature of teaching in the hospital. To resolve the crisis, the house committee asserted that 'it had better still be referred to them to make their own arrangements on that head, and the appointment of Lecturers be avoided by the Governors'. Over the choice of demonstrators and student discipline, the committee was aware that these 'had much better be left to the Medical Gentlemen to arrange and settle, and that the Governors ought not to interfere therein unless called upon'.[87] It acknowledged medical authority and the governors' inability to select teachers. The committee's advice was

---

[86] House committee, 17 August 1825, HA 1/17.
[87] Ibid., 18 January 1827, 28 February 1827, HA 1/18.

accepted; the 1825 resolution was overruled, and Abernethy was allowed to resign his hospital post and continue lecturing.[88]

Victory for the lecturers did not last long. When evidence came to light that Abernethy and Edward Stanley, lecturer in anatomy and physiology, had tried to secure a pledge from Thomas Wormald, the demonstrator of anatomy and pupil of Abernethy, that he would not interfere in the appointment of Abernethy's son 'at any future period', a further crisis developed.[89] Abernethy was keen to blame Stanley, but Wormald insisted that it was Abernethy who had pressured Stanley to sign a bond whereby Stanley would forfeit £14,000 'if Mr. Abernethy's son was not co-lecturer with him'. Nepotism was widespread in London's hospitals, but this seemed too much for the governors after the struggle for authority the year before.[90] Although Abernethy's skill as a lecturer was acknowledged, the governors found his actions scandalous. They felt that such conduct militated 'against the only plan upon which the real use of the Charity must depend that of electing its Medical Officers upon the Ground of professional merit alone'. This was an ideal rarely applied in practice, even at St Bartholomew's. The governors insisted that staff be appointed on 'ability, humanity, and steadiness', ruling that to prevent a repetition of events 'all such appointments be submitted to the House Committee for confirmation'. The lecturers were reminded that the hospital provided considerable funds for their benefit and expected them to bear this in mind.[91] It was a thinly veiled threat. Where Abernethy had secured control for the lecturers, his actions over his son limited this power, giving back to the governors some of the authority they had lost over appointments. The organisation of teaching remained under the control of the lecturers, but the events in the 1820s strained relations with the governors and limited the lecturers' sphere of action.

A slow evolution

By the 1820s, London's medical schools had become the dominant institutional form for medical education, though other modes of training through apprenticeship, private schools and universities continued. New regulations devised by the College of Surgeons – in which staff from St Bartholomew's played a key role – strengthened the position of the London teaching hospitals. Between 1821 and 1824, the College of Surgeons passed a series of resolutions that recognised only those anatomy courses conducted in hospitals by a College examiner. Limitations were placed on

[88] Special committee, 14 August 1827, HA 1/18.
[89] Special general court, 22 August 1827, HA 1/18.
[90] Lancet xii (1826/7), pp. 658, 662.
[91] Special committee, 24–5 August 1827, HA 1/18.

hospital practice that damaged private and provincial schools, and favoured those in London. The resolutions preserved the 'very lucrative teaching monopoly of the consultants in larger hospitals' and were violently attacked by Thomas Wakley, editor of the newly formed *Lancet*. Wakley stamped the journal with his own radical personality and used it as a vehicle to attack the corruption he saw in the medical establishment. The *Lancet* transformed earlier criticisms of the royal colleges and hospitals into a bitter controversy characterised by 'heart-burning and quarrels'; 'personal attack and . . . nicknames'.[92] The resolutions were the first part in a long battle. It was a calculated move taken by the examiners who taught at the very schools the restrictions were designed to benefit. Although the restrictions were removed in 1831, they had already strengthened the London hospital schools and contributed to the decline of the private anatomy schools. In the process, they had helped confirm the status of St Bartholomew's as one of the leading teaching institutions.

However, why did a school at St Bartholomew's take so long to emerge? It was not because the hospital lacked the clinical material for demonstration. It was one of the largest and most reputable hospitals in London and as such attracted apprentices and 'younge Doctors', possibly from its foundation. Neither was it because those working at St Bartholomew's were uninterested in teaching. Staff contributed to the growing vernacular medical literature and wrote textbooks that disseminated their understanding and clinical experience, while Harvey, Terne and others had taught anatomy at the College of Physicians. Although St Bartholomew's had the facilities and staff to teach, it was not until the eighteenth century that a climate existed outside the hospital that favoured the institutionalisation of medical learning within the hospital environment. The creation of a school at St Bartholomew's before the eighteenth century would have been at variance with how medical knowledge and medical learning were constructed in Britain.

Other forces were at work that discouraged the early development of a medical school at St Bartholomew's. Susan Lawrence has argued that the hospital's endowments freed it from the subtle restrictions on practice that the voluntary hospitals experienced with their constant need to solicit funds from the public. She considers that this helped a school to develop.[93] However, St Bartholomew's was a conservative institution. The governors expressed their faith in traditional academic methods and the hospital was part of the medical establishment. Harvey was committed to the College of Physicians where he lectured, a connection that became stronger after 1643

---

[92] Cited in Jean and Irvine Loudon, 'Medicine, Politics and the Medical Periodicals, 1800–50', in *Medical Journals and Medical Knowledge: Historical Essays*, ed. W. F. Bynum, Stephen Lock and Roy Porter (London, 1992), p. 61.
[93] Lawrence, 'Entrepreneurs and Private Enterprise', pp. 187–8.

when he was dismissed from St Bartholomew's for his royalist sympathies. Other staff held influential positions in the College of Physicians and at the United Company. This provided an arena for teaching external to the hospital, while the hospital's status, along with the relative lack of institutional competition until the eighteenth century, ensured a ready supply of pupils and apprentices. The governors might have complained about the presence of apprentices in the 1660s, but they did not prohibit them or directly obstruct staff using St Bartholomew's for teaching. With posts paying an honorarium and virtually guaranteeing a large and distinguished private practice, the financial incentive to lecture was reduced.

Why did this situation change? By the mid-eighteenth century restrictions on teaching were being removed, demand rose and the traditional nature of medical learning was breaking down. The medical guilds were no longer seen as providing appropriate surroundings for the new approach to learning that favoured anatomico-clinical medicine and observation. The privileged position St Bartholomew's held as one of few hospitals in London was also being challenged by the voluntary hospital movement at a time when new avenues for teaching were emerging. Staff at the hospital were influenced by these changes. Nourse and Pott were educated in a different medical tradition from their predecessors and this led them to stress the importance of the bedside and observation. Abernethy was appointed when medical incomes were already under assault because of the growing level of competition. Teaching provided a solution to this problem and his popularity encouraged others to follow. They worked within an environment where the governors were willing to let them advance their teaching and even provided financial assistance.

The growth of a school at St Bartholomew's illustrates how external and internal forces merged. It highlights the interplay between governors and staff, entrepreneurial effort and changes in medical thought that was important in encouraging the development of a hospital medical school. At no point was it an inevitable process.

2

Rise and fall of the 'Abernethian' school

Under John Abernethy, St Bartholomew's had firmly established itself as one of London's leading medical schools by the mid-1820s. Teaching had developed at a time when a growing concentration of entrepreneurial provision encouraged a shift in medical education towards an institutional model. During the late eighteenth and early nineteenth centuries hospital training emerged as an important feature of a qualified and regular practitioner's training as demand for practical learning grew. The traditional universities had turned their back on professional training and new institutions were established to fill the gap. New subjects from the seventeenth-century scientific revolution were gradually incorporated into a curriculum that was undergoing systematisation as practitioners struggled to become the custodians of an authentic knowledge, and as pressure for radical political and medical reform intensified. Common ground was found in the importance ascribed to anatomy and physiology, and in the need for rational or scientific understanding. These debates infused medical education. However, the expense and intensity of these changes had already led some contemporaries to fear that all 'you can expect of a student at his graduation is, that he shall be qualified to *learn* the practice of his art'.[1] While medical reformers thundered against the monopoly of the licensing bodies and called for minimum uniform standards, London's medical schools endeavoured to offer the courses which students and examining bodies demanded.

In this volatile market, St Bartholomew's was able to establish a 'complete' school. Biased towards surgery, teaching was neither dull nor pioneering. However, the College's ability to attract students and prominent lecturers concealed deficiencies and tensions that became more pronounced after the death of Abernethy in 1830. Without Abernethy, the College went into decline just as medical education was undergoing a further period of rationalisation. Attempts were made to limit competition and 'modernise' teaching, but although reforms placed the College on a firmer footing, by 1843 St Bartholomew's had reached a low point.

The rise of the hospital student

When Abernethy started teaching, a shift was already underway in the nature of students attending London's hospitals. Apprenticeship and pupilage based

---

[1] *Lancet* i (1829/30), p. 42.

on personalities and patronage was in decline as medical education was institutionalised. A new type of student was emerging: the hospital student. By Abernethy's death in 1830 apprenticeship and pupilage had been largely replaced. In the process, hospitals in London were transformed. The presence of lecturers and a large body of students made them into centres of learning, which had a dramatic impact on patients' experiences as students crowded round the bedside.

Students had first entered St Bartholomew's as apprentices of the surgical staff or pupils of the physicians. It was one of the privileges of holding a hospital appointment; few doctors practising at a London hospital failed to take on pupils, encouraged by the large fees which supplemented otherwise honorary hospital posts. Pupils and apprentices were tolerated provided they did not disrupt the working of the wards. By the mid-seventeenth century their presence had become a normal feature of the routine at St Bartholomew's. With no quota set on the number a surgeon or physician could train at any one time (unlike Guy's or St Thomas's), teaching was free to expand.[2] However, the nature of apprenticeship and high fees restricted access to the wards, in effect limiting the numbers that used the hospital to train.

In return for training, apprentices promised obedience, loyalty, secrecy and to work for their master. Access to the wards and some responsibility for patient care was by implication an integral part of an agreement based on personality and patronage. This implicit arrangement made apprenticeship to a hospital surgeon attractive despite the high fees.[3] The high cost was a premium for personal attention and helped equip the apprentice to enter society and secure wealthy patients. With St Bartholomew's having a comparatively large and distinguished staff, it offered a certain lure for those seeking clinical experience or contacts. Percival Pott and Abernethy were both able to place their apprentices in hospital posts, or aid them in establishing profitable practices. Apprenticeship not only affected students' future careers but also their experiences of the hospital. Abernethy was not easy to work with: he had difficult relationships with his apprentices that often left a legacy of ill feeling. Pott had a temper, was inclined to vanity and was fickle with his pupils. According to Ludford Harvey, an aspiring apprentice of Pott's, the 'fair fabric of my hopes' was 'reduced to ruins' when another pupil, James Earle, 'terminated the . . . virginity of Miss Pott' after a 'courtship of one fortnight'. Earle's marriage to Pott's daughter gave him 'an aspiring surgeon for his son in law, whom for the last 10 years the whole family had most cordially ridiculed and abused'. Pott transferred his

[2] E. M. McInnes, *St Thomas's Hospital* (London, 1963), p. 76.
[3] See Joan Lane, 'The Role of Apprenticeship in Eighteenth-Century Medical Education in England', in *William Hunter and the Eighteenth Century Medical World*, ed. W. F. Bynum and Roy Porter (Cambridge, 1985), pp. 57–103.

patronage to Earle, leaving Harvey in an unfavourable position.[4] Other apprentices' diaries point to different frustrations, but these were more than counterbalanced by the potential rewards of an apprenticeship to a hospital doctor.

The growth of hospital schools challenged the need for rigid agreements between students and hospital staff, contributing to a breakdown in the apprenticeship system. To fill the gap, other means of gaining hospital experience emerged to offer post-apprenticeship training to students eager to extend their experience. When Abernethy started teaching in the late 1780s, students desiring to hear lectures and walk the wards who had already served an apprenticeship already outnumbered pupils. Pressure was mounting to break medicine's links with the craft and trade activities associated with apprenticeship, which appeared increasingly unsystematic, obsolete and reactionary. By the 1800s the system was breaking down, despite the insistence of the Society of Apothecaries under the 1815 Apothecaries Act that a five-year apprenticeship was required for their diploma. Apprentice-ship agreements that had traditionally tied students to their masters for up to five years were relaxed, allowing students to leave the apprenticeship early to spend some time at a London hospital. Post-apprenticeship study at a medical school became increasingly common for those seeking subtle advantages in the medical market. With an apprenticeship often 'dull, and at times tedious and apparently useless', the greater degree of freedom and opportunities for learning offered by hospitals made them attractive locations for study.[5] They promised something apprenticeship could not: 'intense exposure to surgical conditions and operations not only seen less frequently in private practice, but also diagnosed and performed with the most current methods'.[6] Access to the wards for a fee allowed those who could not afford an apprenticeship to a London practitioner to watch the staff at work. This greatly extended the number of students who could use St Bartholomew's for part of their training. Unlike apprenticeships, hospital students were not tied to any one practitioner, school or lecturer, although the high cost of training curtailed students' ability to attend a variety of hospitals. For Ivan Waddington, this movement into hospitals ensured that students came under the clinical and ethical control of an elite group of teachers. A more intense period of professional socialisation followed, which 'fostered a sense of professional community that asserted the primacy of professional rather than lay values'.[7]

---

[4] Journal of Ludford Harvey, ff. 48–9, X54/1.

[5] Stephen Paget, ed., *Memoirs and Letters of Sir James Paget* (London, 1902), p. 19.

[6] Ivan Waddington, 'General Practitioners and Consultants in Early Nineteenth Century England: The Sociology of an Intra-Professional Conflict', in *Health Care and Popular Medicine in Nineteenth Century England: Essays in the Social History of Medicine*, ed. John Woodward and David Richards (New York, 1977), p. 169.

[7] Ivan Waddington, *The Medical Profession in the Industrial Revolution* (Dublin, 1984), p. 203.

By the 1820s, St Bartholomew's had acquired a central place for students seeking a medical career. Although staff continued to offer prestigious pupilages to those who could afford them, this had ceased to be the main means through which students attended the hospital. Student numbers had increased dramatically since the 1790s, forcing new ways of learning as students sought to 'fulfil their own expectations about the education necessary for successful practice'. For Susan Lawrence, such attendance came to mark a doctor 'as a practitioner with an appropriate background'.[8] Either students could pay to visit the wards or, if they wished, more experience could be secured by an appointment as dresser to one of the surgeons. These appointments were a hybrid of traditional apprenticeships that recognised the need for cheaper and more informal arrangements between practitioner and student. Students were usually introduced to one of the surgeons through the network of informal and formal contacts that existed between hospital staff and their qualified pupils. Family connections and patronage remained important, since it was at the surgeon's discretion whether or not to take a student on. Apart from the high premium, no other qualification or examination was required.

To meet the requirements of the licensing bodies, dressers were appointed for twelve months and often split their attendance between two surgeons to increase their experience. After the death of an 'accident patient' on his discharge from the hospital in 1822, the governors intervened. They insisted that all dressers had to have 'the experience of a regular attendance as a Pupil of the Hospital for twelvemonths at least'.[9] The decision in theory reduced the teaching staff's control over who was appointed and limited dresserships to senior students. No opposition was offered because the new regulation ensured that some students would now spend at least a year at St Bartholomew's raising the amount of fees to the College. In practice, these students did most of the work in the hospital. Governors accepted their presence as a necessary evil and a source of 'indispensable free work'.[10] Dressers rarely gained any credit and were 'brutally insulted' by the house surgeons, who treated them as ignorant and inferior.[11] The position was worth the trouble and high fee however. It allowed students to gain privileged access to the wards and acted as a stepping stone to a post.

---

[8] Susan C. Lawrence, 'Educating the Senses: Students, Teachers and Medical Rhetoric in Eighteenth Century London', in *Medicine and the Five Senses*, ed. W. F. Bynum and Roy Porter (Cambridge, 1993), p. 157; Susan C. Lawrence, *Charitable Knowledge: Hospital Pupils and Practitioners in Eighteenth-Century London* (Cambridge, 1996), pp. 135–6.

[9] House committee, 20 September 1822, HA 4/17; John Wrottesley and Samuel Smith, 'St Bartholomew's Hospital', *32nd Report of the Charity Commissions*, Part vi (London, 1840), pp. 71, 56–7.

[10] Lawrence, *Charitable Knowledge*, p. 127.

[11] Robert Christison, *Life of Robert Christison*, 3 vols (London, 1885/6), Vol. 1, p. 190; *Lancet* viii (1825), p. 183.

An imperfect education?

The idea that medical students should spend part of their training in a hospital had become a central feature of European medical education by the 1820s. In Britain, the College of Surgeons demanded at least a year (or six months after 1828) at a London hospital from 1812 before a student was allowed to sit for a licence. The Society of Apothecaries introduced similar regulations in 1815. Ironically, this reduced the time spent at a hospital to close to the minimum requirement. Leeway existed in the enforcement of these requirements, but the decision was a codification of what had become an established practice; one that helped confirm the authority of the London hospitals.[12] There was still room for argument, however. If walking the wards had become the norm, the degree of emphasis given to practical hospital training remained a source of friction. While the medical press made their recommendations, London's hospital schools advertised the facilities they offered.

The medical regime adopted at St Bartholomew's made it attractive to students. It offered the potential for observation and hands-on experience characteristic of Parisian hospitals that was felt to be lacking in many London hospitals. Unlike the voluntary hospitals founded in the eighteenth century, St Bartholomew's had a comparatively liberal admissions policy. Rules requiring an admission fee were abolished in 1821 and only smallpox cases were excluded. In theory, patients had to be recommended by either a governor or a City magistrate, but the hospital also admitted accident cases 'at all hours without any order'.[13] Students could therefore see the full range of medical and surgical cases and were present at all parts of the admission process. After the patient had been washed, dressed and sent to the wards, students who had paid for the privilege accompanied the physician or surgeon during the initial examination. Students could also attend daily ward rounds and, with surgeons visiting on different days, a wide variety of practice could be seen. After 1826, students' access to the hospital was extended when they were permitted to visit at any time.[14] This and the possibility of a private conversation with one of the medical staff outside the ward round was prized by students.[15] Similar freedoms did not exist elsewhere: at St George's, students were only admitted from ten in the morning to two in the afternoon, while they were barred from the wards at the Westminster.[16]

What advantage students took of the 'valuable knowledge' offered at St Bartholomew's was left entirely to them. In their repeated stress on the

---

[12] Susan C. Lawrence, 'Entrepreneurs and Private Enterprise: The Development of Medical Lecturing in London, 1775–1820', *BHM* lxii (1988), p. 57.

[13] Wrottesley and Smith, 'St Bartholomew's', pp. 56–7.

[14] *Lancet* ix (1825/6), p. 20.

[15] Lawrence, *Charitable Knowledge*, p. 149.

[16] *Lancet* x (1826), pp. 724–5.

importance of observation, lecturers were clear that 'it would be the students' fault if they [did] not profit by the opportunities that were before them'.[17] Contemporaries were less charitable to the hospital. Thomas Wakley, founder of the radical *Lancet*, was disparaging of the opportunities available at St Bartholomew's. Although he found fault with all London schools, he was sceptical of the teaching arrangements at St Bartholomew's, especially after a heated quarrel with Abernethy over the publication of his lectures.[18] After the dispute, the *Lancet* became an enthusiastic critic of the hospital, delighting in every opportunity to condemn teaching or Abernethy. Although the journal agreed that 'much valuable information may be culled' from the wards, it felt that this was 'principally of the negative kind and showing what ought to be avoided, rather than what ought to be performed'.[19] Problems did exist. Surgical students rarely visited the medical wards unless they were also a pupil of one of the physicians. They therefore relied on the 'few crumbs they might pick up now and then during the medical treatment of surgical cases'.[20] Surgeons and physicians at every London hospital skipped cases, hurried from bed to bed, and often made only superficial examinations. Ward rounds were little more a combination of *mêlée* and race. Diligent students had to '*catch what we can*', and what an individual learned depended on his ability to work and push to the front.[21] The situation at St Bartholomew's was no different. Seventy to eighty students regularly attended the wards, making observation difficult. In the operating theatre the front row was reserved for dressers obscuring the view for other, less privileged students. With students relieving the tension with 'hideous yells' and jeering, it was also often impossible to hear what was going on. Critics referred to the assembled crowd as the 'Smithfield mob' and the College quickly became renowned for the problem of witnessing operations. Overcrowding became so bad that the surgeon Henry Earle suggested having bars around the operating table, and in 1837 all 'strangers' who interfered with the comfort of the 'regular students' were excluded to ease congestion.[22]

Teaching was also haphazard. Although hospitals provided an ideal environment for clinical instruction, allowing the 'oral culture of the wards' to become a central element in training, interest in bedside teaching varied with individual teachers.[23] It was not unknown for doctors to ignore students in the wards. Even in the 1830s, when the importance of bedside teaching had been acknowledged, there was a general unease about clinical

---

[17] Ibid., i (1838/9), p. 146.

[18] For dispute, see John Thornton, *John Abernethy: A Biography* (London, 1953).

[19] *Lancet* i (1823/4), p. 761.

[20] Christison, *Life of Robert Christison*, vol. 1, pp. 191, 193; *Lancet* xii (1826/7), pp. 536–7.

[21] *Lancet*, iv (1824), pp. 159, 216.

[22] Medical College, 29 September 1837, MS 15.

[23] Lawrence, *Charitable Knowledge*, p.154.

instruction. At the Westminster staff failed to offer any teaching at the bedside; at Guy's the irregular attendance of the surgeons ensured that tuition remained a novelty.[24] Although the situation was not as bad at St Bartholomew's, there was little systematic attempt until the mid-1820s to provide bedside teaching. Pott's enthusiasm for clinical instruction was not shared by his successors.[25] The surgeons Henry Earle and John Vincent often failed to explain cases. Vincent almost ran through the wards, covering seventy to eighty patients in just over an hour and seldom attempting to 'give any thing in the shape of clinical instruction'. Earle was wary of bedside teaching, believing it impractical.[26] Others at St Bartholomew's shared his assessment and students were forced to rely on their eyes rather than their ears when on the wards. Clinical teaching was deficient in other respects. For some, the way the College organised its teaching appeared 'calculated to prevent the progress and repress the ardour of the student'. Anatomical demonstrations were scheduled at the same time as ward rounds.[27] With few accurate clinical records, students did not have 'the opportunity of becoming acquainted with the medicines which are prescribed during the treatment of each patient'. Interesting cases were observed largely by chance. Despite the considerable stress placed on clinical records as a means of learning, a certain malaise continued to exist at St Bartholomew's that hampered the collection of clinical information.[28]

The appointment of Peter Mere Latham in 1824 as lecturer in the practice of medicine started a gradual process of change. A student of Oxford and the hospital, and the son of the respected John Latham who had taught at St Bartholomew's, Latham was both professionally uncontroversial and a medical gentleman. Believing that 'every mode of lecturing has been unduly exalted above clinical lecturing; and every place where knowledge is to be had, or is supposed to be had, has been unduly preferred to the bed-side', he worked to build up teaching in the wards.[29] An enthusiast for physical examination, Latham was part of a new generation of hospital physicians for whom ward teaching and clinical lectures were vital for the emerging concept of clinical medicine. His *Lectures on Subjects Connected with Clinical Medicine* extolled the virtues of bedside teaching, and in so doing helped stimulate clinical teaching at St Bartholomew's and at other London hospitals. Latham claimed that the demands placed on students gave them too little time in the wards. His solution was to discourage a slavish adherence to lectures, and to

[24] *Lancet* i (1840/1), p.28.

[25] Wellcome: Percival Pott, 'Lectures on Surgery' (c.1770), MS 3957.

[26] *Lancet* i (1829/30), p. 124.

[27] Ibid., 21 May 1825, p. 222; ibid., ii (1827/8), pp. 348–9, 558–9.

[28] Ibid., ix (1825/6), p. 20; ibid., x (1826), p. 724.

[29] Peter Mere Latham, *Lectures on Subjects Connected with Clinical Medicine* (London, 1836), p. 30.

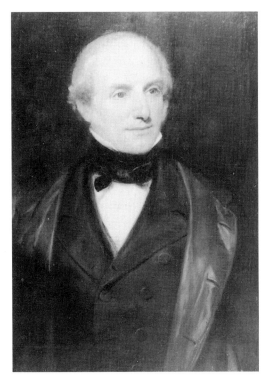

Plate 2.1 Peter Mere Latham, physician to St Bartholomew's

make teaching more clinical and suggestive to guide students to learn the realities for themselves. He also advised them on how to use their senses and on how to perform a physical examination that would elucidate the signs and symptoms of disease.[30] A growing faith in physical examination and signs stimulated by Laennec's work on auscultation encouraged this trend. Under Latham's influence, regular clinical lectures were started. In comparison to European schools, clinical teaching was at first sporadic or impersonal, but by the mid-1830s the importance of clinical lectures had been recognised and a clinical component added to courses.

The encouragement given to clinical teaching by Latham was only part of the answer to deficient clinical instruction. However, the situation at St Bartholomew's was probably no worse than that facing other hospital schools. A concentration on profitable lecturing ensured that teaching in the wards was often neglected. Every London hospital school was attacked during the 1820s when the medical establishment was facing intense criticism.

---

[30] Peter Mere Latham, *Lectures on Subjects Connected with Clinical Medicine, comprising Diseases of the Heart* (London, 1846), p. v; Latham, *Lectures* (1836), pp. 30–7.

Reformers determined to challenge existing monopolies included hospital schools in their denunciations as attention focused on how doctors were trained and licensed. The *Lancet*'s difficult relationship with Abernethy ensured that problems at St Bartholomew's were highlighted given Wakely's belief that 'the instruction of the student has been shamefully sacrificed to the private interests of two or three individuals'.[31]

Rage for dissection

Hospital schools were not only valued for the opportunities they offered for observing the living; they were also important forums for examining the dead. Changes in the medical gaze in the late eighteenth century and the development of an anatomico-clinical approach stressed the importance of dissection in understanding disease. The promise of dissection became a powerful tool in attracting students. By the start of the nineteenth century a student's education was considered defective if it did not include some morbid anatomy. It undermined old uncertainties and helped confirm a new way of looking at the body.

Post-mortems were a socially constrained activity that had some legitimacy when used to investigate the cause of death. The use of dissection to learn about anatomical structures had to be treated more carefully however. If doctors were certain that anatomy was vital to understanding disease, the public was not so easily convinced. Dissection was seen as a fate worse than death, reserved in law since the mid-sixteenth century as an additional punishment for certain cases of murder. In depriving the subject of a grave it was a practice that was feared, leading to riots when surgeons tried to take the bodies of criminals for dissection. With the legal supply of bodies from the gallows limited to six per annum, secret arrangements were encouraged that became associated with the practice of bodysnatching.[32] Anatomy teachers, 'fearful of punishment, riot, prosecution, and damage to their reputations', increasingly delegated the task of supplying corpses and paid for the privilege. Mass graves and the poor state of most churchyards made the practice relatively straightforward. The discovery of Burke and Hare's murderous exploits in Edinburgh in 1828 was merely the most public example of an established trade in cadavers.[33]

Given the public anxiety that surrounded grave robbing, those running London's charitable hospitals were anxious about what happened to the

[31] *Lancet* xii (1826/7), p. 625.

[32] See Ruth Richardson, *Death, Dissection and the Destitute* (London, 1989) for a full discussion of dissection and medicine.

[33] Ruth Richardson, '"Trading Assassins" and the Licensing of Anatomy', in *British Medicine in the Age of Reform*, ed. Roger French and Andrew Wear (Cambridge, 1991), pp. 76–7.

corpses of the poor. The governors at St Bartholomew's were no exception. Their insistence that the beadle supervise all dissections, that they be undertaken in the presence of one of the staff, and that the body be sewn up and placed in a coffin, guaranteed some lay supervision. It also, as Susan Lawrence suggests, 'presumably deterred staff and students from taking away obviously large portions . . . for further dissection'.[34] There was always room for manoeuvre. In 1796, Owen Evans, a student at St Bartholomew's, referred to going 'into the Dissecting rooms to hear Demonstrations'. Private and hospital schools internalised the principles of anatomico-clinical medicine and placed considerable stress on the importance of first-hand dissection. Evans was able to help 'Mr Abernethy's Man get the Subject ready for Lecture' and it seems clear that he was not the only student to do this. Students increasingly saw it as their 'right' to attend and undertake dissections.[35] By 1805, the College had publicly recognised this. It advertised 'Practical Anatomy' classes, a euphemism for dissection, and in 1822 Edward Stanley as demonstrator of anatomy published a manual to help students in their labours.[36]

Staff at St Bartholomew's used anatomy and dissection in their publications to assert their credentials as 'working men of science', although they were circumspect about where the bodies came from.[37] Staff believed that dissection was 'a dirty source of knowledge', but this did not stop them encouraging students to dissect.[38] 'Nothing in life', according to Abernethy, could ' . . . be considered as more important' than anatomy: 'it is the foundation of all medical knowledge.' He suggested to the 1828 select committee on anatomy that students should not only see regular dissections but also practise operative technique on cadavers.[39] William Lawrence and Stanley as Abernethy's demonstrators shared his views and actively encouraged students to dissect.

Despite the rhetoric, students were not given the opportunities desired. Few could be certain of practical dissection experience and, if bodies were secured, they were treasured for as long as they lasted. In winter, students at St Bartholomew's were literally frozen out of the dissecting rooms. Dissections remained poorly regulated: post-mortems were rarely announced and attendance at them was largely a lottery until criticism led to notices

[34] House committee, 19 December 1750, HA 1/12; Lawrence, Charitable Knowledge, p. 196.
[35] John M. T. Ford, ed., A Medical Student at St Thomas's Hospital 1801–2: The Weekes Family Letters, Medical History Supplement 7 (1987), pp. 34–5.
[36] Edward Stanley, A Manual of Practical Anatomy, for the use of students engaged in dissections (London, 1822).
[37] John H. Warner, 'Idea of Science in English Medicine', in British Medicine, ed. French and Wear, pp. 136–64.
[38] Cited in Richardson, Death, Dissection and the Destitute, p. 95.
[39] SC on Anatomy, PP (1828) viii, pp. 1, 28, 30–1.

being placed informing students when they would occur. Problems remained. The physicians rarely attended, and dissections continued to be carried out at all hours of the day without students being informed.[40] Poor students were placed at a further disadvantage by a sixpenny charge for admission to a post-mortem, and prices for 'subjects' were considered 'exorbitant' by the late 1790s. Although admission charges were finally abolished in 1826 in response to student pressure, prices for cadavers continued to rise, since they became notoriously scarce as the vigilance of the public and the fear of bodysnatchers increased.[41] In Edinburgh, the Monros had to rely on models to teach anatomy. St Bartholomew's probably had a more plentiful supply. Cadavers were furnished from the hospital's burial ground and bodies from the wards were used. It was not unknown for students to be involved in such activities. Often it was a race between the students and the family to see who could get to the body first.[42] Like surgeons at other hospitals, staff frequently used bodysnatchers to supplement corpses from the hospital and students readily complained of financial hardship as the high cost of bodies was passed on to them.[43]

The difficulties and expense of obtaining bodies for dissection were considered to have become a national disgrace by the 1820s. 'The need to obtain an alternative source of corpses . . . other than by "violating the dormitories of the defunct"' had been widely recognised since the 1780s. Schemes for encouraging the bequest of bodies were suggested, and medical reformers argued that the Parisian system should be emulated to provide an abundant, cheap and legal supply.[44] After two doctors were prosecuted for disinterring and examining bodies in 1828, more serious moves were made. Unlike the more famous case of Burke, Hare and Robert Knox, the two doctors had the sympathy of the profession, since the judgment made anatomists just as vulnerable as bodysnatchers.[45] In response, a select committee was established. From the start, it was convinced of the value of dissection. Many (including Abernethy) repeated proposals outlined in a draft act devised by the utilitarian reformer Jeremy Bentham two years earlier. Interested in the issue through his active involvement in the foundation of the London University, Bentham had suggested that bodies might be supplied from the large number of friendless paupers dying in institutions, emulating the French system. It was an effort to decriminalise dissection, not a con-certed bid to eliminate bodysnatching.[46] Notwithstanding the revulsion

---

[40] *Lancet* i (1827/8), p. 767; ibid., i (1833/4), p. 564.
[41] Ibid., i (1825), p. 222; Ford, *Medical Student*, p. 35.
[42] Christison, *Life of Robert Christison*, pp. 192–3.
[43] *SC on Anatomy*, pp. 30, 106; *Lancet*, 19 October 1823, pp. 95–8.
[44] *London Medical and Physical Journal* lx (1828), pp. 373–83; *London Medical Gazette* ii (1828), pp. 406–13.
[45] *Medico-Chirurgical Review* vii (1827), p. 286; ibid., ix (1828), pp. 161–4.
[46] *SC on Anatomy*, pp. 28, 32.

generated by the revelations surrounding Burke and Hare's activities, legislation was delayed by turbulent debates over parliamentary reform. The confession of the 'London Burkers', Bishop and Williams, to the murder of three 'poor street folk' in November 1831 and the furore that surrounded their actions reinvigorated debate. Ten days after Bishop and Williams had been hung and dissected an Anatomy Bill was presented to Parliament. It passed in the face of petitions and extra-parliamentary riots shortly after the 1832 Great Reform Bill. The Act ignored other alternatives and encapsulated Bentham's earlier ideas, recognising that the trade in bodies was no longer acceptable to the public or suitable for the medical schools.[47] It transformed a punishment reserved for certain crimes into a possible legal consequence of poverty.

The provisions of the 1832 Act increased existing hostility to doctors. Angry mobs continued to challenge private schools, and the poor strove to secure a decent burial or worked to delay a pauper funeral to prevent dissection.[48] Private lecturers also were not enthusiastic. In creating an anatomy inspectorate, the Act established a precedent for later state inspectors but for lecturers they were a challenge to their teaching. Nor was the Act wholly effective. After initial success, the number of bodies provided to schools was 36 per cent lower in 1842 than it had been in 1832. Each school felt aggrieved and the central administration responsible for implementing the Act came under attack. Bodysnatchers were marginalised, but other illegal arrangements emerged to overcome continuing scarcity of subjects, despite high workhouse mortality. Informal agreements were made with local parishes, and doctors were prepared to turn a 'blind eye to (sometimes gross) breaches of decency and of the Act's regulations, so long as the public was kept in ignorance and the dissection tables supplied'.[49]

At St Bartholomew's, the 1832 Act did not lead to immediate improvements. The dead house remained 'a miserable kind of shed'. It was damp and dirty, and examinations were usually made in the roughest and least instructive way unless a physician was present. Many felt inconvenienced by these hurried investigations. Although Stanley as lecturer in anatomy promised students a 'plentiful supply' of cadavers, St Bartholomew's like other schools had trouble in obtaining them.[50] Deals with local parishes and an illegal supply of bodies through the hospital did not solve this problem. Under these conditions, staff continued to overlook the Act's regulations to secure a regular supply of bodies to meet the demand for dissection.[51] The

---

[47] Richardson, '"Trading Assassins"', pp. 77–88.

[48] Richardson, *Death, Dissection and the Destitute*, p. 218.

[49] Ibid., p. 255; M. J. Durey, 'Bodysnatchers and Benthamites: The Implications of the Dead Body Bill for the London Schools of Anatomy, 1820–42', *London Journal* ii (1976), pp. 212–7.

[50] Paget, ed., *Memoirs*, p. 42.

[51] Records of dissections, MS 81/1–2.

continued lack of opportunities led to renewed accusations from students that dissections were being conducted in secret. In response, it was decided that regular post-mortems should be undertaken and a record made for those students unable to attend.[52]

Shortages of corpses also led to changes in teaching methods. More attention turned to preservation of cadavers and manuals recommended more procedures per body. At St Bartholomew's, cadavers were increasingly dissected over a one- to two-week period.[53] Although some lecturers at other schools had started pathology courses before 1832, interest in the College remained subdued. Morbid anatomy was barely considered until demonstrations distinct from medicine and surgery were established in 1840 in an effort to diffuse the problem of the lack of cadavers.[54] Encouraged by the work of the demonstrators, staff began to take an increased interest in morbid anatomy and to incorporate it into their way of explaining disease, and became less reluctant to attend dissections. Not all were enthusiastic. Latham worried that an undue emphasis on morbid anatomy would lead to explanations that were 'brief, barren and unprofitable'.[55] Although pathological signs were included in lectures, Latham's fears were not realised. Morbid anatomy remained ancillary until the 1840s. Cadavers remained scarce but a partial legitimisation of supply ensured that the teaching of morbid anatomy had become more organised.

Abernethy's disciplines

Attendance in the dissection room, walking the wards and rudimentary clinical instruction were not the only forms of learning that distinguished the growing number of medical students from 'irregulars' or quacks. Orthodox practitioners were also defined by the knowledge they acquired through lectures. Lecturers offered what the licensing bodies considered to be appropriate knowledge and the success of individual schools depended on whom they could attract to teach. Students from across Britain and America flocked to hear able and prominent men who became a school's greatest asset and expense.

Between 1760 and 1819, according to Susan Lawrence, hospital lecturers began to take on the characteristics of an academic and professional hierarchy. They saw themselves as medical gentlemen, defining their position

[52] *Lancet* i (1833/4), p. 756; Medical College, 27 September 1834, MS 15.
[53] Records of dissections, MS 81/1.
[54] Thomas N. Bonner, *Becoming a Physician: Medical Education in Britain, France, Germany, and the United States, 1750–1945* (New York, 1995), pp. 147–9; William Girling Ball, 'The History of the Medical College of St Bartholomew's Hospital' (1941), p. 23.
[55] Latham, *Clinical Medicine, comprising Diseases of the Heart*, p. xiii.

by publication, teaching and the role they played in the medical establishment.[56] However, for most, teaching was a part-time occupation, sandwiched between hospital work and private practice. Drawn from professional or aspiring middle-class families, most had a university education or had been apprenticed to a hospital surgeon. Those teaching at St Bartholomew's conform to this pattern. Of the thirteen physicians who held posts in the hospital between 1780 and 1842, seven were active in teaching. Of these, three came from medical families; the rest were from legal, clerical or mercantile backgrounds. All had a university education and maintained lucrative private practices and posts at other metropolitan hospitals. Five were active fellows of the Royal College of Physicians. A similar picture existed among surgical staff. If their family and educational backgrounds were not as prominent, their positions in the Royal College of Surgeons made them an influential part of the surgical elite. These doctors were not Inkster's 'marginal men' using the hospital to gain social capital and acceptance, as a post at St Bartholomew's already confirmed their position as one of the medical elite.[57]

Despite the position hospital doctors secured in the professional hierarchy, students were advised to be cautious. They were repeatedly reminded to choose their school carefully and to judge whether its staff had achieved their posts by merit or connection. Nepotism and favouritism were an integral part of the structure of hospital staffing in the early nineteenth century. The ladder of professional advancement followed a general pattern: apprentice/pupil/dresser, demonstrator, surgeon, lecturer, followed by appointments to the various professional bodies and medical corporations. Defenders of the system argued that it favoured former students precisely because their characters and abilities were known. Critics attacked arrangements which appeared to be based on the assumption that the ability to pay was synonymous with 'a head full of brains'.[58] At St Bartholomew's, nepotism was central to how teaching posts were filled. Lecturers and demonstrators were appointed at a personal level based on a system of patronage that favoured those who had studied or worked in the hospital. Of the thirty-seven appointments between 1787 and 1843, fifteen had studied at St Bartholomew's and eight had already worked at the hospital when they started teaching. Under Abernethy, this system of nepotism was at its height. He took a personal hand in many of the College's appointments; his friends and relations were pushed forward and eight of his apprentices were promoted. Abernethy frequently tried to play parties against each other,

[56] Lawrence, *Charitable Knowledge*, p. 254–9.

[57] Ian Inkster, 'Marginal Men: Aspects of the Social Role of Medical Community in Sheffield, 1780–1850', in *Health Care and Popular Medicine in Nineteenth Century England*, ed. Woodward and Richards, pp. 128–63.

[58] *Lancet* i (1830/1), p. 597.

often with little success, and antagonised his pupils and staff. He was finally attacked in 1826 for his 'low intrigue and dirty bargains' over appointments.[59] Changes were made to prevent nepotism, avoiding the problems encountered at other hospitals where similar situations had spilt the institution.[60] Fourteen years later, Paget could still complain 'for, though there had not been a clear admission of the rights of apprentices, it had been made certain that they would be upheld by those who were much stronger than I was ever likely to become'.[61]

Lecturers, demonstrators and members of the surgical staff were not the only members of the hospital or College responsible for students. House surgeons and physicians bridged both worlds, offering the potential for personal and professional ties reminiscent of apprenticeships. Modelled on the 'house pupil' system established at St George's in the 1730s, these posts were officially recognised at St Bartholomew's in 1813. The house surgeon/physician was neither a pupil expected to pay a fee nor a full member of staff. Chosen from students already studying in the College, he was a newly qualified practitioner expected to work in the wards and provide care when the surgeons were absent. An unofficial responsibility was the supervision of students, particularly in the outpatients' department.[62]

The quality of the teaching staff at St Bartholomew's varied considerably. Stanley, known to students as 'the inspired butterman', had the habit of reciting badly parts of nursery rhymes in his lectures. Students objected that his frequent 'jabbering' offered no benefit and complained that he shunned original ideas.[63] Stanley was not the only member of staff singled out for criticism. The lectures of Clement Hue, lecturer in the practice of medicine, and of Charles Wheeler, lecturer in chemistry, were described as 'trash', while Skey and Thomas Wormald were felt to be lame anatomy demonstrators only pushed into position by Abernethy.[64]

These harsh judgements were often one-sided, voiced by an antagonistic *Lancet* with its agenda for medical reform, or by disgruntled students. Although there was a tendency to repeat the same lectures annually and the structure of the courses rarely changed even when they were taken over by new staff, teaching was not uniformly poor. The appointment of Richard Owen as lecturer in comparative anatomy in 1824 gave 'public renown to the hospital'.[65] Owen's popular lectures were not the only successful ones. Although initially hesitant and reserved, Pott developed a lucid style that

[59] Ibid., xii (1826/7), pp. 660–1, 690.

[60] See H. C. Cameron, *Mr Guy's Hospital, 1726–1948* (London, 1954), pp. 145–6, 162–74.

[61] Paget, ed., *Memoirs*, p. 83.

[62] Lawrence, *Charitable Knowledge*, pp. 129–30.

[63] *Lancet* viii (1825), p. 21; ibid., i (1832/3), p. 61.

[64] Ibid., ix (1825/6), p. 20.

[65] Nicholaas A. Rupke, *Richard Owen: Victorian Naturalist* (New Haven, 1994), p. 91.

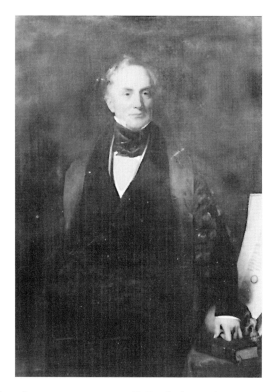

Plate 2.2 William Lawrence, surgeon to St Bartholomew's

'communicated his thoughts with eloquence and ease'.[66] He brought students into the hospital. Other lecturers were equally charismatic. Lawrence held his audience. Although students felt he was 'not warm', his lectures were always full and he was often greeted with a 'burst of applause' when he started talking.[67] According to one student,

> his person, gestures, countenance, and voice were dignified, impressive and persuasive. . . . There was a clearness of method, a terseness of expression, without being epigrammatic . . . a perspicuity in his discourse, that made it a pleasure to follow him.[68]

Students valued other lecturers and demonstrators' skill and attitude towards them, even if their lecturing technique was seen as poor. After eight years as a demonstrator, Skey was regarded as 'the pupil's friend'. Attendance at his

[66] James Earle, ed., *The Chirurgical Works of Percival Pott* (London, 1790), pp. xxii–iv.
[67] Paget, ed., *Memoirs*, p. 45.
[68] *Gentleman's Magazine*, August 1867, p. 245.

classes increased because of the 'facility with which he imparted anatomical knowledge'. Even Stanley's ability to make students realise the value of mundane facts became appreciated.[69]

However, it was Abernethy's fluid and lucid style that most encouraged students to attend. According to one student, he 'excited and exemplified a more scientific investigation and treatment of surgical disease' and 'taught us to extend our views beyond the narrow limits of local causes and remedies'. Abernethy fixed his students' attention, entering the lecture room

> his hands buried deep in his breeches pockets, his body bent slouching forward, blowing or whistling, his eyes twinkling beneath their arches and his lower jaw thrown considerably beneath his upper. Then he would cast himself into a chair, swing one of his legs over an arm of it and commence his lecture in the most *outré* manner.

It was an abruptness that 'never failed to command silence, and rivet attention'.[70] A harsh examiner, Abernethy preferred straight answers and displayed rigid ideas that seldom extended beyond a mechanical Hunterian approach. At first nervous and attracting only a small number of students, Abernethy believed in laying down broad principles, generalising on the facts he had acquired through observation. As he established himself attendance quickly improved. His only self-professed aim was to 'endeavour to excite in the minds of the students the same enthusiasm which he felt himself for the prosecution of a noble science'. Abernethy's lectures were punctuated with stories, and they were admired for their drollery. They were regularly drawn on by lecturers at other schools, though by the 1820s he was attacked for lacking in originality and recycling knowledge fifty years out of date.[71]

The personalities of Pott, Lawrence, Abernethy and the other lecturing staff shaped the nature and popularity of teaching at St Bartholomew's. They gave the College its character and reputation. Their presence had required a reconceptualisation of charitable care that built on the growing number of pupils and students who found it necessary to walk the wards.[72] However, what they offered was linked closely to the licensing requirements of the medical corporations and the demand students generated for hospital knowledge. Lecturers may have shaped their course in terms of style and content, but they were working within an increasingly defined curriculum that in many respects dictated what, if not how, subjects were taught.

[69] *Lancet* xi (1826/7), p. 82; ibid., ii (1832/3), p. 828; Paget, ed., *Memoirs*, p. 45.
[70] Thomas Joseph Pettigrew, *Medical Portrait Gallery*, 2 vols (London, 1838–40), Vol. 1, pp. 4–5; cited in Bonner, *Becoming a Physician*, pp. 80–1.
[71] *Lancet* i (1829/30), p. 33; ibid., 8 May 1824, p. 181; ibid., v (1824/5), p. 7.
[72] Lawrence, *Charitable Knowledge*, p. 188.

Hospital knowledge

Between the late eighteenth and early nineteenth centuries the stress on practical experience was undermined by a growing emphasis on underlying principles gained through the didactic lecture. Influential teachers became more matter-of-fact as the number of institutional lectures increased and courses became shorter. Although lectures were criticised as 'only a method of looking at objects through another person's spectacles', they used a technical terminology that provided the student with a framework by which to understand diseases.[73] They combined instruction with entertainment, helping London's scientific community develop an institutional structure. Information not too different from that found in medical texts formed the core of these courses, which avoided difficult moral and philosophical questions to concentrate on observed 'facts' and scientific study.[74] If Pott encouraged students to be sceptical of routine surgery, he still advocated accepted treatments.[75] Those teaching in London's hospitals were only too aware that examiners preferred the orthodox. This growing stress on the value of the lecture combined with an emphasis on observation to underpin the development of teaching at St Bartholomew's. It was, after all, lectures and those who delivered them that were the main attraction for students.

Instruction was often more relevant to practice than critics of the existing structure of metropolitan medical education wanted to suggest. From the start, teaching at St Bartholomew's was tailored to focus on what experience had proved 'to be the most successful'. Courses dealt with the 'frequent' rather than the unusual and aimed to equip students with knowledge that would fit them 'for all the duties which [they] will have to perform'.[76] Even Abernethy's flamboyant lectures could be readily distilled into notes that would provide a guide for general practice.[77] More theoretical courses on forensic medicine, chemistry, botany or medical physics were also included, based on Scottish efforts from the mid-eighteenth century to incorporate the new sciences into the study of medicine. Abernethy's interest in chemistry and botany helped encourage teaching in these fields. Although it was believed that these subjects contributed little to practice, and they were relegated to the summer session when opportunities for dissection were limited, they did reflect medicine's scientific aspirations and desire for certainty.

---

[73] *Provincial Medical and Surgical Journal* iv (1842), p. 441.

[74] Lawrence, 'Educating the Senses', pp. 154–78.

[75] Wellcome: Student notebook, fl.84–5, MS 6922.

[76] *College Calendar* (1835/6).

[77] Wellcome: Notes of Andrew Thynne's midwifery lectures, MS 4788; Notes of Mr Abernethy's lectures, MS 5600; Notes of lectures on anatomy, physiology, etc. delivered by Mr Abernethy, MS 5606.

Lecturers linked 'sound knowledge . . . with what the pupil *saw*', or should see or feel. They extolled the benefits of direct experience, and used specimens, preparations, skeletons, models and demonstrations to give their classes relevance.[78] Students were told that the 'first business of the medical student' was to learn 'the structure of the body and its living actions'. Once this had been mastered, they were expected to observe diseases and 'watch the circumstances under which they arise', connecting 'these changes with their appropriate signs or symptoms' and necessary treatments.[79] To reflect the realities of practice, medicine and surgery were linked. Pott told his students that physic and surgery were 'really inseperable [*sic*]'. He warned that a physician unaware of surgery would often find himself 'perplexed and deceived', and a surgeon 'ignorant of the use of medicine' might be puzzled and 'may sometimes lose his patients'.[80] Pott's stance was part of an emerging trend and was embraced at St Bartholomew's, where a catholic approach made teaching ideally suited to those seeking to enter surgery or general practice.[81] It was an attitude that reflected the blurred boundaries between practitioners. Medical reformers, struggling for changes in the medical corporations, seized on the idea, and the College of Surgeons began to incorporate a more unified model into its licensing requirements.[82] Medical schools followed in an attempt to make institutional training relevant for the physician, surgeon and emerging general practitioner without having to provide a large number of specialist lectures.

Lecturing at St Bartholomew's was part of the 'helter-skelter' sandwich of courses that Bonner has seen in London.[83] The timetable was arranged to suit the lecturer and not the student, whose duty it was to attend. Although this matched a general London lecturing timetable and provided opportunities to attend lectures at other schools, it did make for a long day. Owen Evans, a student in 1796, described a typical day in October:

> at 10 O Clock Dr Roberts Lectures on the Practice of Physic and Materia Medica, at 1 O Clock we go into the Dissecting rooms to hear Demonstrations, at 2 O Clock Mr. Abernethy begins his Anatomical Lectures . . . half past 5 Dr Clarke on Midwifery, 7 Dr Powell on Chemistry & during the Winter there will 3 times a week a 8 O Clock in the evening Mr. Wilkinson on Experimental Philosophy.

---

[78] See Lawrence, 'Educating the Senses' (pp. 155–78) for the knowledge students received through hospital lectures and the emphasis placed on the 'senses' and 'observation'.

[79] *Lancet* i (1829/30), p. 35.

[80] Wellcome: Student notebook, fl.114–15, MS 6922.

[81] Robert Kirkpatrick, 'Nature's Schools: The Hunterian Revolution in London Hospital Medicine, 1780–1825' (unpublished Ph.D. diss., Cambridge, 1988), p. 225.

[82] *SC on Medical Education*, PP (1834) xiii, pp. 171, 112, 126, 134, 177, 188.

[83] House committee, 17 August 1825, HA 1/17; Bonner, *Becoming a Physician*, p. 82.

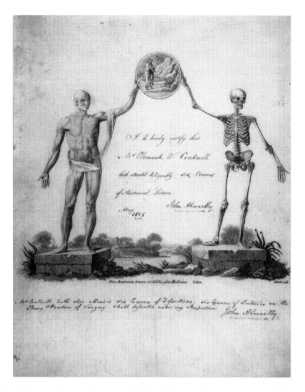

Plate 2.3 Certificate of attendance at John Abernethy's anatomical lectures, 1805

Conscientious students complained that they 'hardly ever get to bed before 12 or 1 0 Clock & sometimes later', criticisms that were not limited to St Bartholomew's.[84] Critics argued that the demands placed on students revealed the assumption that they were 'all ear – all memory – or nothing but LOCKE's blank sheet of paper for lecturers to blot, blurr, and write upon'.[85] The governors' insistence that only staff from the hospital be employed in teaching led to a more organised if no less demanding timetable.

By the 1830s, the College was able to offer one of the most comprehensive courses in London. The timing of some surgeons' ward rounds did occasionally lead to clashes but by 1840s all staff agreed to visit the wards after midday, so that students had the afternoons for hospital practice. Unlike other teaching hospitals, St Bartholomew's mirrored the private schools and offered lectures in all subjects three times a week. Anatomy and physiology

[84] Ford, *Medical Student*, pp. 33–4; Lawrence, 'Entrepreneurs and Private Enterprise', p. 181.
[85] *Lancet* i (1838/9), p. 126.

were the exception. The perceived importance of these subjects meant that they were taught throughout the week and demonstrations were held daily. Changes were constantly made and teaching facilities were improved to take account of them. Theoretical lectures needed little more than a room, or a lecture theatre if large numbers attended, but with the College starting to offer demonstrations and practical lectures different teaching facilities were required. In 1835, the governors agreed to pay for more demonstration space for anatomy teaching. In the following year, a chemical theatre where experiments could be undertaken was built in Long Row, and a theatre for *materia medica* and botany lectures was added. A larger pathological museum was also built to replace the room adjoining the carpenter's shop behind the west wing, which had previously been used.[86]

However, St Bartholomew's remained an essentially conservative, responsive institution wedded to the medical establishment. Although Latham helped establish the importance of clinical lectures, his colleagues were not Peterson's innovative teachers. She has argued that with medical men dominating surgical and medical teaching they were able to define 'the expanding curriculum of required and elective professional studies'.[87] This was not the case at St Bartholomew's. Staff matched the courses they offered to student demand, changes at other schools and to the licensing requirements. With five out of every six students in London working for the LSA, the main forces shaping teaching were the requirements of the College of Surgeons and Society of Apothecaries. A licence was not required for practice until after the 1858 Medical Act, but as it conferred advantages on the practitioner, and as London's hospital schools were well aware of the medical corporations' licensing requirements, the licence provided a loose structure to otherwise *ad hoc* teaching. After the 1815 Apothecaries Act this structure became more pronounced. There was a shift from demand-led courses and individualistic instruction to a more standardised curriculum for non-university practitioners. Flexibility remained, but in determining the appropriate number of lectures and stipulating the subjects to be covered, the licensing bodies regulated the structure of medical education in response to changing professional and social expectations.[88]

This was not always beneficial. Little attempt was made to extend midwifery teaching at St Bartholomew's once it had been established in the 1780s, or to provide additional beds for practical teaching. With attendance at midwifery lectures uniformly low across London, and the subject not fully

[86] Medical College, 25 June 1836, MS 15; House committee, 10 March 1835, HA 1/18.
[87] M. Jeanne Peterson, *Medical Profession in Mid-Victorian London* (Berkeley, 1978), p. 64.
[88] Elizabeth Haigh, 'William Brande and the Chemical Education of Medical Students', in *British Medicine*, ed. French and Wear, p. 190; Susan C. Lawrence, 'Private Enterprise and Public Interests: Medical Education and the Apothecaries Act, 1780–1825', ibid., pp. 45–7.

integrated into the medical curriculum, midwifery – even when it covered diseases of women and children – was seen as an ancillary to training.[89] With no apparent demand, lectures continued as an alternative to practical experience. Midwifery was not the only subject to suffer. New opportunities for science lecturing outside the hospital saw some courses being stopped. Natural philosophy was not offered between the 1790s and 1830s and teaching in the subject was only resumed when it became clear that other schools were offering instruction in physics. A course on comparative anatomy was introduced for the same reason in 1834, although Abernethy, James Macartney and Lawrence had included it in their lectures. It was believed that the addition of these courses would 'complete the arrangements of the Medical School'.[90] Courses on other subjects were opposed. St Bartholomew's did not follow other schools and introduce instruction on phrenology, which was being popularised by its 'inventor' Franz Joseph Gall and his assistant Johann Gaspar Spurzheim.[91] Abernethy's initial view that phrenology, which represented a break from earlier writings on brain and generated considerable popular and medical interest, was socially and religiously dangerous matched wider concerns and made efforts to include any discussion of the topic at St Bartholomew's difficult.[92]

Subjects were gradually subdivided and new ones added as the requirements of the licensing bodies altered, and demand fluctuated (see Table 2.1). Courses on forensic medicine and medical jurisprudence, for example, were offered in response to several forces. Rising interest in public health made forensic medicine important in providing a new class of medical witnesses, while concern about medical uncertainty and fraud encouraged the medical press to campaign for medical jurisprudence. Influenced by these ideas, the Society of Apothecaries made forensic medicine a prerequisite for examination in 1830. The changes immediately established the field in medical education.[93] *Materia medica* similarly benefited from a shift in stance by the licensing bodies. In response to changes in the 1815 Apothecaries Act in 1829 and the College of Surgeons' decision to include *materia medica* in its requirements, the College's course on the practice of medicine was divided and lectures were started on *materia medica*. Before this, students had relied

[89] See Irvine Loudon, *Death in Childbirth: An international study of maternal care and maternal mortality, 1800–1950* (Oxford, 1992).

[90] J. N. Hays, 'London Lecturing Empire, 1800–50', in *Metropolis and Province: Science in British Culture, 1780–1850*, ed. Ian Inkster and Jack Morrell (Philadelphia, 1983), p. 101; House committee, 14 October 1834, HA 1/16.

[91] See Roger Cooter, *Cultural Meaning of Popular Science: Phrenology and the Organisation of Consent in Nineteenth-Century Britain* (Cambridge, 1984).

[92] John Abernethy, *Reflections on Gall and Spruzheim's System of Physiognomy and Phrenology* (London, 1821).

[93] Catherine Crawford, 'A Scientific Profession: Medical Reform and Forensic Medicine in British Periodicals of the Early Nineteenth Century', in *British Medicine*, ed. French and Wear, pp. 203–30.

Table 2.1 Number of lecturers in individual subjects

Subject	1740s	1750s	1760s	1770s	1780s	1790s	1800s	1810s	1820s	1830s
Anatomy and physiology	1		1	1	1	1	2	1	2	2
Surgery		1	1	1	1	1	1	1	2	2
Practice of medicine					1	1	−	−	2	3
Midwifery					1	1	1	1	2	1
Chemistry					1	1		1	2	2
Physics					1	1	−	−	−	1
Comparative anatomy							1	1		1
Materia medica									1	1
Botany										1
Forensic medicine										2
Medical jurisprudence										1

Source: College Calendar

on the variety of biological lectures in London, informal herborising expeditions provided by the apothecary, or taken advantage of the opportunities offered by the Chelsea physic garden. Interest in botany had increased during the 1820s and it came to be considered as an important 'accessory science of medicine' that was in need of 'cultivation'.[94] The course at St Bartholomew's was a belated reaction.

With the expansion of the College more lecturers were needed, and with Abernethy's death in 1830 the opportunity was taken to expand teaching. Anatomy and surgery were separated whereas Abernethy had taught them together. Lectures on pathology were introduced and separate courses on comparative anatomy and physiology were developed.[95] However, medicine was still taught in one two-part course that aimed to 'give a General View of the Theory and Practice of Physic, a detailed account of the Symptoms and Progress of Disease, of the Variations which most frequently occur, and to describe the Modes of Treatment which are found by experience to be most successful'.[96]

Despite these modifications to the structure of teaching, little could challenge the importance ascribed to anatomy. Private medical schools and the early hospital lecturers had institutionalised anatomy teaching and built

[94] *Medico-Chirurgical Review* viii (1828), p. 177.
[95] William Lawrence, *Lectures on Surgery, Medical and Operative* (London, 1832), p. 2; *Lancet* i (1830/1), pp. 412–13; Medical College, 6 June 1840, MS 15.
[96] *College Calendar* (1835/6); Medical College, 6 June 1835, MS 15.

their success on it. Anatomy's empirical vocabulary became part of everyday practice during the eighteenth century.[97] While Pott warned his students about the 'absurd custom of measuring the motion of a surgeon's hand as jockeys do that of the feet of a horse, viz., by a stop-watch' without anaesthetics, the speed of an operation was vital. This made an accurate knowledge of anatomy 'indispensable to the treatment of many surgical cases'.[98] By the late eighteenth century, anatomy was accepted as central to training. Students were increasingly expected to be thoroughly familiar with 'scientific language of the body' and hospital anatomy lectures were one of the main vehicles through which this was achieved. If students were prone to forget the minutiae of anatomy, they were constantly reminded of its importance.[99] Anatomical lectures at St Bartholomew's upheld this view and retained a strong surgical bias. Taught in conjunction with physiology until the 1840s, anatomy was seen as the structure in repose, physiology the structure in action. It was believed that the two were inextricably linked, although a utilitarian approach to physical signs made physiology subservient to anatomy.[100] Abernethy and Lawrence, despite their influence on the development of English physiology, remained anatomical surgeons and taught students accordingly.[101] Only under Paget was greater emphasis placed on physiology when he started lecturing on the subject in 1843.

Although anatomy remained central to a student's education, the subdivision of existing courses and the addition of new ones expanded the medical curriculum and gave it a more scientific emphasis. Courses remained optional as the choice rested with the student. However, with licensing bodies introducing these subjects into their requirements and demanding evidence of attendance, students were in effect left with little choice. The result was an increased emphasis on academic study and hospital attendance. In response, there was a shift from one year spent at a hospital school to, typically, two years attending lectures and visiting the wards. At St Bartholomew's, staff were all too aware that this added to the strain and expense of studying.[102]

---

[97] See Russell Maulitz, *Morbid Appearances: The Anatomy of Pathology in the Early Nineteenth Century* (Cambridge, 1987); Susan C. Lawrence, 'Anatomy and Address', in *The History of Medical Education in Britain*, ed. Vivian Nutton and Roy Porter (Amsterdam, 1995), pp. 199–228.

[98] *Chirurgical Works*, p. 176.

[99] *College Calendar* (1835/6); *Lancet*, 19 October 1823, pp. 95–8.

[100] L. S. Jacyna, 'Principles of General Physiology: The Comparative Dimension to British Neuroscience in the 1830s and 1840s', *Studies in the History of Biology* vii (1984), pp. 47–92; Gerald L. Geison, 'Social and Institutional Factors in the Stagnancy of English Physiology, 1840–1870', *BHM* xlvi (1972), pp. 30–59.

[101] See John Abernethy, *Surgical and Physiological Essays* (London, 1793); Lawrence, *Lectures on Surgery*.

[102] George Burrows, *Introductory Lecture to a Course on Forensic Medicine, delivered in the Anatomical Theatre of St Bartholomew's Hospital* (London, 1831).

Mischievous rivalry

The central role played by Abernethy in the College was both an immense benefit and a problem. His difficult, frequently confrontational manner did not lead to open hostilities but did strain relations, reducing the College's ability to achieve stability in the decade after his death. Abernethy was believed to be 'constantly grumbling', 'finding fault' with how other surgeons performed their duties. As he got older he became 'very unpleasant to assist'. Lawrence was unable to work with him and transferred his lectures (if not his clinical teaching) to the Aldersgate School, the College's major competitor, depriving St Bartholomew's of a dynamic teacher. A very public dispute erupted in 1817 between Lawrence and his former teacher when he challenged the Hunterian views Abernethy had embraced. This further strained relations, as did Lawrence's initial support of medical reform.[103] Lawrence was not alone in the problems he encountered with Abernethy. By 1827, Abernethy's favouritism and opposition to some staff had brought St Bartholomew's into disrepute and nearly resulted in a student riot.[104]

Abernethy's resignation did not see an end to friction. When Paget joined the College in 1834, he noted that the 'constant dissension and mischievous rivalry among the teachers' had existed for some considerable time. The situation was made obvious by the absence of anyone willing to take a leading managerial role.[105] Although Abernethy had created difficulties, he had also kept the College together. After his death, a period of turbulence followed in which the physicians, often allied with the governors, opposed the surgeons. This was part of Abernethy's legacy. The strong surgical bias he had given the College created difficulties, while the events surrounding his attempted resignation between 1825 and 1827 strained relations with the hospital (see Chapter 1). During the 1830s no member of staff emerged to replace Abernethy as a coherent administrative force or dynamic and popular teacher. Lawrence was too unpopular at the College of Surgeons and with the profession, given his initial support for medical reform, to provide any concerted influence. Latham disliked administration and 'hated all disputes'. Stanley tried to play a leading role. Despite his troubled relationship with Lawrence, he worked to diffuse tensions but was too timid and easily ridiculed to take control. The creation of a school committee in 1834 did not see an immediate solution. Differences spilled over into staff relations with students and opposing fractions formed.[106]

It was Hue, physician and lecturer in the practice of medicine between 1823 and 1860, who was largely to blame for fostering a divisive atmosphere.

---

[103] See Lawrence, *Charitable Knowledge*, pp. 327–32.
[104] *Lancet* xii (1826/7), p. 625; ibid., i (1827/8), p. 19.
[105] Paget, ed., *Memoirs*, pp. 40–1.
[106] Medical College, 17 September 1834, MS 15.

Hue was a scholarly but conservative physician who had little faith in new methods of clinical teaching. Although his uninspired lectures meant that he had little influence with students, his views held considerable sway with the governors. As the senior physician, he 'was the chief force on one of the sides in the disputes by which the school was being damaged' and sided with the governors against his colleagues.[107] His relationship with Stanley was particularly strained. In 1836 he accused Stanley of 'trafficking in dead bodies by receiving from the pupils for the purchase of subjects brought from the wards a sum larger in amount than the expenses incurred by him and appropriating the surplus to his own use'. Although Stanley had obtained exclusive use of the dead for the College from one large parish by paying high 'fees' to an undertaker, he proved Hue wrong. Hue went on to antagonise other staff by repeatedly opposing appointments.[108]

Internal conflict frustrated reform, weakening the College's position at a time when attacks in the *Lancet* made teaching appear outdated and, in some cases, inept. Under these conditions the College became less able to ignore competition. Instead of relying on its status to attract lecturers and students, it became more aggressive in its attempts to reduce rivalry. By the 1820s, the expansion of entrepreneurial medical teaching, and an unfettered market for medical education had started to threaten the profitability of hospital lecturing. A dearth of cadavers and fears that private anatomists were encroaching on hospital surgeons ensured that antipathy between these two groups was pronounced.[109] Those working in London's medical schools defended themselves, pressurising the Royal College of Surgeons between 1821 and 1824 to adopt regulations to limit competition. With the College dominated by those holding London hospital posts, the *Lancet* felt that those framing the by-laws were nothing more than 'bats', feasting on nepotism, incompetent, somewhat 'toad-like' and prone to brainless activity.[110] The 'infamous, cruel, tyrannous and ignorant' by-laws only strengthened the position of the London hospitals. Regulations adopted in 1813 requiring students to produce evidence of a year's study at a hospital were extended. Attendance at a London hospital was made compulsory and an insistence on three winter anatomy courses made private summer courses unnecessary for qualification.[111] Critics felt that the additional burden placed on students beyond their apprenticeship was not only unjust but also financially crippling.[112] A reform movement around the *Lancet* extended the debate. It accused the College of Surgeons and the London hospitals of being narrow,

[107] Paget, ed., *Memoirs*, p. 48.
[108] Medical College, 18 August 1836, 1 May 1837, 27 July 1841, MS 15.
[109] Maulitz, *Morbid Appearances*, p. 149.
[110] *Lancet* i (1831/2), pp. 2–3.
[111] Ibid., 29 May 1824, p. 268.
[112] Waddington, *Medical Profession*, p. 33; *Lancet*, 1 May 1824, p. 129.

contemptible bodies that failed to recognise the needs of the profession, calling into question the monopoly of the licensing bodies and the structure of medical education. The court of examiners at the College of Surgeons expressed the same concern for medical education, but used this in a different way. It argued that the new regulations were designed to tighten educational requirements and make them complementary to the 1815 Apothecaries Act. For the court, the best way this could be achieved was by strengthening the London hospitals.[113] It was no coincidence that seven members of the court held hospital posts, with staff from St Bartholomew's forming one of the largest groups. Here the interests of the College and those of the medical establishment were seen as the same. Only Lawrence, teaching at the Aldersgate school, proved an initial dissenting voice, widening the rift with Abernethy.

The College of Surgeons could not entirely prevent competition. Private schools were damaged but continued to limp on. Unlike other hospital schools, St Bartholomew's appeared less able to outface competition. It was at the centre of one of the most overcrowded districts in London for medical courses. By 1831 it was facing rivalry from six private lecturers within a mile of the hospital. The College was also competing with the Middlesex hospital, the Theatre of Anatomy in Giltspur Street, and the Aldersgate School. Only the Middlesex, facing competition from private lecturers and from London University, Little Windmill Street School, and the Westminster Dispensary, was in a similar position. Although the number of schools near St Bartholomew's had diminished by the 1840s, constant criticism of the teaching offered by the College from the *Lancet* made these other institutions appear more attractive, threatening student numbers.

It was competition from the Aldersgate School that was initially perceived to be the main problem. Opened in 1825 by Frederick Tyrrell, surgeon at Guy's and St Thomas's, the Aldersgate School had attracted distinguished teachers.[114] These lecturers contributed to the school's success and until the mid-1840s it was the main rival to St Bartholomew's. Abernethy's death only strengthened the 'sharp opposition' between the two. This adversity was freely acknowledged even by the governors, anxious that it might damage the hospital.[115] The *Lancet* even advised students in 1829 to mix their clinical studies at St Bartholomew's with instruction in medicine, chemistry, pharmacy, midwifery and anatomy at Aldersgate.[116] While students took the journal's advice, staff saw the issue as one of competition not cooperation: in a bid to boost St Bartholomew's position they went to considerable lengths to

---

[113] Zachary Cope, *Royal College of Surgeons of England* (London, 1959), p. 43.
[114] Zachary Cope, 'The Private Medical Schools of London (1746–1914)', in *The Evolution of Hospitals in Britain*, ed. F. N. L. Poynter (London, 1966), pp. 99–109.
[115] Paget, ed., *Memoirs*, p. 40; House committee, 18 January, 28 February 1827, HA 1/18.
[116] *Lancet* i (1829), p. 47.

persuade lecturers to transfer their courses to the College, often with little success.[117]

Competition from other hospital and private schools placed St Bartholomew's in a difficult position. Attacks in the *Lancet* and internal rivalries led to additional problems that seriously damaged the standing of the College. The effect was to reduce student numbers, preventing the College from achieving any stability after Abernethy's death. Once it became clear that student admissions were falling as they were lured to other schools, the teaching staff became even more concerned with the need to limit rivalry. A failure to reduce competition through the College of Surgeons or by poaching staff from other institutions encouraged a change in strategy. When a new threat arose in 1835, the College became more aggressive and political but at the same time the challenge forced St Bartholomew's to implement limited reforms.

In 1835, the lecturers and governors felt forced to take concerted action against what the lecturers were convinced was a common enemy, the London University, that 'godless institution of Gower Street'. The University, which was to become University College London in 1835, had been founded as a limited company in 1825. Modelled on Edinburgh and the German universities, a faculty of medicine was included, although University College Hospital was not opened for clinical training until 1834.[118] Attempts to acquire a charter for the new University had been resisted since 1831 by Oxford and Cambridge, and when it was decided to include medical degrees in proposals for a charter London's hospitals entered the fray. The established schools already distrusted the University and their hostility merged with concerns about the institution's association with utilitarianism and dissent. They distrusted the University's emphasis on science, and were alarmed by its reformist intentions and efforts to mimic Edinburgh. It did not help that the University's fee for anatomy and dissection was considerably lower than charged elsewhere. In their defence, hospital schools argued that the University 'overrated' its value 'as a seat of medical learning' and tried to dismiss it.[119]

When another attempt was made to secure a charter in 1834, opposition mounted. The College of Surgeons added its support and petitioned the government, worried that a charter would interfere with its functions. Others accused the University of attempting to secure exclusive privileges.[120] Hue

[117] Medical College, 28 June 1836, MS 15.

[118] See W. R. Merrington, *University College Hospital and its Medical School: A History* (London, 1976).

[119] *Lancet* i (1830/1), pp. 26–7.

[120] *Medical Gazette* vi (1830), pp. 377–9; ibid., xiv (1834), pp. 147–51; *Lancet* ii (1833/4), pp. 201–3.

and Lawrence at St Bartholomew's played an important role in organising this opposition. Meetings were held in February 1834 at Hue's home and a subcommittee was formed to draw up a petition.[121] The reaction at St Bartholomew's followed a similar course. A growing spirit of cooperation between the hospital and College saw both bodies agree that proposals to grant 'the Power of conferring Medical Degrees' to London University was a threat. Opposition was hardly surprising. Staff opposed anything that would give the University an advantage, especially as the University was able to offer a more extensive course than the one at St Bartholomew's. Anxieties about the Aldersgate School and falling student numbers made the situation appear more desperate.[122] For the College, there were considerable advantages in securing the governors' assistance. Through its connections with the City St Bartholomew's had influential supporters in government. The College was excluded from this arena, and with the debate about the University's charter occurring at parliamentary level the governors' support was seen as crucial.

The memorandum devised by Hue and Lawrence's subcommittee the year before provided the basis for the joint committee's deliberations. Dismissing the University's contribution to medical education, the petition argued that the opportunities offered at St Bartholomew's had been crucial in establishing London as 'a School of Medicine'. It implied that any further competition would reduce the quality of medical education. Overlooking anxieties about inadequate accommodation in their own hospital, staff asserted that the University was not 'superior' to St Bartholomew's. There were some grounds for this view. Clinical teaching in the new University had been restricted to the North London Dispensary since 1828 after an agreement to provide access to wards at the Middlesex broke down. It was therefore felt that the University failed to offer the clinical facilities doctors saw as so important to 'practical instruction'. This had been a criticism of the University from the start. Drawing on the University's challenge to the monopoly of Oxford and Cambridge and its aim of removing obstacles to higher education, the lecturers turned the University's rhetoric against itself. They argued that to invest even the best of the London schools 'with the exclusive Power of conferring Medical Degrees' a monopoly would be established 'most injurious to the Public, directly at variance with the principle on which the institution called the London University was established'. In defence of the existing system, the petition noted that any bid by the University to grant medical degrees would 'destroy that honourable and useful rivalry' that existed in London.[123] The underlying desire to reduce competition was overlooked.

---

[121] Ibid., pp. 699–700.
[122] Special general court, 21 March 1835, HA 1/18.
[123] Medical College, 9 March 1835, MS 15.

Under pressure, the proposal to include medical degrees was not included in the charter. St Bartholomew's welcomed the move. A compromise was reached in 1836. The University was renamed London University College and a separate board of examiners, with a similar function to the Senate at Cambridge, was established.[124] It was this second examining body that was called the University of London.

The debate over the charter raised important questions about the nature of teaching at St Bartholomew's. During discussions, recommendations had been made that teaching should be extended from April to July and divided into two. Although this was a challenge to the College of Surgeons, which had regulated against summer courses, it was in line with evidence presented to the select committee on medical education the year before. In an open letter to the medical profession, staff argued that change was vital to overcome an overcrowded curriculum, give more time to instruction, and limit competition from the private schools. The decision to extend teaching was in part a reaction to mounting concerns about competition and a response to external pressure.[125] When Guy's began to offer summer courses, staff at St Bartholomew's decided that similar courses in chemistry, *materia medica*, botany and midwifery should be set up.[126] The decision provoked immediate hostility from Hue and pressure was brought to bear on him after King's College followed Guy's. Attempts were made to persuade Hue and evidence was presented that students were leaving St Bartholomew's and going elsewhere (particularly to the Aldersgate School) precisely because the College failed to teach during the summer. Reluctantly, Hue agreed that the chemistry theatre could be used during the summer.[127]

With these changes it was deemed important to reaffirm the practical, clinical character of the College. A handbook issued in 1835 explained that lectures in medicine were 'illustrated by *Clinical Observation* on the Cases of Patents in the Hospital'.[128] However, practice did not match the College's claims. Old attitudes to observation persisted and 'there was very little active practical teaching'. One student remembered that it was still customary in the mid-1830s 'to think it sufficient to give opportunities for learning to those who could learn by looking-on and by occasional rather casual talking about the cases'. Clinical teaching remained essentially 'self-guided'.[129]

[124] Negley Harte, *The University of London, 1836–1986* (London, 1986), pp. 73–4.
[125] Medical College, 21 March 1835, MS 15.
[126] Ibid., 28 May 1835, MS 15.
[127] Ibid., 30 May 1833, 6 June 1835, MS 15.
[128] *College Calendar* (1835/6).
[129] Paget, ed., *Memoirs*, pp. 40, 60.

A failed school?

By 1837 the College had reversed its earlier hostility to the University. Falling student numbers had increased anxiety, and with The London, the Middlesex and St George's already affiliated to the University, a decision was made to petition the Senate to admit St Bartholomew's as a school. With the University having no power of inspection or control, affiliation was not seen as a threat to independence. Two years later, the Senate supported the College's application and St Bartholomew's became part of the University.[130] Like the other affiliated schools, it continued as an 'isolated teaching institution', dominated by its clinical staff. However, affiliation did encourage the College to reorganise its teaching to match the University's examination requirements.[131]

Reforms did not at first actively stimulate student numbers. Although St Bartholomew's had shared in the rapid increase in students from the 1780s, without Abernethy student admissions declined and the College became less able to manage internal divisions and external competition. By 1841 it had fallen behind, having been overtaken by University College. Despite reforms, the *Lancet* made teaching in the College appear outmoded, expensive and limited, ensuring that the College had a poor public and professional reputation. The medical press seemed to revel in revealing the College's deficiencies, even when conditions were often no worse, and sometimes much better, than those at other hospital schools.

To some extent Abernethy was to blame. Between 1780 and 1842 teaching in the College had become more clinical and scientific, with a closer association of medicine and surgery. New subjects were included in a curriculum that proved responsive not only to demands made by licensing bodies but also to student pressure. However, the system that Abernethy had bequeathed and the central role he had played in teaching for so long left a legacy of hostility that frustrated change. His conflict with the *Lancet* soured relations, while the hospital's prominent position in the medical establishment made it appear conservative. Conflicts between other staff in the College and their frequent reluctance to change teaching deepened these problems. Although this analysis may ascribe an undue emphasis to the role of personalities, in an institution where it was the lecturers just as much as the facilities that were important, those teaching had a major impact on the College's fortunes.

By 1842 St Bartholomew's had certainly reached a low point, but it had not failed. Reform and the need for new dynamic lectures had become essential, but there was never any question that the College should close. It was time for change, to modernise teaching, and to break with the system established under Abernethy.

---

[130] Medical College, 25 May 1839, MS 15.
[131] L. P. Le Quesne, 'Medicine', in *The University and the World of Learning*, ed. F. M. L. Thompson (London, 1990), p. 129.

3

'A wise and liberal desire to improve'

Mid-Victorian medical education

For William Lawrence, surgeon at St Bartholomew's, the years 1830 to 1858 were a time of 'noisy meetings, and angry discussions' that culminated in the 1858 Medical (Registration) Act.[1] Characterised as an age of reform, it was during the first half of the nineteenth century that the shape of medicine as a profession became recognisably modern. Pressure for reform came from within and from individuals, aided by legislative change that gave a more defined structure to medical education, a legal supply of bodies for dissection, and recognition to the role of the general practitioner.[2] It was during this period that hospital medical schools were consolidated and private schools pushed out, a transition that contributed to the development of shared professional values among doctors. At the same time, the licensing bodies started to issue stricter guidelines on what they expected students to learn. By the 1850s the importance of the bedside and the clinical lecture had become firmly established. However, in medical education the middle years of the nineteenth century have (all too often) been ignored because they lie between the triumph of the London hospital schools and anatomico-clinical medicine, and the 'laboratory revolution'. In Britain, the period has been described as one of stagnation, with a shift in medical advance from the Parisian clinic to the German laboratory.[3] The old corporate order was breaking down but continuities remained.

The 1858 Act was a 'bitter disappointment' to contemporaries, failing to outlaw quackery or institute a single portal of entry by rationalising licensing qualifications. As a piece of protectionism, it gave the emerging medical profession considerable autonomy and an external appearance of unity that poorly disguised intra-professional divisions.[4] Educational reform had been

[1] William Lawrence, *Hunterian Oration* (London, 1846), p. 5.
[2] Roger French and Andrew Wear, 'Introduction', in *British Medicine in an Age of Reform*, ed. Roger French and Andrew Wear (London, 1991), pp. 1–8; Irvine Loudon, 'Medical Practitioners and Medical Reform in Britain 1750–1850', in *Medicine and Society: Historical Essays*, ed. Andrew Wear (Cambridge, 1994), pp. 219–37.
[3] Gerald L. Geison, 'Social and Institutional Factors in the Stagnancy of English Physiology, 1840–70', *BHM* xlvi (1972), pp. 30–58.
[4] Irvine Loudon, *Medical Care and the General Practitioner, 1750–1850* (Oxford, 1986), pp. 297–8.

part of attempts to 'modernise' the royal colleges and limit competition to create properly educated regular practitioners. However, although the Act established the General Medical Council (GMC) to regulate training, the stubbornness of the London medical schools and nature of the licensing bodies initially limited its authority. Students had no obligation to sit examinations in medicine, surgery and midwifery until the 1886 Medical Amendment Act, and could qualify after passing an examination in a single branch of medicine, though most continued to seek a dual qualification, forsaking the LSA for the new LRCP. If the broad outline of training was rarely contested, debates over the nature and structure of education outlasted medical reform. Debate focused on raising the general education of entrants to the profession to support doctors' claims to a gentlemanly status, the relative merits of individual subjects, and on how students were examined and by whom. Licensing bodies, students and lecturers were all blamed for what were perceived to be low standards in training and, while some observers felt there were too many lectures, others argued that students spent too much time on the wards.

If the 1858 Act did not settle debates over education, neither was evidence of stagnation immediately apparent. Medical knowledge was being refashioned as more prestige was attached to natural and scientific knowledge. Although practice and theories were enormously diverse, most could agree that scientific knowledge was fundamental to practice. London remained the dominant centre of scientific life in the 1840s and 1850s, a magnet for medical practitioners and students. While this metropolitan dominance declined after 1850 with the rise of the civic universities, in the mid-Victorian period London's medical schools remained educational and institutional leaders. They provided a centre for the medical elite and formed an important part of a higher educational structure that was itself undergoing a process of reform. Only in the 1870s was this position challenged, as greater emphasis was placed on the importance of experimental and laboratory science to medicine.

St Bartholomew's was relatively unaffected by the climate of medical reform. Those teaching in the College supported the establishment and were more worried about the effects of competition from other teaching hospitals. The result was a period of internal restructuring that ran parallel to the reform movement. Inspiration was drawn from debates on the nature of education at Oxford and Cambridge. The 1840s proved a crucial decade and lecturers in the College became convinced that urgent action was needed to prevent further decay. By 1842 a crisis had been reached. Internal divisions were at their worst; competition was intense. Student numbers had fallen since the retirement of Abernethy, and those who did attend were considered to be of a poor standard. It was not a situation unique to St Bartholomew's: other London schools were also trying to cope with falling student numbers at a time when medical education was under attack. To reverse the perceived position of the College, a package of improvements was suggested that aimed to rejuvenate teaching. They addressed the subjects to be taught and method of teaching, and strove to encourage learning and discipline through a system of rewards and punishments. A further, less anxious attempt to modernise teaching was made in the mid-1860s with the addition of new classes and specialist clinical lectures as educational needs came to shape the hospital's clinical environment. When new College buildings were opened in 1881, St Bartholomew's had re-established itself as London's largest medical school.

A 'home' for students

For the governors of the hospital, it was not falling student numbers that created alarm but the conduct of the students. After the disputes of the 1820s, they had been content to leave the organisation of teaching to the lecturers, convinced that it had benefits for patient care. By 1842 the governors started to have doubts, concerned that students were having an unfavourable impact on the hospital. They felt compelled to intervene. Borrowing heavily from the Oxbridge ideal, they suggested opening an institution in which students could live, dine and study as a way of controlling student behaviour. Although the idea of a collegiate institute formed the backbone of European universities, it was building programmes at Oxford and Cambridge between 1800 and 1830 that drew attention to a collegiate system of moral and academic discipline.[5] Discipline was central to the collegiate ideal. At Oxford and Cambridge, walls, gates and ditches restricted movement; regulations stipulated compulsory attendance at chapel and lectures, and detailed offences that would result in suspension or expulsion.[6] No medical school could afford to be this strict: too rigid a regime would discourage students, resulting in a fall in income and prestige. However, with mounting anxiety about student conduct and the image of the medical profession, a similar disciplinary framework was adopted. Numerous witnesses to the 1834 select committee on medical education recognised that a collegiate system developed 'character' and 'moral' superiority.[7] These were values which doctors wanted incorporated into medical education.

Concerns about student welfare and the morally polluting influence of London had been simmering since the foundation of the London University, where it was believed that students were left without moral superintendence. When linked to concerns about student discipline and fears of the morally subversive influence of the city, public and professional anxiety was aroused

---

[5] See Sheldon Rothblatt, *The Revolution of the Dons: Cambridge and Society in Victorian England* (London, 1968).

[6] See Arthur J. Engel, '"Immoral Intentions": The University of Oxford and the Problem of Prostitution, 1827–1914', *Victorian Studies* xxiii (1979/80), pp. 79–107.

[7] *SC on Medical Education*, PP (1834) xiii, pp. 9, 35.

which mirrored that at St Bartholomew's over student behaviour. Several solutions were suggested. However, it was the virtues of grafting residential colleges on to medical schools that focused debate. In London, Benjamin Harrison, treasurer of Guy's, had first suggested the need for a residential college in 1839, but insufficient funds and accommodation ensured that no action was taken.[8] Harrison's idea stimulated interest, especially at St George's, where the chaplain, Revd John North, tried to persuade the governors that a college modelled on Oxford and Cambridge should be built.[9] In all these plans, residential colleges were seen as synonymous with moral education and a solution to student unruliness.

The enthusiasm expressed in the medical press for the collegiate system was matched by interest at St Bartholomew's. The governors supported the need for a residential college, and when they approached the lecturers in 1842 the idea was cautiously welcomed. With the College in decline, those who supported the scheme convinced their colleagues that a residential college would act as an agent of reform. The suggestion was also seen to 'be productive of great benefits to society' by cutting down student unrest. Common interest was found in the problem of student discipline. James Paget, the recently appointed lecturer in general and morbid anatomy, was called upon to advise.[10]

Paget came to provide the leadership and administrative ability that had been lacking in the College since Abernethy's death. In this, and in his reforming efforts, he mirrored the work of his brother George at Cambridge.[11] At St Bartholomew's, Lawrence, as the most senior surgeon, had failed to provide the direction the College needed. The opportunistic Lawrence had shed his earlier radical politics and become part of the medical establishment, holding back the appointment of junior staff. His presence encouraged friction, and when he finally resigned after his first stroke, the *Lancet* noted that it was 'a direct benefit conferred upon the profession'.[12] Lawrence's influence in the running of the College was limited by his unpopularity, and this allowed the aspiring Paget to assert his ideas.

Paget had followed his brother to St Bartholomew's after completing an apprenticeship. He found the College 'not in good working order', but with facilities that rivalled the other London teaching hospitals. Ambitious for success, Paget won a series of prizes and built up close links with the

[8] H. C. Cameron, *Mr Guys Hospital, 1726–1948* (London, 1954), pp. 180–1.

[9] J. B. Atlay, *Sir Henry Wentworth Acland* (London, 1903), p. 89.

[10] General court, 23 November 1842, HA 1/19.

[11] For George Paget, see M. Jeanne Peterson, 'Sir George Paget and Cambridge Medical Education, 1851–1892', in *History of Medical Education*, ed. Teizo Ogawa (Osaka, 1983), pp. 27–54.

[12] *Lancet* i (1867), p. 635.

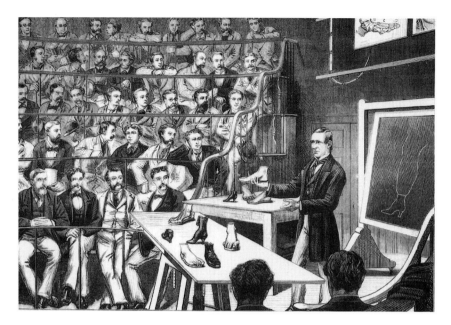

Plate 3.1 'A lecture at St Bartholomew's on a pressing subject' by James Paget. Engraved illustration, *Picture Post*, 25 July 1874

lecturers.[13] After following his brother to Paris, he returned to a post in the anatomy museum at St Bartholomew's. Paget believed it important to remain connected with a 'good school' no matter how low he entered. Although frustrated and constantly worried about money, Paget was popular with the students, but found the College 'dull'. A series of disappointments in securing appointments followed, forcing him to rely on medical journalism to bolster his standing and income, and to offset his disappointment in 'holding the same subordinate offices'. With several staff feeling guilty about not finding him a better post, he was allowed to give demonstrations. Paget used this to improve his position in the College. In 1842, he was finally appointed lecturer after unease had erupted in a conflict between Edward Stanley, the lecturer in anatomy, and his demonstrator, Thomas Wormald. To smooth over tensions, appointments were rearranged and Paget was appointed demonstrator. Paget felt his 'fortune was made'. However, with the College having declined further, he was determined to bolster its status to improve his reputation and income.[14]

[13] Stephen Paget, ed., *Memoirs and Letters of Sir James Paget* (London, 1902), pp. 27, 32, 40–3.
[14] Ibid., pp. 71, 92, 80–4, 105, 117–20, 139.

For the governors, Paget represented an authority on residential colleges. He was engaged to Lydia North, the sister of Revd John North of St George's, and he and North had talked extensively about the need for residential colleges.[15] Paget was also influenced by his brother's experiences as a fellow of Caius College, Cambridge. Contemporaries believed that Paget rarely took a decision without consulting his brother, and he was well aware of the efforts made to reform the collegiate system at Cambridge. Paget's enthusiasm for a residential college encouraged the governors to put aside their doubts and convert six houses in Duke Street to provide accommodation for thirty students with a large room, or 'college hall', built as a breakfast and dining-room.[16] This room gave the residential college its name 'College Hall'. The hospital was not making a sacrifice: Duke Street was 'a dirty little street' and the houses would probably have been demolished as part of an ongoing programme of improvement.[17] The College was not asked to contribute, nor in theory was it given a direct role in how College Hall was managed. No resistance was offered by the lecturers who were keen to avoid any additional burden on falling fees. However, the acceptance that College Hall should be supervised by a warden elected from the teaching staff did secure a role for the College.[18] The post of warden was modelled on the idealised pastoral and disciplinary role of the Oxbridge tutor. A number of Oxford colleges had tightened up the disciplinary functions of their tutors in the 1820s to cope with student unrest. Schemes for residential colleges built on this, and at St Bartholomew's the warden was made responsible for admissions and was expected to play an important part in the students' moral and academic development.[19] However, unlike Oxford and Cambridge, the warden was not responsible for teaching or for fees. This was left to the lecturers, ensuring that they retained control over teaching.

Doubts about the standard of the accommodation saw the governors turning to Paget for advice. With William Peirs Ormerod, a previous pupil of Thomas Arnold at Rugby and the new demonstrator of anatomy, Paget conducted a detailed survey of student lodgings and spending.[20] Ormerod was shy, quiet and industrious, and was believed to exert a good moral influence on the students. A religious man, Ormerod had already abolished smoking and drinking in the dissecting room on the grounds that it interrupted study. Tending to describe rather than analyse, Ormerod was the perfect foil to Paget, who was able to dominate. Using evidence from their survey, Paget and Ormerod put forward their suggestions for how College Hall should be

[15] Ibid., p. 123.
[16] General court, 23 November 1842, HA 1/19.
[17] Paget, ed., *Memoirs*, pp. 123, 145.
[18] Medical College, 1 June 1842, MS 15.
[19] College minutes, 2 February 1843, MS 3.
[20] Ibid., 2 February 1843, 25 February 1843, MS 3.

run. They submitted what they considered to be the best elements of the Oxbridge system combined with the expectations of lodgings in London.[21] By mimicking the Oxbridge system, it was anticipated that a better class of student would be attracted to St Bartholomew's.

The recommendations made by Paget and Ormerod were largely accepted. Although the scale of fees was higher than their estimate of average student expenditure, it compared favourably with the £80 to £100 which grammar schools charged for lodgings and was within the means of the new middle classes.[22] The governors were attempting to provide an attractive and afford-able environment for a class of 'respectable' student that Paget and Ormerod had planned to admit. Once the practical arrangements had been decided, the lecturers were asked to formulate the regulations that would govern College Hall. Character was seen as the key. Preference was given to those likely to complete their training at St Bartholomew's in a bid to increase student numbers. The opportunity was not missed to provide a system of supervision: students were expected to dine in every day and were not allowed to leave College Hall after midnight or stay out overnight without prior permission. Paget was appointed warden to implement the new regulations.[23] As warden, he was able to create the institution he had envisaged. However, Paget quickly became dissatisfied. He believed that for the work he was expected to undertake he had received a 'very bad bargain'.[24]

College Hall was opened in 1843; by October twenty-one students had been given rooms.[25] The governors were pleased with the experiment even though it continued to make a loss until 1869. Although the *Lancet* attacked the 'constant "Does-your-Mother-know-you're-out" sort of *surveillance*', College Hall did encourage the governors to take a 'constant and friendly interest in the School' at a personal and financial level.[26] Difficulties remained (especially when medical education conflicted with patient care), but in cooperating over College Hall the governors had made a further investment. It sealed a model of development established with the opening of the first lecture theatre in 1791, but created a largely one-sided arrangement that benefited the College. The governors were allowed no say in how teaching was organised, and the lecturers continued to use the demands of medical education as a tool to shape the hospital environment.

Under Paget's strict control, College Hall quickly proved a success. Discipline was tightened and students staying in Hall won a large number of scholarships. Students were selected from across the years to ensure balance,

---

[21] Ibid., 9 March 1843, MS 3.
[22] Rothblatt, *Revolution of the Dons*, p. 58.
[23] College minutes, 10 August 1843, 31 August 1843, MS 3.
[24] Paget, ed., *Memoirs*, p. 145.
[25] Residential colleges, June 1901, MS 6/11.
[26] *Lancet* (1842/3), p. 487; Paget, ed., *Memoirs*, p. 126.

but emphasis was placed on those who had distinguished themselves or had come up to London for the first time and had 'no other means of super-vision'.[27] Paget exploited the high demand for rooms to argue for expansion and in 1846 two more houses were added, raising the number of rooms to thirty-eight.[28] Other London medical schools gradually followed the College's lead. Although a scheme to open a hall at the London Hospital collapsed, St Mary's opened one in 1885. The Middlesex followed with a similar scheme in 1887.[29] Where residential halls were established, many were based on the model pioneered by St Bartholomew's.

How influential College Hall was in attracting students is hard to determine. It certainly encouraged a domestic vocabulary in the College's pronouncements. After 1842, St Bartholomew's was frequently described as a 'home' by the medical press, associating it with the collegiate system. This found favour with parents and created the impression of a safe environment that counterbalanced an image of London as the 'modern Babylon'. The association with the style of education offered at Oxford and Cambridge had a powerful appeal. Although doubts were to be expressed in the 1890s about the impact of collegiate establishments on students, Paget believed that the success of the College after 1842 depended 'much on that of the College [Hall]'. Looking back, he argued that College Hall was a new start for St Bartholomew's.[30] College Hall and his wardenship certainly consolidated Paget's position at St Bartholomew's where he was a dominant figure throughout the 1850s and 1860s. The establishment of a residential college also made the College, as the *Lancet* reluctantly acknowledged, very different from other London teaching hospitals. Numbers attending the College consequently rose.[31] In part, this may be attributed to an increase in professional recruitment immediately after the 1858 Act and to moves by middle-class families to favour prolonged education as a response to a demographic shift to smaller families, but the trend had been established in the decade before the Act was passed.[32] On its own, College Hall was not enough to reverse the fall in the number of students coming to St Bartholomew's that had characterised the 1830s. However, as part of a package of reforms it served to make the College a more competitive and attractive institution for students wishing to study in London.

[27] *RC on a University for London*, PP (1889) xxxix, p. 147.

[28] College minutes, 5 November 1846, MS 3.

[29] St Mary's residential college, DH 9/2/22; Regulations of the Middlesex Hospital college, DH 9/2/20.

[30] Paget, ed., *Memoirs*, p. 145.

[31] *Lancet* (1842/3), p. 487.

[32] See Anne Digby, *Making a Medical Living: Doctors and Patients in the English Market of Medicine, 1720–1911* (Cambridge, 1994).

Rewards and punishments

The opening of College Hall was part of an effort at St Bartholomew's to raise educational standards. Changes in the curriculum reinforced the importance of anatomical investigation over experimental methodology. Stanley took the lead in instituting this new emphasis. He had travelled extensively in Europe in the 1830s observing how medicine was taught. With the College at a low point, he was able to persuade his colleagues to introduce a more continental style of teaching he had observed to break from Abernethy's legacy.[33] An enthusiast for morbid anatomy, Stanley added new classes on surgical anatomy, and on general anatomy and physiology.[34] He also encouraged the creation of a course on practical pathology but initially classes were held only when 'opportunities occur'.[35] With anatomy considered to be 'the pillar and backbone of . . . medical and surgical studies', these changes were designed to modernise teaching and retained its practical and clinical utility.[36] Clinical staff who had deserted St Bartholomew's to teach at the Aldersgate School (see Chapter 2) were encouraged by these improvements and returned to the College, thereby boosting its status. Existing staff whom students were seen to dislike were persuaded to resign on the grounds that they were 'highly injurious to the interests of the Medical School'.[37] New lecturers were appointed, allowing further alterations to be made.

Despite these changes, continuity existed with the pattern of teaching that had been established in the 1820s. Outside anatomy, no new subjects were added and moves to raise the educational status of the College shifted to the students. It was not only the provincial medical schools that worked to adopt more stringent academic standards.[38] Mechanisms were established at St Bartholomew's in the 1840s and 1850s to reward the able, provide more guidance and monitor performance. The aim was to improve discipline and encourage study in answer to the pressures of the University of London's MB and the GMC's guidelines.

The development of a system of scholarships, which built on earlier efforts by those connected to the hospital to found prizes, was an important component in achieving this transition. The origin of what was to become an extensive system of scholarships and prizes was influenced by the practices of Oxford and Cambridge. The initiative was taken once more by the governors. In 1834 the president of the hospital, Matthias Prime Lucas, resolved to

[33] Notebook of Edward Stanley, X 5/16.

[34] Medical college, 15–19 April 1843, MS 15.

[35] *College Calendar* (1845/6), p. 15.

[36] *BMJ* (1859), p. 835.

[37] Medical Council, 23 January 1851, MC 1/1.

[38] Stella V. F. Butler, 'A Transformation in Training: The Formation of University Medical Faculties in Manchester, Leeds, and Liverpool, 1870–84', *Medical History* xxx (1986), pp. 118–32.

donate an annual prize to the best student. In response, the lecturers agreed that prizes and honorary distinctions should be awarded annually. In 1842, Samuel Wix, hospitaller (chaplain) and vicar of St Bartholomew's-the-Less, presented £200 to the hospital to found a further prize. Several months later, James Bentley, treasurer to the hospital, matched this contribution. Bentley was a generous benefactor and pressed for a prize for 'encouraging the study of Medicine and Surgery and the advancement of the Medical School'. His gift was invested and it was decided that the interest be used to create an annual prize for the student with the best case notes.[39] Others followed.

The creation of scholarships at St Bartholomew's was part of an extensive philanthropic network but evolved in part because of the hospital's anomalous position in the metropolitan benevolent economy. Reliant on endowed income from property and investments, by 1891 the *Daily Telegraph* could confidently report that St Bartholomew's was 'one of the richest, most reputed and oldest hospital . . . in England'.[40] As such, it functioned outside the benevolent economy and the only money donated to the hospital came from 'strangers invited by the governors to the annual hospital dinners'.[41] Careful management had produced a rental income that by the 1890s was larger than the total income of most other hospitals. This removed the need to court charity. Those who wished to donate money therefore tended to give to the College but directed their gifts through the hospital. Scholarships formed relatively unobtrusive acts of benevolence attracting little attention outside the schools they benefited. In a society where voluntarism was both fashionable and a social duty, those founding scholarships were working in a climate of charity that was integral to their view of society. Although scholarships did not attempt to reform morals, stave off social unrest or promote thrift, and do not easily fit within the models of philanthropy historians have constructed since the 1960s, they did serve a purpose.[42] Those founding scholarships were undoubtedly influenced by a sense of human-itarianism and a social ethic of philanthropy, but scholarships were also an effective form of posthumous self-aggrandisement that the College was keen to encourage. Each scholarship had a name attached reminding the recipient of the founders' generosity. They could act as a memorial for departed friends or relatives, prolonging their name out of love or perhaps guilt. For those connected to St Bartholomew's, a scholarship also offered a commemoration of their work. Elizabeth Baly, for example, gave £1,900 to found the Baly

[39] House committee, 12 July 1842, HA 1/19.
[40] Cited in SC *of the House of Lords on Metropolitan Hospitals etc.*, *First Report*, PP (1890) xvi, p. 171.
[41] John Wrottesley and Samuel Smith, 'St Bartholomew's Hospital', *32nd Report of the Charity Commissions*, Part vi (London, 1840), p. 47.
[42] For a discussion of historical interpretations of charity, see Alan J. Kidd, 'Philanthropy and the "Social History Paradigm"', *Social History* xxi (1996), pp. 180–92.

Scholarship in memory of 'my said brother', William Baly, and did so because he had studied at St Bartholomew's and been 'one of the Physicians'. Scholarships also allowed the benefactor to promote a particular area of study or type of student. When the Shuter Scholarship was established in 1886, Agnes Dodd insisted that candidates had to be arts graduates from the University of Cambridge as her brother James Shuter had followed this path. The scholarship served the dual purpose of providing a memorial to Shuter (fittingly no mention was made that he died of a morphine overdose) and encouraging a class of students which the College was keen to attract.[43] Such charitable gifts formed the basis of the scholarship system.

By 1842 a rudimentary system had been established. The next step was taken three years later by the College in an effort to prevent further decline. The lecturers rejected the creation of more prizes and resolved instead that 'it is desirable to establish Scholarships, with primary advantages to be conferred on those students of this school', who, 'after open examination are judged the most worthy of them'.[44] They saw these scholarships as a way of promoting the best students, of encouraging hard work, and of securing a degree of learning in those entering. A disciplinary function was included: all those competing for a scholarship were expected to conduct themselves in an 'appropriate' manner. Later they were used to 'elucidate an all round or "educative" grasp of a subject or subjects'.[45] Three scholarships were founded to cover anatomy and physiology; chemistry, *materia medica*, botany and medical jurisprudence; and medicine, surgery and midwifery. In the 1860s, the terminology was changed: the scholarship in anatomy, physiology and chemistry became the junior scholarship, with the senior scholarship covering medicine, surgery and midwifery. Although those studying at St Bartholomew's were entitled to enter both, the senior scholarship was designed primarily to attract students from Oxford and Cambridge. Each scholarship was awarded annually unless the minimum pass mark had not been reached.[46]

Scholarships were a good investment and an advertisement for the College. The high cost of medical education in London made scholarships financially and professionally attractive. Although they aimed to attract gentlemen into the profession, their main purpose was to raise the status of the College and students, the latter by appealing to 'an honourable as well as to an inevitable sense of rivalry'.[47] Some doubts were initially expressed, but it was felt that scholarships encouraged a 'spirit of emulation' that merged with College Hall to attract students. By 1889 the warden, Norman

[43] Trust funds, MS 73/12.
[44] Scholarships, MS 11.
[45] Memorandum, 23 February 1967, DF 106.
[46] Callender to College, 9 June 1864, DF 115.
[47] Samuel Squire Sprigge, *Physics and Fiction* (London, 1921), p. 153.

Moore, could confidently claim that scholarships were primarily a form of 'encouragement'. Where they were not established schools saw a fall in student numbers, so that by the late 1860s every medical school in London had started to offer prizes.[48] The incentives to study at a particular school created by scholarships became an important factor for students in deciding which school to attend. By 1872 the *BMJ* was sufficiently worried to warn students not to choose schools purely on the number of scholarships available.[49] St Bartholomew's was a clear beneficiary.

The scholarship and prize system was refined slowly. Greater efforts were made to reward 'practical work in the dissecting rooms or in the wards', and by the 1870s each scholarship had been divided in recognition of rising student numbers.[50] Alterations were made between 1868 and 1874 to reflect changes in the entrance requirements of the University of London and this further boosted admissions. The junior and senior scholarships were adapted and money was found to support four entrance scholarships. These were designed to improve the 'general culture' of the students and promote a liberal education. The status of the senior scholarship was taken over by two new scholarships, one named after William Lawrence; the other after Hannah Brackenbury, medical philanthropist and benefactor of Manchester Medical School.[51] Additional scholarships followed: when the Board of Education investigated the College in 1913, it found fifteen scholarships and ten prizes. Of these, the most prestigious were the Brackenbury Scholarships, which formed the basis of the College's examination system and developed subsidiary prizes designed to reward clinical skill.[52]

Scholarships were only one part of the bid to raise educational standards. The admission of St Bartholomew's as a school of the University of London in 1839, following a period of intense opposition to the institution and its predecessor, allowed students to prepare for the MB (Bachelor of Medicine). Pressure to make the University into an examining body had in part come from the medical community and the MB was the 'first comprehensive medical qualification available to students at the London schools'. However, it was six years before a student from St Bartholomew's took the examination; it was not until the mid-1850s that more than one student per year sat the MB. Although the majority of students at St Bartholomew's (and at other London schools) continued to qualify through the easier and more traditional routes provided by the royal colleges and Society of Apothecaries, this placed the College at a disadvantage. While it could boast extensive clinical facilities and embodied the British emphasis on clinical training, the level

---

[48] *RC on a University for London*, p. 147.
[49] *BMJ* ii (1872), pp. 285–6.
[50] Meeting of medical officers and lecturers, 10 May 1862, MS 12/1.
[51] Baker to College, 15 January 1874, DF 115.
[52] Application to the Board of Education, DF 184.

of theoretical teaching offered was insufficient for most students to pass the MB. Failure rates for the MB, which were due to inadequate science teaching and the poor standard of secondary education, remained high throughout the nineteenth century. In response, a more straightforward examination was introduced in the 1850s. Although this changed in 1861 with the introduction of a preliminary science examination, the College believed throughout the 1850s that its students' poor performance reflected on teaching, especially as those from Guy's, King's and University College dominated pass lists.[53] This prompted Paget, a supporter of the University and future vice-chancellor, to press for the appointment of a resident tutor.

The tutorial system was closely associated with Oxford and Cambridge. Private tutors and coaches had become an established feature of the higher education environment by the eighteenth century and had links with the system of cramming for examinations. At Oxford and Cambridge, tutors had responsibility for the education, discipline and welfare of the college pupils.[54] Interest in the role of the tutor grew in the early nineteenth century as concern mounted about the limited teaching conducted by college Fellows. Reformers criticised teaching at the ancient universities and pressed for separate royal commissions, which were appointed in 1850. Bound up with the issue of religious toleration and political moves to remove 'abuses', reformers looked to private coaches and tutors as the model for a better system of instruction and moral guidance. Tutors were also believed to offer intellectual stimulation and preparation for examination.[55] Paget was aware of these changes through his brother George, who was an important force in the reform of medical education at Cambridge. In addition, the appointment of the two royal commissions in 1850 focused debate. Although the tutorial system was later to prove limiting to science teaching, Paget took the reformist ideas current at Cambridge and Oxford and applied them to St Bartholomew's. Such borrowing from Oxbridge had a profound influence on the development of higher education in Britain.

Monitoring of students' progress had originally been part of the warden's duties, but with Paget appointed lecturer in general and morbid anatomy in 1843, and then professor of anatomy and surgery at the Royal College of Surgeons four years later, he felt constantly overworked. Paget argued that a

[53] A. L. Mansell, 'Examinations and Medical Education: The Preliminary Sciences in the Examinations of London University and the English Conjoint Board, 1861–1911', in *Days of Judgement: Science, Examinations and the Organisation of Knowledge in Late Victorian England*, ed. Roy MacLeod (North Humberside, 1982), pp. 90–1.

[54] Peter Searby, *A History of the University of Cambridge*, 3 vols (Cambridge, 1997), Vol.1, pp. 118–31.

[55] M. C. Curthoys, 'The "Unreformed" Colleges', in *The History of the University of Oxford: Nineteenth Century Oxford*, ed. M. G. Brock and M. C. Curthoys (Oxford, 1997), Vol. 6, pp. 148–52; Rothblatt, *Revolution of the Dons*, pp. 190–209; T. W. Heyck, *Transformation of Intellectual Life in Victorian England* (London, 1982), pp. 72–3, 164–70.

tutor was needed to raise standards. Howard Marsh remembered that when he entered St Bartholomew's in the 1850s most of the students sat only two examinations: the preliminary (or matriculation) examination and the final examination. Between these two many 'idled away until a few months before examination'.[56] To make matters worse, most first-year students received only limited teaching. Paget had had a similar experience and was aware that, for most, study was largely self-determined, leaving plenty of time for coarse 'pleasures and amusements'.[57] A tutorial system was designed to prevent this without removing the need to transfer teaching from the clinical staff. William Scovell Savory, a former student, was therefore appointed medical tutor in 1850. Savory was an ideal choice: he had been an outstanding student and was one of the few to take honours in medicine at the University of London. He was initially paid £50 per annum: £20 from the College and £30 from the warden 'in consideration of the assistance which he will receive'.[58] The arrangement proved temporary. A year after Paget's retirement, the financial responsibility was switched from the warden to a fee raised from those students preparing for a university degree.[59] With the move, emphasis shifted from moral to academic guidance.

High failure rates in the MB led to calls for the widespread adoption of the tutorial system. By 1878 the *BMJ* noted that the presence of tutors in London's medical schools had become common over the 'last twenty years'.[60] Contemporaries felt that under the tutorial system students at St Bartholomew's were 'drilled' but they also noted the 'disquietingly successful results' achieved.[61] Gradually the authority of the tutor was extended to those students preparing for the MRCS and LRCP to give 'pupils the amount of information necessary for their examinations' and to 'teach them to study in a thorough and rational method'.[62] In 1865, with pressure from students, it was decided to appoint two additional tutors.[63] Anxious about the loss of authority, senior staff resented the move and quickly took control from the tutors, ensuring that more emphasis was placed on the medical and surgical staff providing tutorials. Although contemporaries began to wonder if the tutorial system was grinding under another name, this did not dull students' apparent enthusiasm. Numbers attending classes at St Bartholomew's rose, so that by the 1880s there were seldom fewer than forty students in tutorials. However, no regulations stipulated how many tutorial classes students should attend and tutorial sessions remained *ad hoc*.

---

[56] *A Memoir of Howard Marsh* (London, 1921), pp. 8, 10.

[57] Paget, ed., *Memoirs*, p. 355.

[58] Minutes of the medical officers and lecturers, 21 September 1850, MS 12/1.

[59] Ibid., 3 January 1852, MS 12/1.

[60] *BMJ* i (1853), p. 1075; ibid. (1878), p. 791.

[61] Cameron, *Guy's*, p. 226.

[62] Moore to College, 22 October 1873, MS 13/27.

[63] Minutes of the medical officers and lecturers, 22 April 1865, MS 12/1.

Demand forced the College to rethink arrangements. With no fixed room for teaching, Samuel Hatch West, the medical tutor, found it difficult to provide the level of instruction envisaged. West complained that he had neither the time nor strength to cope with the rapid rise in the numbers attending his classes and argued that 'it is clearly beyond the powers of any one man to do it all satisfactorily'. He pressed for a return to the system established in 1865 and for a list of students nearing examination so that he could limit his teaching to those preparing for examination. New guidelines were drawn up and an assistant tutor was appointed in 1881.[64]

The move to a tutorial system and the introduction of scholarships forced the development of a more formal examination system. Written papers gradually supplemented *viva voces* as lecturers struggled to develop examinations that were more rigorous. In traditional universities, this move had begun in the eighteenth century and interest in competitive examinations grew in the first half of the nineteenth century. For the historian John Roach, examinations were 'one of the great discoveries of the nineteenth century Englishman'.[65] Faith in them became unshakeable. As part of the middle-class reform of education and its institutions, examinations were constructed in the mid-nineteenth century as an agent of progress, a solution to favouritism and an encouragement to hard work. Interest was furthered by the honours system at Oxford and Cambridge, and by moves in the Civil Service after 1853 to open posts to competition and merit. A combination of political and psychological arguments was asserted to confirm the role of examinations, and they were quickly integrated as an important factor in academic professionalism and the maintenance of professional standards.[66] Examinations also had a disciplinary function: written papers were believed to promote sustained study around an organised body of knowledge that matched the imperatives of the licensing bodies. These were precisely the values lecturers at St Bartholomew's wanted to incorporate.

The creation of a number of scholarships forced moves to develop a series of internal examinations, with all students 'who show superior knowledge' receiving a testimonial. Tutors were also expected to test students regularly. Wormald had started routine examinations as demonstrator of anatomy in the 1850s. He would place a skull on the table during his lectures to announce that questions would be asked. Unfortunately, many students often left at this point and regular examinations caught on slowly until an 'excessive' number of failures in the University of London's preliminary science examination forced staff to act. The GMC was also pressing for greater stringency in examinations. The College was sensitive to these

---

[64] West to Shore, 24 January 1881, MS 14/1; Minutes of the medical officers and lecturers, 18 March 1882, MS 12/2.

[65] J. P. C. Roach, *Public Examinations in England, 1850–1900* (Cambridge, 1971).

[66] See Harold Perkin, *The Rise of Professional Society: England since 1880* (London, 1989).

changes and the need to promote more disciplined learning. By 1860 all first-year students were examined on a weekly basis. Optional tests on anatomy and physiology were introduced for those preparing for the LRCP, LSA, MRCS and MB. These were supplemented in 1871 by compulsory examinations. The idea provoked considerable discussion, but in 1872 similar tests were started in *materia medica*, botany and chemistry.[67] The practice was extended to clinical study in 1876 to prepare clerks for work on the wards.[68]

The adoption of regular examinations marked a shift in the internal assessment criteria of the College. It also placed St Bartholomew's at the forefront of educational thinking. Calls for the widespread adoption of regular assessments to prevent last-minute cramming were voiced alongside concerns that examinations might strait-jacket students into a tyranny of tests. 'Exam-phobia', prevalent in educational, medical and public debate by the 1880s, did not however find expression in the College. Here faith was maintained in examinations as the answer to accusations of patronage and favouritism believed still to be rife in medicine.[69]

Changes to the curriculum, the appointment of tutors and the intro-duction of scholarships did not immediately reduce tension or stem criticism. Throughout the 1840s conflict between staff frequently flared, especially over appointments. The *Lancet* continued to attack what it saw as the 'comparative inefficiency of medical teaching' in the College and claimed that the lecturers were defrauding the students. Individuals were singled out for censure but no other changes were made and the students found responsible for spreading rumours were effectively excluded.[70] Systematic teaching remained inadequate: many of the staff were regularly late to the wards and to lectures. However, greater stability had been achieved by the mid-1850s at the price of a more bureaucratic system and the establishment a supervisory framework. Efforts were made to avoid quarrels, which were felt to interfere with the 'efficient teaching of the students', by developing a more inclusive administration in which conflict could be resolved.[71] Although management remained in the hands of the senior staff (and especially the surgeons), a committee structure gave the impression of a more homogeneous institution. However, the system was far from democratic and junior staff played only a minor role.

Under the influence of these reforms student numbers increased. Standards rose, so that by the mid-1850s Paget felt that the College was attracting

---

[67] Minutes of the medical officers and lecturers, 18 December 1871, 27 March 1872, MS 12/2.

[68] West to Shore, 24 January 1881, MS 14/1.

[69] Roy MacLeod, 'Science and Examinations in Victorian England', in *Days of Judgement*, ed. MacLeod, pp. 11–12.

[70] *Lancet* i (1853), pp. 180–1; ibid., ii (1854), p. 452.

[71] Minutes of the medical officers and lecturers, 24 March 1860, MS 12/1.

'a better sort of men' and depending more on its reputation than on 'old connections' for pupils.[72] Closer links were established with the University of London which influenced teaching, a view that runs contrary to the belief that the University 'did not affect the position of the [London] medical schools'.[73] After the introduction of the preliminary science examination, the MB was widely recognised as the hardest route for qualification. Although the University became the most important examining body in the country, many teachers in London's medical schools felt that it was 'so far out of sympathy with the actual needs and circumstances of students, that it hinders a great number of men who would be worthy of its degrees from seeking them at all'.[74] Students preferred the easier MRCS and LRCP (or the Conjoint Diploma after 1866) and, with London's medical schools feeling excluded or inadequate, pressure for reform mounted. However, unlike other schools, St Bartholomew's came to see the MB as a benchmark. This attitude was due largely to Paget. Paget was on the University Senate and supported the MB, encouraging his colleagues to become university examiners.[75] Under his influence, courses were modified throughout the 1850s and 1860s to reflect the University's requirements and stress was placed on preparing students for the MB. Although the bulk of the medical profession criticised the University for making a 'fetish' of exams and setting standards that were too high, many outside the profession believed that it offered 'the best school of medicine in this country' and provided an academic education.[76] St Bartholomew's wanted to be associated with this image.

To improve performance in the MB and other professional qualifications, efforts were made to enforce attendance. London's teaching hospitals had long provided certificates to their students as proof of attendance for the examining bodies. At St Bartholomew's the system had been in force since at least 1794. By the 1860s interest had shifted from certificates as a verification of study as pressure grew for medical schools to establish a better system of internal registration to improve discipline and monitor fees. The movement was supported by the GMC and Royal College of Physicians. Registration was believed to prevent idleness, guide students as to the best course of study, and ensure that every student was educated to a standard considered appropriate by the teaching hospital concerned. Problems of forgery confused the issue and a counter-movement argued that compulsory registration and delays by lecturers in signing schedules of attendance put undue pressure on students.[77]

[72] Paget, ed., Memoirs, p. 166.

[73] Rosemary Stevens, Medical Practice in Modern England: The Impact of Specialisation and State Medicine (Harvard, 1966), pp. 20–1.

[74] BMJ ii (1880), p. 853.

[75] Negley Harte, The University of London, 1836–1986 (London, 1986), pp. 93, 105.

[76] BMJ ii (1859), p. 392.

[77] Ibid., i (1874), p. 753; ibid., i (1878), p. 217.

However, these attacks ran against a strong current of opinion which argued that standards of training and conduct could be raised only by ensuring that students attended lectures. How this should be achieved at St Bartholomew's and forgery prevented initially created problems. To promote the 'good order and discipline' of the College, staff were required from 1862 to register 'such gentlemen who shall have regularly attended your lectures and Hospital practice' at the end of each session. An attendance book was started and a careful eye was kept on students to ensure that they did not miss classes.[78] Considerable store was placed on attendance and examination performance, and with the formation of the Discipline committee in 1862 regular checks were made on students, imposing the lecturers' definition of what constituted minimal competency.

That the problem of discipline and performance had re-emerged shows that College Hall was not as effective as hoped. Interest in discipline at St Bartholomew's was not unusual however. Concerned about the image and status of the medical profession, many of the London teaching hospitals were beginning to pay more attention to policing their students. The creation of a Discipline committee at St Bartholomew's was part of this trend.[79] However, where students in the College in the mid-nineteenth century lived up to contemporary claims that medical students were rowdy, the main concern of the committee was with attendance and performance, not moral conduct. It would appear that behaviour could be overlooked provided that students worked hard. In the lecturers' minds there was some overlap: students who failed to attend classes and did badly in examinations were also believed to be dissolute. Initially, the committee was concerned with stamping its authority on the students and with improving standards in anatomy and physiology, but membership was extended in 1880 to include the entire teaching staff.[80] The warden, especially the authoritarian Moore, played a prominent role. With mounting apprehension about the level of 'supposed delinquents' in the College, a 'purge' was made of those considered 'idle or injurious to their fellow students'. After the purge, the committee's attention turned to dealing with idleness and poor attendance.[81] In 1874 it was decided that all those students who did 'not have a fair chance of passing' the qualifying examination should not be entered, and it became policy 'never to allow a student to continue his studies unless he is working'.[82] Monthly audits were

[78] Meeting of the medical officers and lecturers, 10 May 1862, 11 January 1868, MS 12/1.
[79] *RC on a University for London*, p. 73. For a discussion of the work of the Discipline Committee, see Keir Waddington, 'Mayhem and Medical Students: Image, Conduct and Control in the Victorian and Edwardian London Teaching Hospital', *SHM* xv (2002), pp. 45–64.
[80] Discipline committee, 10 November 1880, MS 32/1.
[81] Meeting of the medical officers and lecturers, 18 October 1873, 28 October 1876, 7 December 1878, MS 12/2.
[82] Ibid., 7 February 1874, MS 12/2; *RC on a University for London*, p. 147.

made of the attendance registers: those who 'did not give satisfactory' attendance were disciplined.[83] Parents or guardians were advised when students were not performing well in the hope that pressure would be applied; in serious cases students were suspended or expelled. Most were 'admonished and advised to work', however. Students who confessed to their idleness and 'promised to attend more regularly in future' were typically given 'a fair period of time' to improve with the insistence that the course (or courses) be repeated, committing the student to further time and expense.[84] The financial basis of the College and its need for fees conflicted with the staff's attitudes on attendance and behaviour. Consequently, several warnings were given before pressure was applied. Staff did not intend to be draconian, only to raise standards.

The work of the Discipline committee illustrates how important attendance and examinations came to be for St Bartholomew's by the 1880s, a view shared by many of the London teaching hospitals. During the mid-Victorian period the work of the Discipline committee was at its height. A system of punishments and rewards was created linked to scholarships and tutorials that assumed students did not wish to learn, or at least had to be pressed into doing so. It was a system that had clear parallels with traditional and civic universities: by the 1870s it came under attack from educational reformers who compared it unfavourably with universities in Germany.[85] However, it did produce highly favourable results for St Bartholomew's. No further attempt at reform was made, and the framework of scholarships, examinations, attendance registers and tutorials persisted as the framework of teaching into the twentieth century.

The art of hearing and seeing

Tutors and scholarships could only encourage students to achieve higher standards in the examinations they chose to sit. The Discipline committee was constrained by the same framework. Choice of examinations and licensing body rested with the student, and the College had to respond accordingly. Although the 1815 Apothecaries Act encouraged the develop-ment of a systematic programme of lectures, some of the flexibility that had characterised the free market in training of the late eighteenth century remained. Students at St Bartholomew's in the 1840s could still attend lectures and courses when and as often as they pleased provided they paid, although pressure from the licensing bodies ensured that they were at least

---

[83] Subcommittee, 9 March 1885, MS 34/1.

[84] Discipline committee, 16 October 1895, 22 February 1886, 13 February 1880, MS 32/1.

[85] M. C. Curthoys, 'The Examination System', in *History of the University of Oxford*, ed. Brock and Curthoys, p. 367.

expected to attend certain courses. Most adhered to the minimal time the licensing bodies expected them to study at a London hospital, with between only 5 and 15 per cent spending more than two years at St Bartholomew's. By the 1860s this flexibility had been largely eroded under the influence of the 1858 Medical Act. In 1867, the GMC defined a recommended course of study guided by the traditional pattern of training associated with physicians, and by the system of clinical study that had developed in London.[86] Standardisation gradually replaced the type of training earlier students had chosen voluntarily to meet examination requirements as more subjects were added. Increasingly, students spent three years at a medical school following the curriculum stipulated by the GMC. By the late 1870s four years had become the norm, with the expectation that students would have received a general education before starting to study medicine.[87] For the BMJ, this led to too 'rigid' a system, reflecting fears that the medical curriculum was becoming overcrowded and students overburdened with knowledge, concerns that were to resurface repeatedly in debates about the nature of medical education.[88]

An emphasis on the importance of didactic lectures, formalised and expanded to form a loose curriculum in the 1820s and 1830s, continued to dominate teaching at St Bartholomew's in the mid-nineteenth century. Although clinical lectures and classes were added to the timetable to reflect new ways of looking at disease, the overall structure of teaching remained stable. Only in the 1870s was the number of practical classes increased and greater attention given to the pre-clinical sciences. For much of the mid-nineteenth century, lectures combined with attendance on the wards or in the outpatient departments continued to be the main means through which students received their training. This was linked to practical experience in the post-mortem room, visits to the anatomy museum and limited work in the chemical laboratory. It was a traditional system, attacked by critics. They belittled lectures and complained that most lecturers seldom took 'sufficient care' that the information they piled on their students was understood.[89] These attacks did not dull the importance which medical schools invested in lectures.

Although lectures and observation were considered vital to students, problems existed at St Bartholomew's in ensuring that certain types of lecture were given. Despite the College's reputation for providing opportunities for clinical study, many of the teaching staff remained reluctant to give clinical

[86] Mansell, 'Examinations and Medical Education', p. 89.

[87] Register of students, MS 52; ibid., MS 53/1; Susan C. Lawrence, 'Private Enterprise and Public Interest: Medical Education and the Apothecaries' Act, 1780–1825', in British Medicine, ed. French and Wear, p. 66.

[88] BMJ ii (1862), pp. 365–6.

[89] See William T. Gairdner, On Medicine and Medical Education (Edinburgh, 1858); BMJ ii (1868), pp. 14–16.

lectures. This was particularly clear among the physicians. In 1853, staff had to be reminded 'that the delivery of regular Courses of Clinical Lecturers in the manner required by the several examining boards, and in accordance with their regulations is a necessary part of the instruction to be provided for the students in the Hospital'. Some of the lecturers were outraged, and believed that no one had the right to define the 'duty of the Physicians'.[90] Only gradually did a change in attitude see more clinical lectures introduced, but only a few lecturers could command the full attention of the students. Lectures were regularly interrupted, and a 'subdued disturbance' continued through most which, provided it 'was not too audible', did not 'move the lecturer'.[91] This was hardly surprising: contemporaries felt that 'St Bartholomew's was a school of philosophers' where stately gentlemen lectured in a grand manner 'clothed . . . in choice language' with a 'habit of quoting from the Classics'.[92] It was therefore no surprise that students found Paget's energetic style refreshing and they came out of his 'lectures in great excitement'. Even with Paget's popular lectures, students found most lectures monotonous and would rush to the operating theatre to watch surgeons at work to avoid attending.[93]

Balance was called for between lectures and the operating theatre, post-mortem room, and the ward, but it was in the wards that students were expected to see 'every disease that you will have to treat'. In a repetition of claims familiar to the early nineteenth century, staff continued to advise students that only by watching disease could they learn about treatment.[94] All students 'irrespective of their year or the work upon which they were engaged were earnestly advised to "go round" with one of the surgeons'. Stanley in particular had a large following. He was renowned for his eccentric manner and in some cases would carry out a mini dissection while operating. Overcrowding remained a problem, and such was the press of numbers that surgeons frequently found it difficult to move from bed to bed because the students were packed in so tightly.[95] The haphazard system was replaced in 1864 when all first-year students were divided into four classes. Each class rotated round the surgeons 'so that each Surgeon may be held responsible for seeing after the attendance of the pupils in his wards'. In the following year,

[90] Minutes of the medical officers and lecturers, 9 July 1853, 5 August 1853, 27 September 1853, MS 12/1.

[91] Alfred Willett, 'Our Medical School as I First Knew it', *St Bartholomew's Hospital Journal* (January 1911), p. 53.

[92] Ibid., May 1928, p. 118.

[93] *Lancet* i (1855), p. 228.

[94] Andrew M. McWhinnie, *Introductory Address delivered at St Bartholomew's Hospital on the Opening of the Medical Session, October 1st, 1856* (London, 1856), p. 9; Frederick Farre, *On Self-Culture and the Principles to be Observed in the Study of Medicine* (London, 1849), p. 34.

[95] Alfred Willett, 'The Surgical Side of the Hospital Fifty Years Ago', *St Bartholomew's Hospital Journal* (October 1910), p. 4; Willett, 'Our Medical School', p. 51.

students were appointed as either clerks or dressers to the assistant physicians or surgeons 'whom shall specially instruct in practical details'. Additional clerks were selected to work in the casualty department and post-mortem room. Students were expected to pay for the privilege: free posts were given only to those 'who shall most efficiently discharge' their duties.[96] Part of a phenomenal growth in student hospital posts, the move improved clinical instruction and patient care, and had an important effect in shaping the future careers of successive students.

Students were told to overcome their shyness and ask questions if they did not understand, but were frequently rebuffed by the clinical staff.[97] The viewing of operations was not always possible and many of the lecturers remained aloof. Students regularly complained that staff had to be pressed into making remarks, and they were rarely asked for a diagnosis or treatment.[98] Savory limited his bedside teaching to a few questions or instructions and was irritated by the need to teach basic principles. William Church, lecturer in comparative anatomy, was better at professional administration than teaching. At the bedside he was uncommunicative and tended to overawe students with his brusque manner.[99] Others were as remote, and some liked to trick their students. On the medical side in the 1850s, the *Lancet* believed that only George Burrows, the lecturer in medicine, 'really rendered students . . . sound, enlightened and useful practitioners'.[100] Staff could prove difficult and awe-inspiring. Their mannerisms and interest in private practice created obstacles to practical learning that reduced the effectiveness of teaching. However, this appeared to do the College little harm.

The introduction of surgical consultations in 1868 (on Paget's advice) marked a change in teaching style. The idea was to stimulate learning and direct treatment. They were first held on Thursday afternoons in the wards but due to their popularity and the impossibility of students hearing and seeing everything presented, patients were seen in the operating theatre. This also allowed for a more systematic examination. Consultations covered not only rare cases but also 'what may be called everyday cases, which . . . present especially well-marked or typical signs and symptoms'. William Walsham, the demonstrator of comparative anatomy, believed that through these consultations the student enjoyed 'the advantage of hearing what may be said from various points of view, and is able to enter into and appreciate the

---

[96] Minutes of the medical officers and lecturers, 3 December 1864, 17 December 1864, MS 12/1.

[97] Farre, *On Self-Culture*, p. 32.

[98] *BMJ* ii (1869), p. 404.

[99] *St Bartholomew's Hospital Journal*, June 1928, p. 132.

[100] *Lancet* ii (1854), p. 362.

difficulties that the diagnosis or treatment may present'. This concealed the often violent controversies that erupted.[101]

It is difficult to determine how 'modern' clinical teaching was at St Bartholomew's in the mid-nineteenth century. Considerable differences existed between lecturers in a period when new tools, symbolised by the stethoscope and microscope, were placed at the doctor's disposal. Faith in pathological anatomy strengthened the emphasis given to physical diagnosis, yet this did not mean that tensions over the accuracy or need for new methods were reduced. Greater emphasis was given to physical examination over the patient's interpretation, but although more up-to-date practitioners embraced new medical technology as diagnostic aids, those teaching in London's hospitals were not always quick to embrace change. With the royal colleges forming what one contemporary described in 1851 as the 'rear-guard of the medical body', this was not always a problem.[102] Students at St Bartholomew's were taught the epistemological importance of physical examination, but many of the lecturers continued to stress methods of seeing and touching that had emerged in the late eighteenth and early nineteenth centuries. What might be labelled scientific or technical methods of visualising disease were only slowly incorporated.

The approach favoured by the lecturers at St Bartholomew's seemed to suit the large number of students who increasingly chose to study at the College. The hospital acquired a reputation for conservatism and later for empiricism, but for many students this was more than counterbalanced by the fact that St Bartholomew's was able to offer opportunities that outstripped many of its rivals. The hospital could boast 710 beds in 1878, all of which were available for clinical teaching. The situation was very different at other London medical schools: the London had 800 beds but only thirty were for clinical instruction; Guy's had 695 and forty for clinical teaching.[103] In this respect, it did not always matter that teaching at St Bartholomew's was not the most 'modern' available, especially as this could be rectified by a period of study in France or (increasingly) in Germany.

Changes were made to the type of medicine taught at St Bartholomew's, but these often occurred gradually. Growing interest in the finer structure of the body saw doctors looking more closely at tissues and cells. The microscope became a vehicle through which this finer anatomical knowledge was constructed, producing an expanding body of work on histology, embryology and morbid anatomy, and helping doctors to visualise healthy and diseased tissue in a new way. However, in the 1830s and 1840s, despite technical improvements, few students had any 'personal experience in the

---

[101] William Walsham, 'Our Surgical Consultations', *St Bartholomew's Hospital Report* xxiv (1888), pp. 273–4.
[102] *Provincial Medical and Surgical Journal* (1851), p. 139.
[103] *BMJ* ii (1878), pp. 707–14.

use of a microscope or other laboratory instrument'.[104] At St Bartholomew's, Savory hoped to inspire students with 'microscopic and other illustrations' in his lectures, while the Lloyd Prize was established in 1850 to encourage the use of microscopes. Such examples had little immediate impact on the students when a number of influential staff remained hostile to microscopes. Although scepticism over microscopic work had lessened by the 1840s, their views were coloured by early nineteenth-century suspicions about their use and accuracy. For example, Frederick Skey as lecturer in surgical anatomy told students that microscopes offered 'no support to the judgement of the surgeon' and that any knowledge gained through them 'is too often delusive'.[105] Students did not borrow popular texts on the use of microscopes from the library, and although a small number owed their own microscopes, 'fewer still . . . kept them after qualifying'.[106] Attitudes did begin to change in the mid-1860s in recognition of the growing contribution the microscope was beginning to make to clinical medicine through the work of such men as Virchow and Cohnheim. The BMJ started to counsel students that a 'cheap, usable microscope' was an essential tool for study, and in 1864 it was decided to appoint a demonstrator in microscopy at St Bartholomew's to take account of this, eleven years after the first class was started in London. However, it was not until 1866 that a suitable candidate was found to fill the post. It took a further ten years for the College to provide students with microscopes.[107]

The growing use of the microscope in the College marked the first move towards a pedagogical shift in the nature of medical education through the laboratory. In the 1830s and 1840s more doctors were emphasising the importance of approaching disease through a laboratory investigation of the body's fluids. Chemistry grew in importance for the study of disease and the College used the services of a number of leading chemists, including William Thomas Brande and Edward Frankland to teach students. However, despite the importance given to theoretical and organic chemistry in lectures, and the role of chemistry secured in physiology, most of the practical laboratory work was limited. Frankland believed that most chemical laboratories in England were 'adapted for beginners rather than for serious study' and the laboratory at St Bartholomew's was no different.[108] Work was confined to examinations of urine and little effort was made to examine blood or train students in how to do this until the late 1880s, despite growing interest.[109]

---

[104] Thomas N. Bonner, *Becoming a Physician: Medical Education in Great Britain, France, Germany and the United States, 1750–1945* (New York, 1995), p. 231.

[105] Frederick Carpenter Skey, *The Principles and Practice of Operative Surgery* (London, 1858), p. 494.

[106] Library borrowers, DF 141; W. F. Bynum, *Science and the Practice of Medicine in the Nineteenth Century* (Cambridge, 1994), p. 123.

[107] Minutes of the medical officers and lecturers, 3 December 1864, 24 March 1866, MS 12/1; ibid., 28 October 1876, MS 12/2.

[108] *Nature* iii (1871), p. 445.

[109] Stanley J. Reiser, *Medicine and the Reign of Technology* (Cambridge, 1990), pp. 127–35.

For much of the period, although valuable work was undertaken on clinical medicine and surgery with new procedures devised and refined, St Bartholomew's never saw itself as an institution committed to expanding medical knowledge. Doctors throughout London were sceptical of the value of new clinical instruments and their application, seeing them as a 'potential threat to the mysterious clinical art' which English clinicians were so anxious to defend. Staff at St Bartholomew's were part of this patrician class and were uneasy about using new technology or adopting new methods of physical examination to achieve a diagnosis.[110] Like many institutions, St Bartholomew's was far from monolithic, but an environment existed whereby an empirical view of medicine, strong in clinical teaching and upheld by a faith in localised pathology, was able to dominate. Teaching in the College therefore remained conservative, based on visible symptoms, oral histories and the experiences of the post-mortem room. Response to changes in medical knowledge and practices were slow. St Bartholomew's defined itself by a largely empirical approach: a stance that found favour with a body of practitioners who increasingly worried about the impact of science and the laboratory on medicine. The attitudes of the teaching staff reflected tensions in medicine over the introduction of new methods of seeing and quantifying illness. By the 1880s, would-be reformers could characterise such an approach as anachronistic, one that ignored the importance of science to medicine. However, the faith placed in the bedside and a view of medicine as an art was not easily eroded.

'Popular prejudice for specialists'

Teaching could not remain entirely static and in the mid-nineteenth century the College was forced to take account of the impact of specialisation on medicine. Specialisation was not new to the nineteenth century, but it was during Victoria's reign that specialisation seemed to come of age, marking a period of conceptual growth rather than a revolution in medical science. Historians have endeavoured to see its development as an example of professionalisation, as Roger Cooter notes, to 'account for a division of spoils within the existing medical system, or to show, retrospectively how the cake got cut'.[111] Specialist fields had emerged in the sixteenth century and had developed in areas at first outside orthodox practice. By the start of the nineteenth century specialisation had spread beyond these confines, attracting the attention of regular practitioners. Elite practitioners and the

---

[110] Christopher Lawrence, 'Incommunicable Knowledge: Science, Technology and Clinical Art in Britain 1850–1914', *Journal of Contemporary History* xx (1985), pp. 514–17.
[111] Roger Cooter, *Surgery and Society in Peace and War: Orthopaedics and the Organisation of Modern Medicine, 1880–1948* (Basingstoke, 1993), p. 2.

medical press, 'who valued generalism as a gentlemanly ideal', initially regarded specialists as little more than quacks. 'Through public censure, social pressure, and ostracism, the old guard of the profession tried to contain the growth of specialisation.'[112] Such attacks may be seen as part of a shift from the professional instability of the early nineteenth century to the intra-professional hostility of the mid-Victorian period, encouraged by fears of competition and associations with commercial activity that threatened the desired status of medicine. At first outnumbered by generalists, specialists vigorously rejected the association with quackery and sought to carve out a professional domain. In this, they were supported by a public who became enthusiastic supporters of specialist institutions, encouraging their growth. A shift in the medical gaze from the body to individual organs as the locus of disease provided some legitimacy for a subdivision of practice, and the invention of new diagnostic tools such as the ophthalmoscope provided a focus. Lindsay Granshaw has shown that there were also clear professional advantages in founding a specialist hospital. They gave outsiders a vehicle for advancement and played a key role in transforming the status of the medical specialist, so that by 1914 'specialists were among the leaders in the profession'.[113]

However, it was a troubled transformation. Throughout the mid-nineteenth century the medical press ran a series of campaigns attacking specialists and their hospitals. Economic and intellectual arguments were put forward against specialists, who were seen as damaging to general hospitals and to general practice. The only acceptable specialist institutions were those that treated patients normally excluded from general hospitals: the epileptic, the consumptive, the feverish or the insane. Hospitals for children gained approval, 'since due attention to the wants of the little sufferers necessitates modifications in the usual hospital arrangement'. Paediatrics could also be construed as general medicine on the young.[114] Others specialist hospitals were seen as a nuisance to the public. Specialists were accused of stealing patients and fees from general practitioners. In an environment where the generalist was supreme, specialisation was shown to narrow the mind and lead 'doctors to diagnose their favourite condition in every patient'.[115] This was dangerous in a climate where it was commonly believed that 'diseases generally are so connected with each other, and a knowledge of one is so

[112] M. Jeanne Peterson, *The Medical Profession in Mid-Victorian London* (Berkeley, 1978), p. 277.
[113] George Rosen, *The Specialisation of Medicine with Particular Reference to Ophthalmology* (New York, 1944); Lindsay Granshaw, '"Fame and fortune by means of bricks and mortar": The Medical Profession and Specialist Hospitals in Britain, 1800–1948', in *The Hospital in History*, ed. Lindsay Granshaw and Roy Porter (London, 1989), pp. 199–220.
[114] *Lancet* i (1867), p. 279.
[115] Ibid., i (1857), p. 650.

necessary to the right understanding of another'.[116] Specialists were attacked by those who saw them as essentially damaging to the profession, to medicine and to the public, but when specialist services were confined within London's general hospitals they proved less controversial.

The growth of specialist institutions raised concerns for medical education. Lecturers worried that specialisation would sway students towards becoming 'narrow-minded' and prevent them from looking at the whole patient. At a more fundamental level, it was feared that by encouraging the public to believe that 'particular classes of disease can be more successfully treated' in specialist hospitals, they attracted interesting cases away from medical schools, robbing students 'of that range of study which is necessary' for instruction.[117] For London's teaching hospitals, this threatened their basis of clinical training. To make matters worse, several specialist hospitals started to offer lectures and invited students to visit their wards. The introduction of a competing or contrary voice in training was feared as specialist hospitals posed the possibility of 'an alternative authority in knowledge of disease, treatment and medical science'.[118] The implication was that students would travel to specialist hospitals to hear lectures on cases no longer being admitted to general hospitals, so undermining the status and income of the London medical schools. To remove the threat, teaching hospitals established specialist services. These had more to do with teaching than with the pursuit of a concept of efficiency, professional interests or patient needs, as claimed by Sturdy and Cooter.[119] The demand of medical education therefore became the vehicle through which specialist services were introduced into teaching hospitals.

Despite attacks on specialisation, many of those working in general hospitals had already established links with specialist institutions. Ambitious young doctors began to seek temporary positions in specialist hospitals and returned this knowledge to teaching hospitals.[120] This facilitated the creation of special departments in teaching hospitals. The model used by the founders of the early specialist hospitals was adopted: services were initially started as outpatient departments before being institutionalised in wards. Those appointed to run them were seen as generalists with a special interest, rather than as specialists. According to Peterson, this allowed the maintenance of the 'supremacy' of general medicine and surgery, while incorporating

---

[116] Cited in Peterson, *Medical Profession*, pp. 273–4.

[117] Ibid., p. 275; *Lancet* i (1863), p. 183.

[118] Peterson, *Medical Profession*, p. 276.

[119] Steve Sturdy and Roger Cooter, 'Science, Scientific Management, and the Transformation of Medicine in Britain, c.1870–1950', *History of Science* xxiv (1998), pp. 427–8.

[120] Lindsay Granshaw, 'The Rise of the Modern Hospital in Britain', in *Medicine and Society*, ed. Wear, p. 207.

specialties into teaching, forcing a reworking of the rhetoric of generalism so that it came reluctantly to stress the need to integrate specialist services within a single, hierarchical system of care.[121] However, moves to create special wards remained problematic. Only gradually did attitudes begin to change as support grew for a compartmentalisation of outpatient departments. General medicine and surgery still dominated, but by the mid-1870s a role could be seen for specialist teaching departments as remedying the 'glaring defects of general hospitals'.[122]

At St Bartholomew's the development of specialisation was driven by teaching, illustrating the extent to which the College was able to shape clinical services. In the mid-nineteenth century, specialisation was still largely unknown at St Bartholomew's. Even progressive teachers like Peter Mere Latham worried that specialisation 'narrow[ed]' views of medicine so that holistic views dominated.[123] What might be labelled specialist practice was undertaken in the general wards as part of the normal running of the hospital, although a ward was reserved for the treatment of venereal disease. Children, for example, were admitted to the medical and surgical wards, as were cases of fever (except smallpox). Staff working in emerging specialist fields largely kept their interests outside the hospital. Holmes Coote, for example, worked at the Royal Orthopaedic Hospital, where he was assistant surgeon, but remained a generalist at St Bartholomew's where he dismissed specialisation as a 'grave error'.[124] Wormald was also curious about orthopaedics through his work at the Foundling Hospital. Although he demonstrated 'doubtful case[s]' to students, most of his teaching at St Bartholomew's was confined to anatomy. Lawrence adopted a similar stance. He was an authoritative figure in the early development of ophthalmology and defended eye hospitals because they remedied 'a deficiency in the existing source of professional instruction'. However, at St Bartholomew's he made no attempt to press for an ophthalmic department. Lawrence argued that medicine could be advanced only by men 'of extensive anatomical knowledge, and of great insight into disease' and adopted the same approach in his teaching.[125] His colleagues in the College tended to agree and put forward a unified, generalist model of medicine.

Just as the development of eye hospitals led to the growth of specialist hospitals, ophthalmic wards pioneered the growth of specialist departments

---

[121] Peterson, *Medical Profession*, p. 277.

[122] *Lancet* i (1867), pp. 571–2; ibid., i (1876), pp. 930–1.

[123] Peter Mere Latham, *Lectures on Subjects Connected with Clinical Medicine comprising Diseases of the Heart* (London, 1846), p. 7.

[124] Holmes Coote, *On Joint Diseases; their Pathology, Diagnosis and Treatment Including the Nature and Treatment of Deformities, and Curvatures of the Spine* (London, 1867), p. ix.

[125] *Memoir of Howard Marsh*, p. 25; William Lawrence, *A Treatise on the Diseases of the Eye* (London, 1844), pp. 2–4, 6.

in London's teaching hospitals.[126] Ophthalmology had been transformed in the first half of the nineteenth century through an epidemic of Egyptian ophthalmia from a field ridiculed for quackery to one of the most successful specialties. Existing on neutral ground between physic and surgery, the subject was 'reinvented' and given legitimacy and respectability.[127] Patients flocked to the new eye hospitals and the eye came to be understood as the 'quintessential organ, both in its health and morbid states'.[128] In adopting a framework that appealed to generalists and with links established with venereal disease, by the 1850s doctors saw it as vital to train students in ophthalmology.

While other London hospitals had established eye departments in the 1850s with the growing popularity of the ophthalmoscope and the greater prospect of treatment, the proximity of Moorfields to St Bartholomew's, and Lawrence's links with the former, kept the number of eye cases admitted to the hospital to a minimum and delayed development. Lawrence's death in 1867 saw a shift occur. With ophthalmic departments already open in seven general hospitals, it was decided to appoint a 'demonstrator of diseases of the eye'.[129] The new demonstrator was expected to teach the 'practical use of the ophthalmoscope' and bring together the treatment of all ophthalmic cases in a department to aid teaching. For the first time, the College was seeking to appoint 'a person of acknowledged standing and eminence' in a specialist field.[130] The appointment of a demonstrator prompted little immediate improvement, however. Beds were not forthcoming and the College was accused of training students who knew dangerously little about 'eye diseases'.[131] Pressure was applied on the governors to establish an eye department, but calls went unheeded until the issue was taken up by the press. Tensions were already running high after a series of disagreements between the governors and doctors over the running of the casualty department. In response to the press's attacks, the governors admitted that they had ignored the lecturers' requests and in 1869 agreed to open an ophthalmic ward. Changes were made to the manning of the casualty department to reduce overcrowding. This was not enough for the *Lancet*. It

---

[126] Richard Kershaw, *Special Hospitals: Their Origin, Development and Relationship to Medical Education; Their Economic Aspects and Relative Freedom from Abuse* (London, 1909), pp. 62–4.

[127] Luke Davidson, '"Identities Ascertained": British Ophthalmology in the First Half of the Nineteenth Century', *SHM* ix (1996), pp. 313–33.

[128] Lawrence, *Diseases of the Eye*, pp. 1–2.

[129] Brian Abel-Smith, *The Hospitals, 1800–1948: A Study in Social Administration in England and Wales* (London, 1964), p. 24.

[130] Henry Power, 'Report of the Ophthalmic Department', *St Bartholomew's Hospital Reports* vii (1871), pp. 19–23; Minutes of the medical officers and lecturers, 9 February 1867, MS 12/1.

[131] *Lancet* i (1869), p. 884.

saw the events as another example of poor hospital management and the rift that existed between lay governors and doctors, rounding on the hospital's administration as corrupt and extravagant.[132]

Moves to improve ophthalmology occurred against a background of efforts in the College to stimulate interest in other specialist subjects that could be shown to have an application to general practice. St Bartholomew's lagged behind many of its contemporaries in the provision of specialist clinics. In an effort to improve clinical teaching, it was decided in 1864 that the 'Assistant Officers of the Hospital' should instruct 'the pupils in certain Medical and Surgical subjects'. Emphasis was placed on orthopaedics and diseases of the skin, ear, nose and throat. These were areas that could be safely combined with general medicine or surgery and had seen clinics established at other hospitals.[133]

Hospital surgeons in the 1860s had started to incorporate orthopaedic surgery via conservative surgery and subcutaneous osteotomy – a technique for cutting and dividing bones without exposing tissue to infection – into their work. Here the emphasis was on the treatment of acquired and inherited skeletal deformities, bolstered by concerns about 'crippled' children. These practices were encouraged at St Bartholomew's by George Callender and Skey. Other staff were also developing an interest in orthopaedics, merging it with a holistic orientation that saw orthopaedics as part of paediatrics and general surgery. This interest, and the large number of accident cases admitted, provided a framework in which orthopaedics could develop in the hospital, giving it a legitimacy that matched growing interest in the field of general surgery.[134] Similar generalist claims were made for dermatology, a flourishing field for private practice, with the first special skin hospital founded in 1863. In the same year a hospital for diseases of the throat had been formed. It gained rapidly in popularity, while the development of the laryngoscope six years before had forced a new way of looking at the throat and nose. Opinions were divided over its benefits, but as the use of the laryngoscope required skilled instruction there was a clear need for training.[135] Students were encouraged to attend such institutions to learn new procedures and ways of looking at disease, challenging the monopoly of the London hospitals in defining illness and lesions. Staff at St Bartholomew's felt threatened by these developments. Efforts were therefore made to attract patients 'suffering from such complaints as Out-Patients', but 'practical instruction' was at first restricted to a 'member of the Medical and Surgical Staff'.[136]

---

[132] BMJ ii (1869), p. 563; Lancet ii (1969), p. 615; ibid., 1 (1870), p. 50.

[133] Minutes of the medical officers and lecturers, 17 December 1864, MS 12/1.

[134] For the rise of orthopaedics see Cooter, Surgery and Society, pp. 14–23.

[135] Peterson, Medical Profession, pp. 261, 266–9; Reiser, Medicine and the Reign of Technology, pp. 52–3.

[136] Minutes of the medical officers and lecturers, 17 December 1864, 9 February 1867, MS 12/1.

New clinical demonstratorships limited to outpatient teaching followed in 1867, spurred on by the resolution made over ophthalmology teaching. These were selected from the registrars and assistant surgeons when it became clear that the existing arrangements were insufficient for the 'good repute and efficient maintenance of the teaching'.[137] In the first wave, James Andrew and the quiet Reginald Southey were appointed to give clinical lectures on diseases of the skin, the first in London. Alfred Willett was placed in charge of orthopaedic teaching, while Thomas Smith was made clinical lecturer on diseases of the ear. In creating these posts, St Bartholomew's quickly gained a leading position in the provision of specialist services, a position that contrasted with its previous lack of specialist care.[138] Specialist outpatient clinics under the control of the new clinical demonstrators were formed, developing specialist care without threatening the generalists' control of beds. However, none of those initially appointed showed a particular interest in the disease they were expected to teach. Southey had studied tuberculosis and kidney disease, having developed an enthusiasm for microscopy after becoming convinced by Virchow's approach.[139] Andrew was working on diseases of the heart; both held appointments at the City of London Hospital for Diseases of the Chest.[140] Neither was particularly committed to diseases of the skin. The same was true of the other post holders. In was only in the late 1870s that doctors started to be appointed who also worked in the field which they were supposed to teach.[141] Despite this, the new specialist teaching clinics became a proving ground for young doctors whose work was otherwise constricted by their lack of control over beds. Positions in the specialist departments allowed them to establish reputations as teachers and practitioners before they moved back into general teaching posts.

Even with the creation of specialist clinical lecturers and outpatient clinics, opposition to specialisation remained. The attitude was summed up by Samuel Gee. Although Gee was appointed demonstrator of diseases of the

[137] Ibid.

[138] Stevens, *Medical Practice*, pp. 28–9.

[139] Reginald Southey, *The Nature and Affinities of Tubercle* (London, 1867).

[140] 'Minute Structure of Human Kidney', *St Bartholomew's Hospital Reports* i (1865), pp. 164–8; James Andrew, 'On the Diagnosis of Systolic Endocardial Murmurs', ibid., i (1865).

[141] These included Henry Butlin, appointed demonstrator of diseases of the larynx in 1880, who worked on cancer of the throat, and Howard Marsh, who started to give clinical lectures on orthopaedics in 1878. Marsh was surgeon to the Hospital for Children with Chronic Diseases of the Joints and, before being appointed to lecture on orthopaedics, had already published on diseases of the joints: see *St Bartholomew's Hospital Reports* ii (1866), pp. 147–55; ibid., xi (1875), pp. 113–25. Marsh was to become an authority on orthopaedics and his *Diseases of the Joints* (London, 1886) became a key text. However, Marsh spent only three years as demonstrator of orthopaedics before devoting his energy to surgical anatomy teaching.

skin in 1869, he believed that 'the name of a specialist' was one that deserved derision.[142] Formal recognition by the licensing bodies of the need to train students in specialist fields was slow to be secured. Without this pressure, the College was less inclined to make further changes. After the drive to create specialist clinical lectureships between 1867 and 1876, the position of the specialist departments remained precarious. Most patients admitted from the outpatient departments continued to be handed over to generalists. Instruction in orthopaedics, diseases of the skin, ear and throat were limited to demonstrations, and although formal lectures were started in ophthalmology in 1870 and dental anatomy in 1871, problems were encountered. Specialist teaching remained on the fringe. William Harmer, a student at St Bartholomew's in the 1890s, remembered that most of the staff were entirely satisfied that they were 'quite capable of dealing with almost any speciality or operation'. The idea of specialist departments was greeted with little enthusiasm after their initial establishment, and medical education at St Bartholomew's was firmly rooted in the 'great triumvirate of Medicine, Surgery and Midwifery'.[143]

Pressure to rebuild

The 1870s and 1880s saw a number of rebuilding projects in London's teaching hospitals that ran in parallel with the building mania which appeared to be engulfing voluntary hospitals. Faced with intense competition, rising student numbers and changes in the structure of medicine, medical schools were under constant pressure to adapt. The need for practical scientific instruction placed new demands on medical schools and required a rethinking of their internal space.

Improvements had been made at St Bartholomew's throughout the 1870s to cope with the increase in student numbers, which rendered existing accommodation insufficient. The dissection room had been temporarily converted for use as a chemistry laboratory each summer when no dissections occurred. In 1865 it was decided to build a new chemical classroom, and in 1870 a new chemical laboratory was opened, including a lecture theatre and preparation room on the site of the old apothecary's shop. However, anxiety over space increased. The lecturers pressed the hospital for more room, only to be told that the governors could not '[appropriate] to the purpose of the School any additional part of the Hospital buildings'.[144] Doubts about the

[142] Cited in Norman Moore, *The History of St Bartholomew's Hospital*, 2 vols (London, 1918), Vol. 2, p. 733.
[143] *St Bartholomew's Hospital Journal*, December 1962, p. 289.
[144] Minutes of the medical officers and lecturers, 22 July 1871, MS 12/2; Medical council, 11 January 1873, MC 1/1.

suitability of the College's accommodation intensified. By 1876 the number of students had reached 436 and accommodation was at crisis point.

The problem of accommodation was highlighted by Sydney Waterlow, treasurer of the hospital. A major city philanthropist with an interest in education, he had been approached by Savory and Andrew with the idea of rebuilding. When appointed Lord Mayor in 1873, he had pressed the City Livery Companies to increase their support for education and applied this interest in education to St Bartholomew's where he was appointed treasurer in the same year.[145] Having listened to Savory and Andrew, Waterlow worried that as many of the existing College buildings were over fifty years old most were outdated or too small. Temporary additional accommodation was suggested and consideration was given to the possibility of rebuilding.[146] Edward l'Anson, the hospital surveyor, was asked to investigate. His preliminary findings pointed to the need for rebuilding. Using this evidence, Waterlow persuaded the governors 'to provide the best possible accommodation for the pupils attending the lectures and demonstrations'.[147] Convinced that rebuilding would benefit the hospital because an increase in student numbers would add to the 'advancement and diffusion of medical and sanitary knowledge', the governors offered to meet the cost.[148]

The new block aimed to double existing accommodation. The hospital provided the funding and Waterlow became closely involved in the planning. L'Anson was commissioned to prepare plans which Waterlow felt should be modelled on Owen's College in Manchester. He had been particularly struck by the teaching facilities there, and Alfred Waterhouse, the aspiring architect behind Manchester Town Hall later responsible for the Natural History Museum, was consulted largely because, like Manchester, the site at St Bartholomew's was constricted. Trained as an architect and surveyor in the family practice, l'Anson had designed the Royal Exchange Buildings in the 1840s, winning repute and contributing to consolidation of his father's City practice. Waterhouse believed that 'whilst he kept in touch with the artistic side of his profession, he was distinguished for his skill and varied practice', and became a leading architect in the design of City office buildings.[149] At St Bartholomew's, building was extended into Giltspur Street and West Smithfield to produce a larger museum and library. It was the first major work to match Gibbs' rebuilding of the hospital in the eighteenth century in terms of scale and ambition. To make more room for the new buildings, the main carriage entrance of the hospital was moved from

[145] Sean Glynn, 'The City of London and Higher Education', in *London Higher*, ed. Roderick Floud and Sean Glynn (London, 1998), pp. 130, 132–3.
[146] House committee, 14 November 1876, HA 1/24.
[147] Ibid., 8 May 1877, HA 1/24; *College Calendar* (1878/9), p. 89.
[148] Order of the Charity Commission, 1877, MS 6/1.
[149] *Chartered Surveyors Weekly* ix (1984), p. 815.

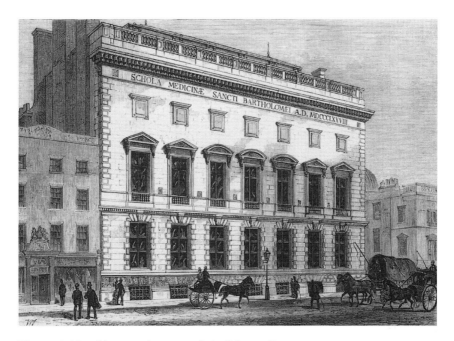

Plate 3.2 New library and museum from Giltspur Street

Giltspur Street to the Henry VIII Gate, and teaching was rearranged until the new accommodation was completed. This allowed the College to continue to function, gradually moving into the new buildings as they were completed.[150]

The opening of the library, museum and physiology workroom in 1879 was seen as 'the first instalment of still larger and more important buildings'. L'Anson's Italianate design was considered admirable. Harmonious with Gibbs' hospital buildings and borrowing some of their elements, the space was both functional and modern. The *Builder* saw the new building as having 'all the vigour, simplicity and refinement of the best Italian work'.[151] The *Lancet* considered it 'beautiful' and believed that once the entire project was completed 'the arrangements for teaching will probably be unsurpassed'.[152] By 1881 the College was in 'thorough working order'. For the *Citizen*, the new buildings embodied the greatness of the College in stone, even if the lecture theatres were felt to be too steep for practical use. Throughout, the 'abundance of space, ventilation, and convenience for students . . . are everywhere perceptible'.[153]

---

[150] Building committee, 20 October 1879, MS 14/3.
[151] *Builder*, 4 February 1888, p. 78.
[152] *Lancet* ii (1879), p. 701.
[153] *Citizen*, 28 May 1881.

Largest school in London

In 1886, there were 439 new entrants to medicine registered in England. Seventy-seven were at St Bartholomew's, making it the largest medical school in the capital and the fourth largest in Britain. Contemporaries believed that this could be explained by the small size of University College Hospital, which restricted student numbers, and by a recent nursing dispute at Guy's which had damaged the hospital's standing.[154] No attempt was made to explain the College's size in terms of facilities or reputation. Few other teaching hospitals could compete with the incentives to study provided by the scholarships offered at St Bartholomew's. Nor could they offer the same facilities for teaching or residential accommodation, despite the extensive programme of rebuilding initiated by most medical schools in the 1870s and 1880s. College Hall, tutors, examinations and a Discipline committee did not make St Bartholomew's an Oxford or Cambridge in London, but they did associate the College with a style of education that counterbalanced the perceived 'dangers' of its metropolitan location. The College's reputation seemed secure by the late 1870s. Joseph Lister, surgeon and pioneer of antisepsis, believed that St Bartholomew's was the leading medical school in London, unlike 'poor King's' where he had moved to from Edinburgh.[155] The *BMJ* came to a similar conclusion: St Bartholomew's approached 'most nearly to a satisfactory type of good teaching and adequate facilities and resources for general study'. The journal felt that 'the excellent organisation of the school, the large material in the hospital, and the *prestige* of some great names' more than justified the large number of students who flocked to St Bartholomew's for their medical training.[156]

Between 1842 and 1881, St Bartholomew's had succeeded in rejuvenating its teaching and its status. The College's position as the largest and most successful in London gave staff a certain self-confidence, but fears of competition lurked beneath the surface. Mid-Victorian reforms had established a structure of medical education that was to prove lasting, encouraging a faith in scholarships, an academic approach and support for the idea of a university of London. Yet, in the rapidly changing environment of medicine and medical education, the College could not afford to stand still for long. New buildings and the creation of specialist clinics proved insufficient to meet the demands placed on teaching by the increasing emphasis given to the experimental sciences and laboratory medicine from

---

[154] Edinburgh with 280 students, Glasgow with 137 and Cambridge with 90 were the three largest medical schools: Walter Rivington, *The Medical Profession* (Dublin, 1888), pp. 677–8. For the nursing dispute at Guy's, see Keir Waddington, 'The Nursing Dispute at Guy's Hospital', *Social History of Medicine* viii (1995), pp. 211–30.

[155] James Matthews Duncan, *Miscellaneous Letters*, p. 35.

[156] *BMJ* ii (1879), p. 703.

the 1880s onwards. Once more, the College began to fall behind. St Bartholomew's remained confident and even arrogant in its approach, believing its methods were best, but throughout the 1880s and 1890s it could not escape from the fact that the nature of medicine and medical education was changing. By 1900 the lecturers were embracing a more scientific and academic approach. Where the mid-nineteenth century had seen a process of internal reform and rejuvenation, the late nineteenth century saw the start of a trend that brought more science into teaching.

Part II

Science and learning 1880–1939

4

Scientific beginnings

The opening of the new College buildings between 1879 and 1881 was an acknowledgement that the College had outgrown the institutional environment bequeathed by Abernethy in the 1820s. St Bartholomew's had firmly established itself as the largest medical school in London; an important part of the elite teaching hospital system that reaffirmed professional divisions and contributed to medicine's professional identity. Under the influence of James Paget, emphasis had been placed on academic performance and discipline through the development of a collegiate and tutorial structure. This encouraged a sense of complacency, so that by 1900 the system of rewards and punishments established in the mid-Victorian period had been relaxed.

A series of attacks between 1820 and 1870 had labelled the College as conservative, a defender of the status quo. There remained some truth to these accusations. It was only from the 1890s onwards that the empirical traditions which dominated St Bartholomew's were challenged. Between 1880 and 1900, staff reacted to a shift in attitudes on the content of medical education taking place at an intellectual and practical level against a background of mounting debate on the role of science in education. It was during this period that 'laboratories and experimental disciplines were becoming central, at least in the ideology of science'.[1] The emergence at Cambridge of research schools in physics and physiology furthered this movement, and a series of royal commissions on technical education highlighted the importance of science to vocational training. Medicine tentatively allied itself with these changes as new ways of looking at disease through the laboratory gained ground. However, if doctors recognised that science and experimentation had always played an important role in medicine, it was the type of science that created problems, first through experimental physiology and then through the laboratory sciences. Alterations were made to the curriculum to reflect the 'spread of science' the public was believed to demand from practitioners.[2] Specialisation and the integration of new medical disciplines and technology required new subjects and techniques to be taught. The greater emphasis placed on science by the examining bodies, and an expansion in the number of subjects covered,

---

[1] John Pickstone, 'Ways of Knowing: Towards a Historical Sociology of Science, Technology and Medicine', *British Journal for the History of Science* xxvi (1993), p. 450.
[2] *St Bartholomew's Hospital Journal*, November 1893, p. 18.

meant that a larger number of students spent between four and five years studying. The General Medical Council (GMC) recognised this change in 1892 when it set the minimal period of study to five years to give greater breadth to science. Change was uneven. Pre-clinical teaching was able to integrate a laboratory-based approach faster than the clinical sciences, where an empirical tradition continued to dominate. Differences also existed between London and the provinces, with the latter quicker to respond to the shift in ideas about medicine and medical education.

St Bartholomew's gradually tempered its empirical stance as experimental and laboratory science was seen as increasingly important to a doctor's training. As such, it was teaching rather than a concern for managerial efficiency or public health that shaped the development of science and laboratory accommodation.[3] Like specialisation, the laboratory was brought into the hospital on educational grounds. The benefits accruing to patients were seen as secondary until the 1890s when the College changed tack, stressing the laboratory's utility to patient care to secure funding from the governors.

The growing acceptance of a limited definition of science in medical education saw the emergence of a more 'modern' style of training. It forced the development of a new type of teaching space – the teaching laboratory – which provided a new discipline and mode of instruction. Apprenticeship had been marginalised by the 1850s in favour of hospital-based study as the practice came under attack, although it was not until 1892 that apprenticeship was finally abolished by the GMC. While support was expressed for a period of study under a general practitioner to expose students to the realities of general practice, only those on the periphery seriously recommended a return to an apprenticeship system.[4] Further changes had become apparent. In theory the fee system, where students paid for the classes they wanted to attend, still allowed a flexible, DIY training. However, under the influence of the GMC a more homogeneous pattern emerged, despite mid-century claims that uniformity would be impossible or detrimental. As the GMC devoted 'most of its active energies to reforming medical education', it exerted a considerable influence on what was taught. By the 1890s, the courses offered by the eleven London schools were the same in principle, differing only in minor details.[5] The trend towards homogenisation saw a decline in the number of students moving between schools.

[3] This contrasts with the view outlined by Roger Cooter and Steve Sturdy in 'Science, Scientific Management, and the Transformation of Medicine in Britain, c.1870–1950' (*History of Science* xxxvi (1998), pp. 421–66), who argued that laboratories first became closely involved in medicine in the sphere of public health.
[4] See James Grey Glover, *The Gaps in Medical Education: Considered in the Light of the Reports of the Inspectors and Examinations of the Medical Council* (London, 1889), pp. 19–20.
[5] Anne Digby, *The Evolution of British General Practice, 1850–1948* (Oxford, 1999), p. 39.

Increasingly they came to spend most of their time studying at one institution, a tendency that promoted greater allegiance to individual institutions.

The 1880s and 1890s proved an important period for medical education. Growing emphasis was placed on the value of the experimental sciences, the period of study was lengthened, and divisions between pre-clinical and clinical subjects were formalised, moves that were linked to new ways of constructing disease. It also saw the establishment of a framework for debates on the locus and nature of medical education that were to dominate the twentieth century. However, it is important not to portray the 1880s and 1890s as decades of fundamental change. Old practices continued at the bedside and in the lecture theatre. Many of the pathological and bacteriological discoveries, later hailed as triumphs, were resisted. Nor did St Bartholomew's wholeheartedly embrace these changes, at least at first. Attitudes and clinical practices were slow to alter. The appointment of Alfredo Kanthack as lecturer in pathology in 1893 therefore marked a watershed. Although there had been no revolution and empirical methods remained strong, a growing interest in pathology as an aid to diagnosis allowed laboratory science to gain ground in the College.

A place for science?

Tensions existed between the interests of those running London's hospitals, who wanted to maintain high standards of care and avoid scandals, and those teaching in them. At St Bartholomew's the governors continued to see patients as suitable subjects for medical charity, while the lecturers had come to see them as objects of care; vehicles for teaching. With seventy-four clerks and dressers working in the outpatient departments and with additional dressers and clerks attached to the specialist departments, there were 920 hospital posts available to students by the 1890s. Before taking up these posts, students received elementary instruction in the duties they would be expected to perform, and were taught how to apply their anatomical knowledge, use instruments and examine urine 'and other Secretions'.[6] Although most of the patients were considered 'uninteresting cases' for teaching, for the lecturers these posts played an important role. If teaching in the wards and outpatient department remained *ad hoc*, and was limited by overcrowding, teaching staff not only defended the students' rights to assist but also stressed the importance of doing so. Their views brought them into conflict with the governors who worried that with 'advanced' students taking 'an equal share of the patients' in the outpatient department patient care was

---

[6] *College Calendar* (1892/3), pp. 32–3, 39; ibid. (1893/4), p. 41.

suffering.[7] The resulting arguments reaffirmed the observational nature of training at St Bartholomew's. Although attempts to limit student numbers on the wards were successfully resisted by the lecturers, the governors became more reticent about supporting schemes that did not have a direct bearing on treatment. In response, teaching staff shifted the language they used. When arguing for new facilities, they started to adopt a rhetoric that stressed the value of improvements to treatment rather than to teaching. However, just as the lecturers were defending students' access to patients and the importance of observation, a different set of debates were highlighting the value of science to medicine.

Thomas Bonner has suggested that the 'stunning achievements in laboratory medicine' in Germany ensured that doctors by the 1870s 'began to talk openly of medicine as a "science", relishing the new authority that came with a term normally reserved for such exact sciences as mathematics and astronomy'.[8] The rhetorical or ideological role which science played in defining and consolidating professional status was important for doctors, even if they assigned science a limited role at the bedside. For many contemporaries, science embodied the essence of modernity. Different constructions of science were integral to the Victorian worldview. Lectures and the press popularised the value of science; museums and public exhibitions made it 'visible'. Herbert Spencer, one of the most influential challengers of traditional liberal education, suggested that science was the knowledge of 'most worth'. Despite the slow progress in incorporating these ideas into education, science became a form of 'cultural self-expression'; part of middle-class discourse.[9] Doctors increasingly co-opted a positivist language of science for their own professional ends, building on a language of naturalism that had come to characterise debates on social issues.[10] However, how laboratory medicine was to be incorporated into training when the laboratory had an ambiguous position in the production of knowledge was a more contentious issue.

By the mid-nineteenth century there were many competing types of scientific medicine and authority. Medicine had never pretended be unscientific and, according to Bynum, the 'alliance of science (however perceived) and medicine was no nineteenth century invention'.[11] Although

---

[7] Bodleian Library: Robert Bridges, Medical Lecture, fos. 17–20.

[8] Thomas N. Bonner, *Becoming a Physician: Medical Education in Great Britain, France, Germany and the United States, 1750–1945* (New York, 1995), p. 252.

[9] J. A. V. Chapple, *Science and Literature in the Nineteenth Century* (London, 1986), pp. 4–12.

[10] See Christopher Lawrence, *Medicine in the Making of Modern Britain, 1700–1900* (London, 1994), pp. 70–1. For the use of science to aid status, see S. E. D. Shortt, 'Physicians, Science and Status: Issues in the Professionalisation of Anglo-American Medicine in the Nineteenth Century', *Medical History* xxvii (1983), pp. 51–68.

[11] W. F. Bynum, *Science and the Practice of Medicine in the Nineteenth Century* (Cambridge, 1994), p. 93.

a broad consensus had been reached in the mid-Victorian period on the need for science in medicine, the type of laboratory science emerging in the late nineteenth century was epistemologically different from the ideas in which many doctors had been trained in the 1850s and 1860s. How and where this was to be included in training sparked controversy and marked the start of a pedagogical revolution in medical education.[12] The role of science in a liberal education was also hotly debated by the likes of Spencer, Thomas H. Huxley, Lyon Playfair and John H. Newman. Pressure was exerted from the emerging scientific community, which wanted to serve its own professional ends by making Britain into a scientific nation. However, although moves were made for greater educational provision for scientific and technical training in schools, by the late 1890s the need for more science in education continued to be preached *ad nauseam*. The controversy surrounding the role of experimental and laboratory medicine formed part of these wider debates and was influenced by them.

The pragmatic nature of the London medical schools, and their self-imposed distance from higher education, ensured that these issues were not coherently debated in a metropolitan educational context until the 1880s. British clinicians had been impressed by advances in France and Germany in the 1850s and 1860s, but had been less motivated to change given the strength of their own educational experience. By the 1880s the situation had altered as pressure grew for the acceptance of German advances. How this new style of laboratory science was to fit with a model of training based on a view of professional status linked to notions of 'gentlemanly' character saw different models of medicine clash. The resulting debates over the position and merit of laboratory and the experimental sciences occurred, according to Mark Weatherall, 'in places over which the profession had most control: in medical schools, on the pages of medical journals, at meetings of medical societies, and increasingly, in hospitals'.[13] For John Harley Warner, medical education was the 'principal conduit' for infusing a new language and interest in science into medicine.[14] The process was far from unproblematic.

Arguments about the value of bedside medicine versus laboratory science, skills versus knowledge, so familiar to twentieth-century discussions on academic medicine, were first fought out over, and confined to, the preliminary and pre-clinical sciences.[15] This reflected advances in the understanding of disease rather than in its treatment, and matched the distinction medical schools made between pure science and the application of science to

---

[12] John H. Warner, 'Science in Medicine', *Osiris* 2nd ser. i (1985), p. 45.

[13] Mark W. Weatherall, 'Making Medicine Scientific: Empiricism, Rationality, and Quackery in Mid-Victorian Britain', *SHM* ix (1996), p. 175.

[14] Warner, 'Science', p. 43.

[15] The preliminary sciences were chemistry, physics and biology, or those covered by the First MB.

medicine. The University of London had encouraged this in 1861 when the revised MB regulations established a preliminary science examination. The GMC had followed in 1877 by suggesting that the preliminary sciences should be studied before the end of the first year. The high level of knowledge required for the MB, which few medical students did well at, intensified debate.[16] Doubts were expressed about whether the preliminary sciences would be better taught at school, university or in a teaching hospital, doubts which merged with discussions about the role of the University of London in medical education. Although there was considerable overlap, two broad strands emerged as rifts developed between clinicians, academic teachers and professional scientists.

According to Christopher Lawrence, groups in the elite 'invoked an epistemology of individual experience' to defend the autonomy of clinical medicine, rejecting applied science in favour of skill and character. These groups used a clinical language that defended their position from 'scientifically minded practitioners and the pedagogic claims of a new generation of basic science teachers'.[17] These men did not reject science, but were 'scientific by other standards' based on clinical empiricism and experience.[18] At first in the majority, this patrician class held influential positions in the medical establishment. They asserted that medicine was an art based on observation and 'incommunicable knowledge', linked to a carefully defined notion of clinical science and character. Thomas Huxley was clear that 'nothing but what is absolutely practical will go down in England', arguing that the experimental sciences were seen to be of dubious value to the practitioner.[19] While it was agreed that medicine should be based on science, it was a science limited to anatomy, physiology or the basic sciences, subjects that did not threaten established practices or status. Those who supported this view, many of whom either taught or held posts in London's hospitals, had been socialised into the profession at a time when Victorians had little confidence in 'medical "science" and serious reservations about medical men's social authority and prestige'.[20] In adopting the view that status in medicine was based on experience, which was a product of individual character, these men felt that status was affirmed through criteria that

---

[16] A. L. Mansell, 'Examinations and Medical Education: The Preliminary Sciences in the Examinations of London University and the English Conjoint Board, 1861–1911', in *Days of Judgement: Science, Examinations and the Organisation of Knowledge in Late Victorian England*, ed. Roy MacLeod (North Humberside, 1982), pp. 90–1.

[17] Christopher Lawrence, 'Incommunicable Knowledge: Science, Technology and Clinical Art in Britain, 1850–1914', *Journal of Contemporary History* xx (1985), pp. 505, 503–20.

[18] Warner, 'Science', p. 57.

[19] Cited in Bonner, *Becoming a Physician*, p. 245.

[20] M. Jeanne Peterson, *The Medical Profession in Mid-Victorian London* (Berkeley, 1978), pp. 38–9, 55.

stressed classical learning and liberality of mind. In doing so, they embraced a liberal education because a 'non-vocational education was seen as morally superior'.[21] Although the notion of a liberal education was in flux, and striving towards more balance between art and science, it was still felt to confer an intellectual and social superiority that was believed to be the key to social acceptance. In medicine, Georgian notions of civility and liberal education as the means of achieving professional status continued to thrive just as they were being questioned in other fields.

These views contrasted with those of a different group of clinicians who strove to make laboratory science the source of clinical authority. For Lawrence, these clinicians were from 'the most self-consciously intellectual faction of the elite, especially the university teachers, notably those associated with University College London, Cambridge University and the Royal Society'.[22] Often in a minority, and cautious about the benefits of laboratory science to medicine, they drew part of their status from the contributions they made to experimental and clinical science. They advocated that clinical medicine should correspond to scientific reasoning, and stressed the value of science and the laboratory to training. A growing emphasis on experimental and laboratory discipline in the ideology of science and changes to medical practice, which placed a greater emphasis on the functional nature of disease, combined to help them articulate these ideas. For them, training in the laboratory represented a series of practical skills that could be learned and a form of polite knowledge that was compatible with notions of gentlemanly status. The laboratory was cast as an important technical and observational space, parallel but subservient to the bedside; one that extended the traditions of hands-on learning present in London's teaching hospitals. As the assistant physician at the Middlesex noted, laboratories are 'absolutely essential for the adequate teaching of the medical man ... for the acquaintance it gave him with the manipulation of instruments of precision and the habits of observation'.[23] While these doctors continued to support the value of a liberal education, they also argued that laboratory training was important because doctors who were not exposed to laboratory knowledge would flounder in 'an aimless fashion, never able to gain any accurate conception of disease' or keep up with advances.[24] Throughout, the emphasis was on practical learning, a stress that meshed with the practical culture of the hospital, and found favour with students dissatisfied with a culture of lectures and with overcrowded and unsystematic bedside teaching.

[21] T. W. Heyck, *Transformation of Intellectual Life in Victorian England* (London, 1982), p. 103.

[22] Lawrence, *Medicine*, p. 72.

[23] *Lancet* ii (1898), p. 1069.

[24] Cited in Roy Porter, *The Greatest Benefit of Mankind* (London, 1997), p. 305.

The contradiction of these two positions was summed up by Patrick Black, lecturer in principles and practice of medicine at St Bartholomew's: 'your profession *demands* from you that you shall possess what is called scientific knowledge, and it is expected from your acknowledged station in society that you should not be wanting in those accomplishments which distinguish the position of gentlemen.'[25] The traditionalists worried that a reorientation of training towards the laboratory would distort clinical judgement. Those who advocated science were shown to be attacking older 'gentlemanly' ideas in favour of meritocracy, a point that alarmed the elite who saw a levelling with laboratory workers and a loss of professional status. The tension between the two views was in part resolved by rethinking the preliminary and pre-clinical sciences to give medicine a firmer scientific footing separate from clinical training. 'Science' and the laboratory could be safely confined to the pre-clinical period, leaving the art of medicine to the clinical years.

There was some support for strengthening science through the preliminary and pre-clinical subjects at St Bartholomew's. It came mainly from those who had travelled to Germany to work in laboratories in Berlin, Vienna, Leipzig and other centres. They brought back with them an interest in research and laboratory medicine. William Savory was an exception. In other areas a conservative, he had had a scientific training through the University of London and insisted on a grounding in science before students started their clinical study. He believed medical schools should become 'scientific workshops' and argued that 'a sound and successful practitioner' was also 'a diligent student of those sciences which investigate our structure and functions in their healthy and natural state'.[26] Thomas Shore, the stern lecturer in biology and future dean, claimed this role for biology, building on the biological and histological constructions that characterised English physiology after 1870. Shore saw science as a way of explaining the body. In linking biology with physiology, he was staking a claim for the experimental sciences at St Bartholomew's. To make his version of medical education less confrontational, Shore stressed that by training students in the 'elementary laws of life' their 'powers of observation' and technical knowledge would be extended.[27] Shore was borrowing directly from assertions made by Huxley and the GMC in their support for preliminary science training. Other preliminary and pre-clinical teachers at St Bartholomew's were to repeat these claims and by the 1890s these arguments had become part of a common rhetoric.

Staff who supported the idea that medical schools should be 'scientific workshops' tended to be in the minority at St Bartholomew's. Defenders of

---

[25] Cited in Lawrence, 'Incommunicable Knowledge', p. 507.

[26] *BMJ* i (1878), p. 791; *St Bartholomew's Hospital Journal*, August 1932, p. 215.

[27] Thomas Shore, 'On the Study of Biology in Relation to Medicine', *St Bartholomew's Hospital Reports* xxiv (1888), pp. 65–82; 'Preliminary Scientific Teaching', ibid., xii (1886), pp. 150–1.

experimentation and vivisection like Thomas Lauder Brunton, a founder of the Physiological Society and leading experimenter, and Edward Klein, pioneer of English bacteriology, did not speak out in committees for a greater emphasis on science in training despite the role they played in popularising medical science. They appeared to be more interested in their own research than in shaping medical education in the College. Many of the older clinicians educated in the 1840s and 1850s saw an elite medical education not just as giving students a technical training but as preparing them for society. Such men dominated St Bartholomew's and ensured that teaching continued to owe much to an 'anatomical-chirurgical' approach. Although not opposed to experimentation or German ideas, they joined debates on medical education firmly on the side of a traditional approach, stressing the need to raise students' general and classical education. These views were reflected in the attitudes of Dyce Duckworth, lecturer in clinical medicine, and Samuel Gee, lecturer in the practice of medicine. The pompous Duckworth was an Edinburgh graduate, a traditionalist and a long-standing treasurer of the Royal College of Physicians. Part of the medical elite and a stickler for etiquette, he saw medicine as an art and dismissed what he believed to be the 'modern side in education'. Duckworth bemoaned the 'decline of letters' in medicine and believed that literature, Greek and Latin gave students a good grounding, and stressed the need for clinical instinct and intuition.[28] Gee was even more adamant. A student of University College Hospital, Gee was a highly respected clinician and teacher who was convinced of the merits of classical learning. An intellectual chauvinist well read in German ideas on bacteriology and pathology yet dismissive of them, he told students to forget their physiology when entering the wards because where physiology was an 'experimental science', medicine was 'an empirical art'.[29] He even 'went so far as to doubt the value of experiment in the natural sciences'.[30] Gee was a self-confessed empiric and taught students accordingly, stressing the painstaking analysis of physical signs. The physiologist Henry Dale, looking back on his time as a student at St Bartholomew's, held that these attitudes still characterised the College at the start of the twentieth century. He asserted that staff 'openly professed their knowledge to be the product of an empirical craft'.[31] Learning at the bedside was one thing; learning from the bench-side was quite another. It threatened the empirical style of medicine linked to clinical experience that was so strong at St Bartholomew's and was therefore to be distrusted.

[28] Dyce Duckworth, *Knowledge and Wisdom in Medicine* (London, 1902), p. 13; *St Bartholomew's Hospital Journal*, October 1893, p. 3.
[29] Cited in Kenneth D. Keele, *Evolution of Clinical Method in Medicine* (London, 1963), p. 105.
[30] Cited in Christopher Lawrence, 'A Tale of Two Sciences: Bedside and Bench in Twentieth Century Britain', *Medical History* xliii (1999), p. 450.
[31] W. S. Feldberg, 'Henry Hallet Dale', *Biographical Memoirs of the Fellows of the Royal Society* xvi (1970), pp. 89–90.

Science shapes the curriculum

During the 1880s, a change occurred in attitudes to the role of science in medical education. As groups in the medical profession became more confident about scientific medicine and its contribution, an 'accord' between scientific and practical teaching was called for.[32] However, although Shore suggested that between 1880 and 1894 the 'method of practical laboratory and clinical teaching' became established in London, it was in the provincial schools that the greatest changes occurred.[33] Outside London, the most active period of university development of the whole century took place as part of wider movements in educational reform.[34] In provincial schools, science, as Sturdy has suggested, was promoted because it could be shown to have practical and financial benefits.[35] Provincial medical schools had grown rapidly, so that by the 1870s they were 'scrambl[ing] to strengthen their offerings in science' by establishing links with civic colleges, which had become the principal location for professional scientists outside London. This was designed to improve their status and to ensure the range of laboratory teaching required by the licensing bodies. Civic colleges tailored their teaching to reflect the needs of medical students by offering instruction in those subjects which medical schools found too expensive to provide.[36] Efforts were also made to improve science teaching at Oxford and Cambridge, although it was Cambridge that took the lead in an effort to catch up with earlier reforms at Oxford.[37] For reformers, these changes marked an 'intellectual revolution' in medicine, but many dismissed these efforts: they looked to London as the barometer of advancing ideas. Here steps 'to build laboratories, appoint full-time teachers, and reorient medical education around a core of scientific study' were slow to emerge.[38]

In this gradual transformation of learning, experimental physiology, which had moved from a focus on structure in the 1850s and 1860s, at first led the way as the model medical science. It was given a firmer public and professional

---

[32] *Lancet* ii (1885), p. 624.

[33] Thomas Shore, 'Evolution of Medicine and Medical Teaching', *St Bartholomew's Hospital Journal*, February 1894, p. 72.

[34] Michael Sanderson, ed., *The Universities in the Nineteenth Century* (London, 1975), pp. 142–3.

[35] Steve Sturdy, 'The Political Economy of Scientific Medicine: Science, Education and the Transformation of Medical Practice in Sheffield, 1890–1922', *Medical History* xxxvi (1992), pp. 125–59.

[36] See Stella V. F. Butler, 'A Transformation in Training: The Formation of University Medical Faculties in Manchester, Leeds, and Liverpool, 1870–84', *Medical History* xxx (1986), pp. 119–25; David R. Jones, *The Origins of Civic Universities: Manchester, Liverpool and Leeds* (London, 1988), pp. 70–3, 159–68.

[37] Janet Howarth, 'Science Education in late-Victorian Oxford: A Curious Case of Failure?' (*EHR* cii (1987), pp. 334–71) offers a balanced view of the relative scientific merits of Oxford and Cambridge.

[38] Michael Foster, *On Medical Education at Cambridge* (London, 1878), p. 4.

identity by advances made in France and Germany and by the antivivisection lobby, which created a large body of doctors in opposition who defended biomedical science.[39] Experimental physiology had a clear laboratory focus that encapsulated the values of science which the self-conscious intellectual elite wanted to incorporate, even if its practical value was doubted. Development depended initially on a group of highly committed individuals. Major advances were first made at Cambridge where Michael Foster created a research school. He was able to rearrange teaching so that students spent as much time in the laboratory as they did in lectures.[40] In London, John Scott Burdon Sanderson at University College pressed for more laboratory accommodation for physiology. University College from its foundation had stressed the role of science to medicine, and Burdon Sanderson followed in this tradition by collecting a group of laboratory investigators and students. Change was less marked in the hospital schools like St Bartholomew's and St Thomas's, where the clinical culture of medical education was at its strongest. 'The high cost of laboratory education, the dependence of the teaching enterprise on student fees and private practice, and the orientation of the hospital toward patient service all contributed to a reluctance to make any but the most necessary changes.'[41] Innovation in providing new courses – if not new knowledge – was slowed further because schools were dissuaded by the institutional structure of medical education from deviating from a curriculum accepted by examiners and demanded by students.[42]

Although the academic nature of medicine had been stressed at St Bartholomew's since the 1840s, the entrenched empirical view of medicine based on anatomy and observation hampered the integration of the experimental sciences. While provision had been made for a chemical laboratory since the 1820s, students were essentially told to look 'at the living body with anatomical eyes', to touch and see in a way familiar to those who had studied in the College in the 1830s and 1840s.[43] A strong sense of individualism ensured that any scientific interests which staff had were seldom channelled into the College. Those who advocated better science teaching, like Henry Armstrong, lecturer in chemistry and prominent educational reformer, held junior posts and were unable to exert much

[39] See Nicolaas A. Rupke, 'Pro-Vivisection in England in the Early 1880s', in *Vivisection in Historical Perspective*, ed. Nicolaas A. Rupke (London, 1987), pp. 188–208.

[40] See Gerald L. Geison, *Michael Foster and the Cambridge School of Physiology: The Scientific Enterprise in Late Victorian Society* (Princeton, 1978); Geison, 'Social and Institutional Factors in the Stagnancy of English Physiology, 1840–1870', BHM xlvi (1972), pp. 30–58.

[41] Bonner, *Becoming a Physician*, p. 275.

[42] See Stella V. F. Butler, 'Science and the Education of Doctors during the Nineteenth Century: A Study of British Medical Schools with Particular Reference to the Development and Uses of Physiology' (unpublished Ph.D. diss., UMIST, 1982).

[43] Luther Holden, *Landmarks, Medical and Surgical* (London, 1876), p. 2.

influence on how teaching was organised.[44] The College's position as one of the largest teaching hospitals in London ensured further that there was little need to promote science as a way of bolstering status. With no links to a multi-faculty college like King's or University College, the emphasis was firmly on what was perceived to be relevant to medical practice. If the College did not rest on its laurels, a large body of students and faith in its standing did encourage conservatism. The lecturers remained cautious of the experimental sciences, concentrating their energy on clinical medicine. Change was initiated instead by the GMC and the licensing bodies.

Although the College tried to resist the GMC's brand of 'uniformity' it was, like every teaching hospital, obliged to offer a similar range of subjects for students sitting one of the many qualifying examinations. When the Royal College of Surgeons introduced revised examination requirements in 1871 that gave a greater role for the experimental sciences, the College responded by appointing a committee to investigate the steps that 'should be taken in the formation of a class in practical physiology'. For Geison, the decision by the Royal College, which was followed by the other licensing bodies, had a considerable impact on medicine and started a trend towards the inclusion of the experimental sciences.[45] University College became the leading model, but St Bartholomew's paid little attention to what was happening there. It was decided to cut the number of physiology lectures from four to three per week and to use the extra time for laboratory classes. A new demonstrator of practical physiology was appointed from the clinical staff, and space was begrudgingly found for laboratory classes in the reading room, reflecting something of the importance initially attached to experimental physiology. The arrangements quickly proved untenable. The reading room was impractical and generated complaints from other students who wanted to use it. Demonstrations were therefore moved to the medical committee room, where by 1887 they were being held three times a week before a new physiology laboratory was opened.[46]

The reluctant acceptance of experimental physiology at St Bartholomew's was reflected in the career of Henry Power. Power was a close friend of Foster and Huxley, professor of physiology at the Royal Veterinary College and an examiner in physiology for the Royal College of Surgeons. At St Bartholomew's, however, he confined his interests to ophthalmic surgery, on which he lectured from 1870 to 1895. Power was not the only member of staff interested in experimental physiology; Vincent Dormer Harris and D'Arcy Power wrote a manual for students on the subject.[47] Klein and Brunton were

[44] Henry Armstrong, *The Teaching of Scientific Method and Other Papers on Education* (London, 1925).

[45] Geison, *Foster*, p. 329.

[46] Minutes of lecturers and medical staff, 15 July 1871, 30 November 1872, MS 12/2.

[47] Vincent Dormer Harris and D'Arcy Power, *Manual for the Physiological Laboratory* (London, 1880).

ardent experimenters, though limited room and complaints from other staff hampered serious research in the College. Klein had come to Britain on the insistence of Sanderson, but quickly damaged the physiologists' cause during the 1875 Royal Commission on vivisection.[48] He remained distanced from the College, where he was disliked by several of the senior staff, and his teaching was quickly diluted in the anatomy and physiology course. Brunton was more closely associated with St Bartholomew's. A passionate defender of animal experiments, he worked with Sanderson and Klein on the *Handbook for the Physiological Laboratory*, which marked 'a watershed in the transmission of Continental methods to British laboratories'.[49] Despite his interest in digestion and secretion, his pharmacological research absorbed most of his energies, and his diagnostic approach (which often appeared to owe more to an interpretation of symptoms based on disordered physiology) was viewed with scepticism.[50] Although he broke with tradition and introduced more lectures on the physiological action of drugs into the *materia medica* course, Brunton did not hold a teaching post in physiology. Whereas he was willing to defend research outside St Bartholomew's, he did little to promote physiology in the College. Harris, as demonstrator of practical physiology, was in a better position, but his junior post and appointments at three other London hospitals gave him little time or leverage. Other promising demonstrators of physiology, such as Walter Pye, whose work with Lauder Brunton attracted considerable attention, quickly left for posts elsewhere.[51]

Further changes to the examination requirements of the University of London in 1883 precipitated a departure from the classificatory model of teaching that had encouraged little more than cramming. Greater emphasis was placed on practical classes: botany and zoology, which were receiving more scientific attention in the 1880s as work was conducted on the chemical aspects of plant physiology and enzymes, were merged and relabelled biology. An effort was also made to increase the laboratory element in physics and chemistry, subjects that were combined easily given the physical basis of English chemistry. In response, courses were started at St Bartholomew's on practical biology.[52] However, with more emphasis on practical teaching pressure increased for laboratory accommodation. As most

[48] His 'unfortunate' and blunt statements about how experimental animals were treated strengthened the claims of the antivivisectionist lobby, contributing to a climate in which restrictive legislation on animal experiments were passed: see *Report of the RC on the Practice of Subjecting Live Animals to Experiments for Scientific Purposes*, PP (1876) xli.

[49] Edward Sharpey-Schafer, *History of the Physiological Society during its First Fifty Years, 1876–1926* (London, 1927), pp. 7–8.

[50] Thomas Lauder Brunton, *Textbook of Pharmacology, Therapeutics and Materia Medica* (London, 1885).

[51] Walter Pye and Thomas Lauder Brunton, 'Action of *Erythrophleum guinense*', *Philosophical Transactions* clxvii (1877), p. 627.

[52] Shore, 'Preliminary Scientific Teaching', pp. 149–50.

London medical schools were pressed for space, suggestions were made that these subjects should be moved to separate special schools. This had been mooted in 1870 and an investigation into the University of London's teaching role in 1893 returned to the idea.[53] It was staunchly resisted by the lecturers at St Bartholomew's who decided to create a separate department for the preliminary sciences.[54] The decision forced the development of laboratories to accommodate the increase in practical teaching, and placed science on a stronger footing.

New guidelines devised by the GMC in 1892 further extended the curriculum and placed more weight on the preliminary and pre-clinical studies. As a representative body, the GMC worked by common consent, but by the 1890s it was exerting a more authoritative voice. This was reflected in the 1892 guidelines, which had already been loosely outlined by the Royal Commission on medical degrees in 1882.[55] No radical changes were made, but the GMC did defend the role of science in training. The University of London responded immediately. It devised a five-year curriculum that left no medical school entirely satisfied. Anxiety was expressed about the uncertainty of the new arrangements and the effect they would have, but even the less intellectually rigorous Conjoint Board (the merged examining body of the royal colleges created in 1884) moved to include the preliminary sciences. Although staff at St Bartholomew's were ambivalent, even hostile to the GMC, they could not resist a shift in examination requirements of the University and Conjoint Board.[56] By 1893, students at the College found that not only had an extra year of study been added, along with a compulsory element in psychiatry, ophthalmic surgery and infectious diseases, but also new courses in the biological sciences. Biology was seen as central to the understanding of disease which the new curriculum aimed to promote. It was felt to lead 'to the better understanding of not only the normal but also the pathological, process' and to prepare students for a style of medicine that was becoming increasingly biological. At St Bartholomew's a separate lecturership in biology was created to take account of this, removing teaching from comparative anatomy. The number of chemistry demonstrators was also increased and less emphasis was placed on the 'laws of Chemical Composition and Decomposition'.[57] Further changes by the Conjoint Board encouraged the introduction of more lectures on organic chemistry. Under these influences, the department was expanded and brought under the

---

[53] *Lancet* ii (1870), p. 544; *RC to Consider the Draft Charter for the Proposed Gresham University in London*, PP (1894) xxxiv, p. 848.

[54] Shore, 'Preliminary Scientific Teaching', pp. 149–50.

[55] *RC on Grant of Medical Degrees*, PP (1882) xxix.

[56] See Peterson, *Medical Profession*, pp. 240–1.

[57] *St Bartholomew's Hospital Journal*, November 1893, 18; Shore to Moore, 27 April 1892, MS 14/5.

control of a subcommittee. Other science departments were quickly placed under similar committees, though no suggestion was made that the clinical departments should move from their ward-based administration.[58] The move to establish pre-clinical subcommittees further defined the departments. They created a new administrative hierarchy in the College that gave departments greater independence and provided a prototype for the boards of studies created in 1905.

A greater educational emphasis on science did not mean that room or money could be found in the College to improve existing accommodation. Rebuilding had set the institutional pattern for the College and, while it was a relatively straightforward process to rearrange lectures or appoint additional staff, it was not as easy to provide the physical framework required for laboratories and workrooms. With a higher proportion of students sitting the less demanding Conjoint Board, there was less incentive to develop science teaching for students who were rarely interested. At Charing Cross, the Middlesex, St George's and the Westminster, this problem was side-stepped by sending students to the Normal School of Science in South Kensington for preliminary science classes. Anxious contemporaries predicted that this would be the trend in medical education, but St Bartholomew's refused to dilute its training.[59] For all this, space and funds for laboratories not directly connected to clinical practice continued to have a low priority. In 1891, Frederick Womack, lecturer in chemical physics, complained that students entering examinations in physics would be at a 'considerable disadvantage as compared with those from other schools' because the laboratories were under-equipped for teaching.[60] In the following year, Shore added further complaints about the rooms for practical biology. He feared 'that unless this department is placed on a satisfactory basis, we shall be unable to maintain out position in competition with other Schools' just at a time when King's, University College and Guy's were all seeking money to improve their laboratory facilities.[61] Anxious about competition, money was finally found for a rudimentary laboratory, which was opened in 1892. The physics laboratory was moved from the basement into better accommodation in 1899 and the physiology laboratory was re-equipped 'with all the most approved applications'.[62] Efforts were made to remodel teaching to match the University's requirements, but this did not stop one University examiner making 'depreciatory' comments about the quality of science teaching at St Bartholomew's.[63]

---

[58] Finance Committee, 28 May 1894, MS 31/1.
[59] Rivington, *Medical Profession*, p. 723.
[60] Memorandum, c.1891, MS 14/5.
[61] Shore to Moore, 18 April 1891, MS 14/5; *College Calendar* (1887/8), p. 45; H. C. Cameron, *Mr Guy's Hospital, 1726–1948* (London, 1954), pp. 279–81.
[62] *College Calendar* (1898/9), pp. 53, 55.
[63] Shore to University, 27 October 1892, MS 14/5.

Table 4.1   University of London preliminary science examination: successful
candidates (%)

	Year	% of candidates successful: All schools	% of candidates successful: St Bartholomew's
July	1885	62.8	65.0
Jan	1886	50.0	66.6
July	1886	51.4	64.3
Jan	1887	60.6	66.6
July	1887	72.8	80.0
Jan	1888	29.6	66.6
Total		61.9	82.3

Source: RC on a University for London, PP (1889) xxxix, p. 253

Despite disparaging assessments, St Bartholomew's did reorganise its
science teaching with greater success when compared to other London
medical schools (see Table 4.1). Concerns about the poor pass rate in the
University's preliminary science examination had been met in part by
the creation of the junior science open scholarship, which aimed to attract
able students to St Bartholomew's.[64] In the intermediate MB examination in
1885, students from the College 'secured nearly as many places in honours as
all the other [medical] schools combined'. Only University College had a
consistently higher pass rate. It was felt that this was 'partly due to the sound
scientific training St Bartholomew's students receive in the earlier part of
their career'.[65] This was an optimistic assessment, but although empirical
attitudes remained strong, they were being challenged. If the experimental
and pre-clinical sciences encouraged a growing acceptance of science in
medicine, general developments in pathology, especially when linked to
bacteriology, and clinical medicine did more to reshape attitudes.

'Temples of clinical science'

Debates over the value of different types of medical science and the
importance of character to medical education underlay arguments about
the role of the laboratory and pathology (augmented by bacteriology) in the
curriculum. The laboratory, rather than being another resource at the doctor's
disposal, was constructed by some as a challenge to the pre-eminent position
hospital medicine had achieved.[66] The laboratory revolution was a difficult

[64] Baker to College, 15 January 1874, DF 115.
[65] Shore, 'Preliminary Scientific Teaching', p. 153.
[66] See Andrew Cunningham and Perry Williams, eds, *The Laboratory Revolution in
Medicine* (Cambridge, 1992).

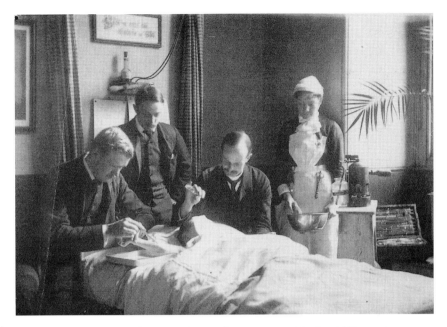

Plate 4.1 Operation under general anaesthesia in a ward bed, *c.*1890

one. Germ theories and what Michael Worboys has defined as 'germ practices' did attract clinicians and became 'carriers of *new meanings for science in
medicine*'. However, they sat uneasily with earlier ideas about medicine,
encouraging a certain clinical ambivalence.[67] Ideas on fermentation,
putrefaction and contagion were reinterpreted first under the influence of
Louis Pasteur and then by Robert Koch to give a new dimension to disease
and contagion. However, practices at the bedside did not change as quickly.
Empirical notions of causation, firmly upheld by a continuing faith in
localised pathology, continued to thrive. Many staff in the College at first saw
little relevance for laboratory and bacteriological analysis. When Frederick
Andrewes entered St Bartholomew's as a student in the early 1880s, 'nobody
seemed at all excited about bacteriology'.[68] Older staff, often sceptical about
the use of theory, were conservative in their approach. This mentality and
faith in empiricism was not unique to the College. Similar attitudes existed at
Guy's, while Robert Young, a student at the Middlesex in 1889, remembered

[67] Michael Worboys, *Spreading Germs: Disease Theories and Medical Practice in Britain,
1865–1900* (Cambridge, 2000), p. 7.
[68] Lawrence, 'Incommunicable Knowledge', pp. 503–29; Frederick Andrewes, 'The
Beginnings of Bacteriology at St Bartholomew's', *St Bartholomew's Hospital Journal*, April
1928, p. 101.

that the main tests were limited to chemical analysis. Young could have been describing conditions at St Bartholomew's.[69]

A delay existed between a growing faith in bacteriology in the 1880s and the need to train students in laboratory methods. In many institutions, this was not successfully realised until the following decade. As Worboys has suggested, it was the clinical and social benefits of germ theory and laboratory science that shaped the 'modernisation' of pathology and inclusion of bacteriology into teaching rather than the intellectual discoveries of Pasteur or Koch.[70] This was hardly surprising in a College where surgery dominated the organisation of learning. Laboratory-based knowledge was given a role in clinical teaching through surgery that was more than 'a preparatory role in a separate pre-clinical curriculum' as Cooter and Sturdy have argued.[71] Staff were less reticent about accepting science where it could be shown to be clinically relevant.

In the 1870s and 1880s, this was still a long way off. When Andrewes joined the College, as 'far as a good deal of the surgical teaching . . . was concerned [Lister] might never have lived'.[72] The methods suggested by Joseph Lister and his disciples continued to be disputed, and many medical practitioners remained indifferent to germ theories. Lister's science, initially espousing Pasteur's approach and then coming to adopt Koch's ideas, proved contested but highly malleable, able to incorporate different techniques so that differences existed between the practices adopted in 1867 (when Lister first published his ideas) and those of 1900.[73] However, based on a complicated technique rather than on a standardised procedure, antisepsis encountered theoretical as well as practical problems, especially after studies in the 1870s pointed to cracks in the theory. Ironically, it was these challenges that stimulated interest in germs.

Opposition appeared entrenched at St Bartholomew's. Senior staff were either sceptical or openly hostile, putting forward alternatives that coloured their teaching. Hostility to antisepsis was widespread in London where traditional approaches to surgery and the understanding of diseases were

---

[69] Cameron, *Guy's*, pp. 279–81; *Fifty Years of Medicine* (London, 1950), p. 283.

[70] Worboys, *Spreading Germs*, p. 7.

[71] Cooter and Sturdy, 'Transformation of Medicine', p. 438.

[72] Andrewes, 'Beginnings of Bacteriology', p. 101.

[73] For Listerism and asepsis, see Christopher Lawrence and R. Dixley, "Practising on Principle: Joseph Lister and the Germ Theories of Diseases', in *Medical Theory; Surgical Practice: Studies in the History of Surgery*, ed. Christopher Lawrence (London, 1992), pp. 153–215; Lindsay Granshaw, "'Upon this principle I have based a practice": The Development and Reception of Antisepsis in Britain, 1867–90', in *Medical Innovation in Historical Perspective*, ed. John V. Pickstone (Basingstoke, 1992), pp. 17–46; T. H. Pennington, 'Listerism, its Decline and its Persistence: The Introduction of Aseptic Surgical Techniques in three British Teaching Hospitals, 1890–99', *Medical History* xxxix (1995), pp. 35–60.

more secure. Many wearied of the details Lister demanded and wanted a simpler approach that did not challenge established ideas and practices as much. At St Bartholomew's this opposition gave the hospital the reputation of an institution opposed to Listerism. Although Thomas Smith, popular and risqué lecturer in clinical surgery, had started to teach students about antiseptic methods in 1876 after a visit to Edinburgh, many of his senior colleagues 'never took cordially to antiseptic surgery'.[74] William Morrant Baker, George Callender and Savory were key proponents of an anti-Listerian mentality. A domineering figure in the medical establishment, Savory had attacked Lister's ideas in a controversial address to the British Medical Association in 1879. He was highly critical of what he saw as Listerians' concentration on external causes, which he felt disregarded 'internal' conditions. Although he accepted that germs could cause sepsis, like many who followed the 'cleanliness school', Savory was vehemently opposed to Lister's methods and believed that 'simpler techniques worked more effectively'.[75] He reportedly teased surgeons interested in antisepsis and excluded from his wards house surgeons who smelt of antiseptics.[76]

Opposition was not uniform. Younger staff (like Butlin, Harrison Cripps, Smith and Alfred Willett) adopted a mixed antiseptic/aseptic approach. Building on research in the 1870s which suggested that germs did not always produce disease, they embraced Listerian methods at a time when they were being portrayed as an adjunct to natural healing. They borrowed a German model of infection and not the earlier disputed theories about putrefaction. However, even the younger staff remained divided, split between antiseptic and aseptic regimes that reflected the accumulation of the 'many small deviations from intellectual and practical routine[s] among the surgical community *as a whole*'.[77]

It was the sarcastic Charles Barrett Lockwood who took the lead in introducing what he defined as these 'modern' scientific methods to his teaching and surgical work. He had trained at St Bartholomew's, and as a student had been sent by Smith to Edinburgh to observe Lister at a time when 'nine surgeons out of ten do not care much' for germ theory. After working at the Dean Street Lock Hospital, Lockwood returned to the College as demonstrator of anatomy in 1881. Lockwood's passion for anatomy had a considerable impact on teaching. With William Bruce Clarke, he started weekly examinations and was a founder member of the Association of British Anatomists, though his ideas were often considered unorthodox. Long hours

[74] Alfred Willett, 'In Memoriam: Morrant Baker', *St Bartholomew's Hospital Reports* xxxii (1896), pp. xil-xlix.
[75] *BMJ* ii (1879), pp. 211–12.
[76] Archibald Garrod, 'St Bartholomew's Fifty Years Ago', *St Bartholomew's Hospital Journal*, July 1930, p. 181.
[77] Lawrence and Dixley, 'Practising on Principle', p. 207.

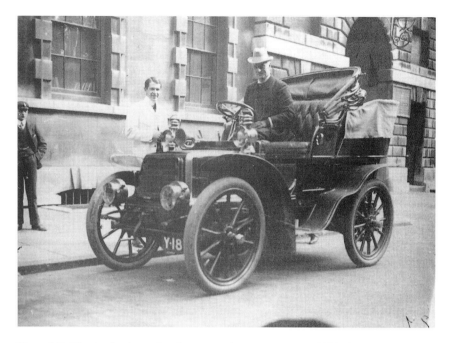

Plate 4.2 Charles Lockwood in his car in the outer court, c.1902–8

in the dissection room damaged his health but did not dull his enthusiasm for practical instruction. Highly critical of text-based study, Lockwood upheld a model of observation and earlier views of anatomy as the 'bed-rock upon which surgery is built'. In his bedside teaching, he exhorted students to be exact and to say 'I know because I saw'. Students often found his lectures a penance, while his caustic and savage approach alienated many. However, his scientific exactitude had a lasting impact on teaching.[78]

Throughout, Lockwood encouraged the 'latest' scientific methods and 'sometimes could not control his feelings from conviction of the truth of his case'.[79] This was clearest in his surgical work where each operation was approached as if it was a bacteriological experiment. At the Great Northern Hospital, where he held the post of surgeon from 1888, he conducted a series of bacteriological studies on wound infection. At St Bartholomew's he applied the same principles.[80] Working with Henry Butlin, who encouraged him, their partnership became known as the 'Aseptic Firm'. Butlin believed that it raised the status of surgery and encouraged patients to seek early treatment. For Butlin, this was particularly important: he stressed the need

---

[78] *St Bartholomew's Hospital Journal*, April 1935, pp. 141–5.
[79] Cited in Pennington, 'Listerism', p. 51.
[80] *BMJ* ii (1890), pp. 943–7; ibid., i (1892), pp. 1127–37.

for the early removal of cancerous growths, having rejected a humoral view in favour of one inspired by Virchow and his idea that disease came from abnormal changes within cells.[81] Lockwood meanwhile struggled to secure asepsis in everything connected to his work and carried out microscope examinations of 'wound products' to look for infection.[82] To further these ideas, Lockwood and Harris started private bacteriological classes in 1889 in the physiology department after they had attended a similar course given by Klein at the Brown Animal Sanatory Institution.[83] Classes were practical and technical, providing lessons that could not be gleaned easily from the growing number of textbooks on laboratory work and bacteriology. They followed Lockwood's view of bacteriology: like many surgeons, he was concerned with the identification of infection.[84] Lockwood's course was not the first. Edgar Crookshank, one of Lister's assistants, had begun an extra-mural bacteriology course at King's College London in 1887. Lockwood's course followed, and others were started as the number of bacteriological laboratories grew.[85]

Lockwood exerted considerable influence over his house surgeons and dressers whom he bullied into adopting his rigorous methods. Gradually even reluctant physicians, won over by the clinical applications of bacteriology, began to see a role for the laboratory. By the mid-1880s, theorising about germs had been replaced by further research and a growing number of clinicians became interested in the emerging science of bacteriology. For them the micro-organism became 'all-sufficient' despite early indications that bacteriology had its limitations.[86] Some lecturers at St Bartholomew's began to offer elementary classes in bacteriology as part of their courses. Butlin, for example, taught students in the throat department about the value of examining patients' sputum for Koch's bacillus. Fitting with expectations that doctors would use microscopes and culture plates to identify disease, he gave his students a printed address on the role of 'poisons' in wound infection.[87]

In other areas, however, bacteriology received less attention. Surgeons were more interested in removing infection than in identifying its origins, and this generally shaped their interests. Although rebuilding had aimed to promote the 'advancement and diffusion of medical and sanitary knowledge', Richard Thorne Thorne, principal medical officer of the Local Government Board

---

[81] Henry Butlin, *On the Operative Surgery of Malignant Disease* (London, 1887), pp. 4–5.

[82] *BMJ* ii (1890), pp. 943–7.

[83] *St Bartholomew's Hospital Reports* xxiv (1898), p. 196.

[84] Subcommittee, MS 34/1; Charles B. Lockwood, *Aseptic Surgery* (London, 1896), p. 15.

[85] W. D. Foster, 'Early History of Clinical Pathology in Great Britain', *Medical History* iii (1959), pp. 180–1.

[86] Cited in Anne Hardy, 'On the Cusp: Epidemiology and Bacteriology at the Local Government Board, 1890–1905', *Medical History* xlii (1998), p. 329.

[87] Abernethian Society, 1876–88, SA 1/12.

(LGB) and lecturer in preventive medicine in the College, was sceptical of bacteriology.[88] He adopted a largely sanitarian approach in his teaching.[89] Thorne Thorne also spent a large part of his time at the LGB. Klein equally showed little interest in developing bacteriology at St Bartholomew's until the 1890s. An Austro-Hungarian, he had come to London from Vienna in 1871 to undertake research at the Brown Institution and two years later was appointed to lecture on histology at St Bartholomew's. His original research on animal diseases and histology was modified as he became increasingly interested in the 'intimate' relation between micro-organisms and infectious diseases. Adopting an antigenic approach, Klein mapped out a view of bacteriology that owed much to the chemical pathology of infectious disease.[90] When appointed at St Bartholomew's he transferred his bacteriological work from his laboratories in Great Russell Street and encouraged students to undertake research. However, most of his work continued to be for the LGB.[91] Although periodically he tried to stimulate interest in bacteriology at St Bartholomew's, he preferred to offer bacteriology classes outside the College at the Brown Institution. Blunt and undiplomatic, Klein was unpopular and a breach between him and Andrewes over typhoid added a personal element that initially limited Andrewes's work to anatomical demonstrations. It did not help that errors were detected in Klein's bacteriological work, which did little to enhance his status and hampered the acceptance of germ theories.[92] Instruction in bacteriology therefore remained patchy, left to individual lecturers to organise.

Efforts had also faltered initially to establish pathology as a separate discipline. It was not until the 1850s and 1860s with a further reductionist turn from morbid anatomy of gross lesions to cellular pathology that the subject was reoriented as pathologists came to concern themselves with the living. The College was slow to adopt these ideas. In the 1840s and 1850s, Paget had held students captive with his lectures on surgical pathology. His enthusiasm and belief that doctors should always keep 'a mind for science in practice' had less impact on teaching, however.[93] Until the 1870s, the dominance of clinical observation in diagnosis and a faith in the College in the morbid anatomy of gross lesions ensured that pathology continued to be seen as part of clinical practice defined through post-mortems.

[88] Order of the Charity Commission, 1877, MS 6/1.

[89] See Richard Thorne Thorne, 'Aetiology, Spread and Prevention of Diphtheria', *Journal of the Sanitary Institute* xv (1894), pp. 7–20; *Annual Report of the Medical Officer of the Local Government Board* (1896), pp. 18–26.

[90] Edward Emanuel Klein, *Micro-organisms and Disease: An Introduction to the Study of Specific Micro-organisms* (London, 1896), p. 1.

[91] Andrewes, 'Beginnings of Bacteriology', p. 104.

[92] Hardy, 'On the Cusp', p. 341.

[93] Stephen Paget, ed., *Memoirs and Letters of Sir James Paget* (London, 1901), pp. 175, 368.

This approach was challenged by Norman Moore and Anthony Bowlby. They wanted to move teaching from the naked-eye pathology of post-mortems with its preoccupation with morbid appearances and treatment to a more histological approach.[94] The interest shown by Moore and Bowlby was not atypical: other staff had belatedly begun to point to 'a rapid advance' in pathology and the need for a 'special course of study'.[95] Although Virchow's work on cellular pathology was criticised in Britain, it did increase the status of pathology as a discipline. Its value to surgery was extended through bacteriology and histology. Koch's identification of the tubercle bacillus and the methods he outlined further stimulated interest and research. At University College Hospital, Victor Horsley, director of the pathology department from 1887 to 1896, was pressing for reform to replace the old conception of pathology as morbid anatomy. The Royal College of Surgeons also started to adapt its examination requirements.[96] As pathology became more specialised under the weight of new discoveries, the duties of the surgeon and pathologist were separated. Moore and Bowlby recognised this trend and in 1887 pressed for reform.

Bowlby, more famous for his work in the Boer War, had been appointed curator of the museum in 1881. Here he had built up the collection of surgical pathology specimens and tried to fill the growing demand for microscopic diagnosis from his colleagues. Microscopy had developed rapidly but required a certain skill in the preparation of slides. To meet an interest from the students, Bowlby had started unofficial classes on morbid anatomy as interest grew in the use of microscopes in the identification of bacteria. In 1887, he published *Surgical Pathology and Morbid Anatomy*, a guide for students that outlined the pathological process as related to surgery. Bowlby was more interested in the clinical characteristics of diseases than in bacteriology, but he did devote a section to 'micro-organisms in their relation to pathological process'.[97] Staff at St Bartholomew's were quick to appreciate his work, citing Bowlby in their textbooks as having given invaluable help with the pathology, although much of their bacteriological content remained dated.

Moore also made his contribution. He had started demonstrations in the post-mortem room in 1883, having been convinced of the merits of pathological observation by Gee (who earnestly believed that morbid anatomy gave meaning to the bedside). Following an approach that had been pioneered in the eighteenth century, Moore believed in following patients through from the bedside to the post-mortem room to uncover diagnosis and prognosis where treatment had not proved effective. Like Bowlby, Moore was

---

[94] A *Memoir of Howard Marsh* (London, 1921), p. 20.

[95] Howard Marsh, *Diseases of the Joints* (London, 1886), p. vii.

[96] *Report of the Department of Pathological Chemistry of University College London*, New Series, 1896–1902.

[97] Anthony A. Bowlby, *Surgical Pathology and Morbid Anatomy* (London, 1887).

aware of the role microbes played in disease causation and sought to integrate this approach into his pathology teaching. To improve students' knowledge of morbid anatomy, he worked with Bowlby to offer classes in microscopic pathology.[98]

Facing growing demand, Moore and Bowlby pressed for a single course on pathology as part of moves to reconsider the appointment structure. The retirement in 1887 of the deeply religious Wickham Legg, who had taught morbid anatomy since 1878, offered the opportunity to rethink 'the whole subject of pathological teaching'. Here Moore and Bowlby were assisted by an influx of junior men who were more open to the application of science to medicine. No attempt was made to copy Horsley at University College. Pathology teaching was reorganised: the lecturer was made responsible for the post-mortem room and a room next to the museum was 'stolen' for teaching. For the first time, those teaching pathology gained control from the clinical staff over post-mortems. However, teaching remained linked closely to surgery and split between various departments until the appointment of Alfredo Kanthack on Moore's resignation in 1893.[99]

At the time of Kanthack's appointment, it 'was the bright morning of bacteriology'. 'New discoveries or new applications of old ones kept rolling in' with pathology cast as the 'science of disease' and the realm of the expert.[100] Chemical pathology was adding an experimental dimension to the morphological identifications of new bacilli that had developed in the 1880s. At the same time, the 'importance of microbes as specific agents of disease was becoming increasingly recognised'.[101] Changes were also being made to the Diploma of Public Health (DPH) that reflected the growing interest in bacteriology and laboratory medicine. The appointment of Kanthack at St Bartholomew's was as much a response to these external changes as it was to the stimulus given by Bowlby and Moore.

The Brazilian-born Kanthack had been educated at University College Liverpool before entering St Bartholomew's as a student. After receiving his FRCS, he went to Berlin to study under Virchow and Koch. Germany inspired his interest in pathology and bacteriology, but when he returned to England, his first post was as midwifery assistant to James Matthews Duncan, lecturer in midwifery and physician-accoucheur at the hospital where he had

---

[98] Norman Moore, *Principles and Practice of Medicine* (London, 1893), p. 27; Norman Moore, *Pathological Anatomy of Disease: Arranged According to The Nomenclature of Diseases of the Royal College of Physicians of London* (London, 1889); Frederick Andrewes, 'Growth and Work of the Pathological Department', *St Bartholomew's Hospital Reports* xxxiv (1898), pp. 195–6.

[99] Minutes of the lecturers and medical staff, 26 March 1887, MS 12/2; Subcommittee, 4 March 1887, MS 34/1.

[100] Andrewes, 'Beginnings of Bacteriology', p. 117.

[101] Keith Vernon, 'Pus, Sewage, Beer and Milk: Microbiology in Britain, 1870–1940', *History of Science* xxviii (1990), p. 295.

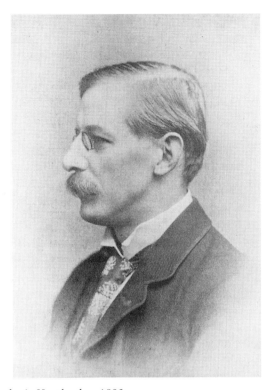

Plate 4.3 Alfredo A. Kanthack, *c.*1890

trained. After working for the Leprosy Commission in India, Kanthack went to Cambridge to pursue pathological research under Charles Smart Roy, professor of pathology. Roy had worked with Foster and was committed to an experimental approach. Under him, Kanthack organised Cambridge's bacteriological work before moving back to Liverpool, where he attracted a large number of students to his bacteriology classes. At the time, Liverpool was 'a convenient port-of-call . . . in careers that owed more to experience gained in London and Cambridge'.[102] Kanthack opposed empiricism and embraced a laboratory methodology. He considered it his 'life's mission to devote all my energy to develop the scientific spirit in medicine', arguing that every student should be taught not only to use percussion and palpation but also to use bacteriological methods to determine disease. Kanthack brought these ideas with him in 1893 when he returned to St Bartholomew's to a poorly equipped department.

---

[102] Stella V. F. Butler, 'Centres and Peripheries: The Development of British Physiology, 1870–1914', *Journal of the History of Biology* xxi (1988), p. 497.

Kanthack immediately set about convincing his colleagues that 'every thinking man' should occupy himself with determining 'what are the substances which cause pneumonia, diphtheria and tetanus? How exactly do they work?'[103] The elementary classes given by Lockwood and Harris were discontinued. After Klein agreed to transfer some of his equipment from his public health laboratory, a new series of bacteriology classes were begun under Kanthack. Modelled on the new guidelines for the London and Cambridge DPH, lectures and three-hour demonstrations were arranged to suit those who wanted to attend.[104]

Kanthack's enthusiasm encouraged a gradual transformation in attitudes in the College. Led by those interested in asepsis, staff began to argue that 'progress in Medical Science has of late been so considerable that the investigation of disease has to a large extent divided itself in to two branches, the examination at the bedside and the investigation of pathological and bacteriological products in the laboratory'.[105] Only a few like Gee remained adamant that the naked eye was better than the laboratory. Demand for expensive laboratory instruction was increasing and, with provincial universities able to offer a higher standard of science teaching than many London schools, lecturers at St Bartholomew's began to worry that it was harder 'to keep in the front rank'.[106] The symbiotic relationship established between provincial medical schools, local industry and academic institutions challenged the position of London. In the 1890s, the number of medical students in London began to decrease. The fee-based system translated this shift in the geography of medical education into financial terms, adding to anxiety in the London schools that had for so long been confident of their superiority.[107] With student numbers at St Bartholomew's having fallen since 1887, local anxieties reflected metropolitan fears. Added to concerns about competition was growing public and professional demand for laboratory facilities. The publicity surrounding the diphtheria antitoxin (announced in 1894 and used at St Bartholomew's within months) emphasised the promise of bacteriology. Local medical officers of health, who wanted to send samples to the hospital for testing, were also applying pressure.[108] However, at St Bartholomew's pressure to undertake pubic health work was of secondary importance in the appointment of a full-time pathologist.[109] Rather, it was a

[103] Alfredo A. Kanthack, 'Science and Art of Medicine', St Bartholomew's Hospital Journal, August 1898, p. 162.
[104] Kanthack and John H. Drysdale, A Course of Elementary Practical Bacteriology: Including Bacteriological Analysis and Chemistry (London, 1895), p. v.
[105] Shore to Lawrence, October 1893, 14/5.
[106] Meeting of the almoners with the medical council, 17 January 1895, HA 6/5.
[107] Butler, 'Transformation in Training', p. 126.
[108] Meeting of the almoners with the medical council, 17 January 1895, HA 6/5.
[109] Sturdy, 'Political Economy of Scientific Medicine', pp. 131–2.

combination of these pressures that forced staff to rethink the role of the hospital and the position of the College.

Encouraged by Kanthack's unofficial diagnostic work in the wards, the lecturers came to believe that the appointment of a pathologist would solve many of their perceived problems. In looking at diseases 'in a way in which they had never been investigated before', Kanthack proved that pathology had a role to play on the wards. It also helped that the growing technical knowledge needed to provide reliable pathological and bacteriological analysis made the skills of a trained pathologist essential.[110] Provincial universities and the newly formed London County Council had already made similar appointments. Other London teaching hospitals were also beginning to develop their bacteriological and public health laboratories. A lack of funds made this difficult at St Bartholomew's. Lecturers' incomes had fallen by two-thirds since the 1860s: the cost of medical education, and the need to employ more pre-clinical staff to meet the demand for science teaching, rose just as student numbers had started to fall.[111] Provincial medical schools had circumvented the problem through alliances with civic colleges and by endowing posts. The need to endow teaching and research in science had gained momentum in the 1870s as part of the university reform movement and debates on the contribution of science to industry. In medicine, endowment was viewed as a way of providing scientific teaching without increasing the burden on individual institutions. By exploiting local industrial needs and civic pride, civic universities and their medical schools succeeded in achieving financial support to fund new laboratories.[112] Some of the London teaching hospitals tried this approach, only to find strong competition from other colleges whose work had greater industrial application. The movement to establish technical colleges and polytechnics, and to provide for the needs of the sick poor, further deflected funding. In this climate, the College felt it had little prospect of endowment given the hospital's reputation as a 'prodigiously and enormously rich' institution. In addition, staff were not prepared to raise fees. The extension of the curriculum to five years had placed an additional burden on students and it was felt that if fees were increased many would go elsewhere. The solution was seen to lie with the hospital. Despite tension between the two, the tradition of seeking support from the governors was still strong. Instead of appealing to the public or to local business and medical interests, the lecturers appealed to the hospital for money to pay a pathologist.[113]

---

[110] House committee, 14 March 1895, HA 1/27.

[111] Meeting of the almoners with the medical council, 17 January 1895, HA 6/5.

[112] See Michael Sanderson, *The Universities and British Industry, 1850–1970* (London, 1972), pp. 62–81; Henry A. Ormerod, *Early History of the Liverpool Medical School from 1834 to 1877* (Liverpool, 1953), pp. 48–9.

[113] Meeting of the almoners with the medical council, 17 January 1895, HA 6/5.

A letter to the hospital's treasurer argued the necessity 'to have working in the Hospital an Officer specially skilled in Pathology and Bacteriology whose *whole* time shall be devoted to the subject and who shall carry on investigations and other original work'. Pathological investigations, it declared, were 'an essential step towards the adequate treatment not only of the patients in general, but also of particular cases actually in the wards'.[114] Initially the governors rejected the suggestion as too expensive, especially as doubts about the College's contribution to patient care made them reluctant to adopt suggestions from the lecturers at a time when finances were strained. News of the diphtheria antitoxin gave the College another opportunity to approach the governors with an offer whereby the lecturers would pay one-third of the cost of the post. Yet a discrepancy of interests existed. The College's proposed contribution was more than the salary of many of the medical staff, threatening the already low salaries the lecturers earned from teaching. Trevor Lawrence, the sympathetic treasurer (and son of the surgeon William Lawrence), used this to apply pressure on the governors. In the course of the negotiations, thinly veiled threats were made by both sides and the College became worried when some of the governors hinted that they should have 'cognisance of the whole thing'.[115] The idea of an endowment was rejected and problems were smoothed over. The governors finally agreed to appoint a pathologist on £100 per annum once they had been convinced that the post would benefit the patients. This was considerably less than the £600 initially suggested. Kanthack, who had been pressed on the governors by the medical council, was the inevitable choice.[116]

The appointment of a full-time hospital pathologist with an associated lecturership in pathology produced an immediate (if not lasting) increase in student numbers, and helped remodel attitudes to laboratory medicine. Kanthack worked to apply new advances to the bedside, adopting a familiar model of developing bacteriological diagnosis as an 'adjunct to clinical methods'. His standing, clinical skill and level of support from leading surgeons in the College ensured that his department was not seen as inferior or lacking in diagnostic authority as were such departments in other hospitals.[117] He believed that when 'symptomatology leaves us in the lurch, the microscope, test-tube, platinum needle and laboratory must come to our aid'.[118] Kanthack strove to raise the profile of pathology and bacteriology in the College. If he heard of an unusual disease, he would rush to the ward

---

[114] Subcommittee, 18 June 1894, MS 34/1.

[115] Meeting of the almoners with the medical council, 17 January 1895, HA 6/5.

[116] House committee, 9 May 1895, HA 1/27.

[117] See L. S. Jacyna, 'The Laboratory and the Clinic: The Impact of Pathology on Surgical Diagnosis in the Glasgow Western Infirmary, 1875–1910', *BHM* lxii (1988), pp. 384–406.

[118] Alfredo A. Kanthack, 'Pathology in its Relation to the Study of Clinical Medicine and Surgery', *St Bartholomew's Hospital Journal*, March 1895, p. 87.

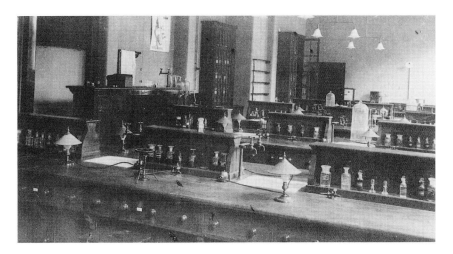

Plate 4.4 Bacteriological laboratory, c.1902–30

without waiting for a formal summons. New courses in pathological chemistry and haematology were started. Bacteriology teaching was unified even if classes were not at first compulsory. The course aimed to be both theoretical (to introduce students to the science of bacteriology) and practical (to teach students how to prepare and test samples). Detailed notes or slips were produced to explain bacteriological tests, but the system quickly became cumbersome and Kanthack replaced them with the first textbook of practical bacteriology. Work focused on German discoveries and the identification of bacilli and, with the course lasting only three months, lessons were intended to be as representative as possible.[119] Kanthack's appointment as deputy professor of pathology at Cambridge after Roy's near nervous breakdown in 1897 did not disrupt the course, which was taken over by J. Stephens, and Kanthack continued to attend St Bartholomew's for three days a week. It was during this period that Kanthack secured the appointment of six pathology dressers to work in the surgical wards to cover his absences. The creation of a new class of dresser, known as 'cutters' because most of their work involved cutting microscope sections, brought students into closer contact with pathology and bacteriology, and encouraged its integration into bedside practices.[120]

Kanthack's death in 1898 was seen as a calamity for science. The responsibility for demonstrating the value of pathology and bacteriology to the clinical staff was taken up by Andrewes, Kanthack's unassuming but witty

---

[119] Kanthack and Drysdale, *Elementary Practical Bacteriology*, pp. vi-vii.
[120] William Girling Ball, 'History of the Medical College of St Bartholomew's Hospital' (1941), pp. 176, 184.

demonstrator who worked well with the clinical staff. Andrewes admitted that such was the extent of Kanthack's organisation that he had little to do when he took over the department. However, he consolidated Kanthack's work and built up links between bacteriology, public health and clinical medicine. Additional staff were appointed, a research scholarship founded, and the department was expanded so that by 1907 it had moved beyond the single laboratory which Kanthack had worked into a three-storey department.[121] Although St Bartholomew's was not immediately transformed into one of Lockwood's 'temples of clinical science', the introduction of pathology and bacteriology teaching did contribute to change in the culture of the College. The subjects provided a focus for laboratory-based medicine and research, blending with an emerging sense of a need to develop academic medicine.

Into the twentieth century

When Paget delivered the Abernethian Society address at St Bartholomew's in 1894, he suggested that 'science and practice seem to some [doctors] incompatible'. Paget thought this 'sheer nonsense', and argued for the application of science to medicine to improve learning.[122] Others disagreed. Speakers at the Royal Medical Benevolent College dinner in the following year, for example, saw medicine and science as already 'hand-in-glove'.[123] Such views were in the majority, reflecting growing professional confidence linked to a faith in bacteriology and pathology. However, Paget's assessment did point to a changing frame of reference. He was suggesting that science was no longer associated with pre-clinical teaching as it had been in the 1880s but had come to be linked via bacteriology and pathology to clinical practice. Kanthack echoed these views four years later. For Kanthack, 'medicine is no longer an empirical art, it is a science'.[124] Many continued to disagree and strove to defend traditional practices. In 1910, Samuel Squire Sprigge, editor of the *Lancet*, in warning about an overcrowded curriculum, continued to point to the dangers of 'an excessive elaboration of purely scientific instruction'.[125] The two approaches highlighted the different views of medicine and medical education at the end of the century. Doctors' rhetorical use of science was not sufficient to oust doubts about its real value.

Medical education at St Bartholomew's was caught somewhere between the two. By 1893, the College taught fifty-three subjects to 498 students with

---

[121] Andrewes, 'Pathological Department', p. 199.

[122] James Paget, 'On the Advancement of Knowledge by the Scientific Study of Disease', *St Bartholomew's Hospital Journal*, December 1894, p. 18.

[123] *Lancet* i (1895), p. 1322.

[124] Kanthack, 'Science and Art of Medicine', p. 166.

[125] Samuel Squire Sprigge, *Some Considerations of Medical Education* (London, 1910), p. v.

a staff of forty-one. New posts and laboratories had been added in physiology, chemistry and pathology, and the syllabuses of several science courses had been rethought to give a greater emphasis to practical work. The clinical courses, in terms of finance and staff, still dominated. Despite a growing interest in the value of pathology to clinical medicine and a greater emphasis on science teaching, the gentlemanly character of the College remained. Reginald Vick, a student at St Bartholomew's just after the turn of the century, remembered that students and nurses were still not allowed to mix. Earlier innovation had been replaced by complacency. He noted that teaching remained largely confined to formal lectures with the 'question-and-answer' style of teaching, which was later to dominate, just starting. Practical classes were often sandwiched into available time and space, although improvements to the pre-clinical laboratory facilities were made in the 1890s. A considerable amount of coaching went on in the museum and provided a valuable source of income for poorly paid demonstrators. A rigid hierarchy was also maintained. Senior staff treated their juniors in a formidable manner, and all staff had to wear frock-coats and top hats.[126]

Beneath this aura of respectability and conservatism, attitudes and ideas about medical education and medicine were beginning to change. A greater interest in pathology and bacteriology had begun to have an effect on the culture if not on the character of the College. If clinical medicine remained strong, it increasingly had to take account of the laboratory and the work of the pathological department. Although some clung to a rigid faith in empiricism, staff (and especially the younger staff) at St Bartholomew's did move towards envisaging a distinct role for science in medical education and clinical practice. By 1893, lecturers in the College were clear that 'the rapid increase in scientific knowledge' had 'greatly enlarged the scope of medical and surgical education'.[127] This view was to become stronger in the first decades of the twentieth century. A more academic model of medical education, influenced by American and German ideas, asserted itself and a greater effort was made to encourage 'scientific' learning.

[126] *St Bartholomew's Hospital Journal*, December 1945, pp. 149–51.
[127] Shore to Lawrence, October 1893, MS 14/5.

5

'Leaders of educational purpose'

The rise of academic medicine

In 1903, Samuel Gee, lecturer in clinical medicine and arch empiricist, warned that St Bartholomew's was facing a 'climactic period'. He predicted that 'greater changes' were 'impending over the Hospital than it had undergone since it was rebuilt' in the eighteenth century. Gee was referring in part to the controversy surrounding plans for a new outpatient department (opened in 1907) that threatened to split the medical staff from the governors, but also to the new system of pathology instruction introduced in 1903. His statement proved prophetic. Gee feared that St Bartholomew's was losing its distinguished position, a recurrent theme in the history of the College. He pleaded for greater emphasis on clinical research and argued that the College should be treated 'not as an appendage to the hospital but [as] an equal'.[1] Ironically Gee was a traditionalist, wary of scientific medicine, but in calling for more research, a school of pathology and greater independence he reflected a growing body of opinion that sought to rethink how medicine was taught.

If the years between 1903 and 1921 were not the 'climactic period' that Gee had envisaged, the intellectual organisation of the College was reformed. More emphasis was placed on research and a clinical academic model was adopted that attempted to integrate laboratory medicine with bedside practice. In 1919, the first clinical units headed by full-time professors were established at St Bartholomew's. Two years later, the lecturers successfully petitioned for a Charter of Incorporation, formally separating the medical school from the hospital and transforming it into the 'Medical College of St Bartholomew's Hospital'.

The formation of two professorial clinical units at St Bartholomew's has been seen as part of a new agenda for medical reform and recognition of the importance of science at the bedside. Between 1900 and 1920, university and medical education in London became a subject of intense debate. Tensions between those who upheld a vocational system of training and those who advocated a more academic, science-based curriculum as part of a university education came to characterise considerations of the structure of medical education. English reformers drew inspiration from Germany and America, but the view that the famous survey conducted by Abraham Flexner in 1910

---

[1] Samuel Gee, *Medical Lectures and Aphorisms* (London, 1902), pp. 349–50.

for the Carnegie Institute ushered in a period of reform has been cast into doubt. Both Ludmerer and Rothstein have suggested that Flexner's *Medical Education in the United States and Canada*, published in 1910, reflected changes that had gathered momentum since the 1890s.[2] The same may be said for Flexner's impact on England. Flexner was an apostle of reform and the Royal Commission on University Education in London, appointed in 1909 under Richard Haldane (later Lord), was influenced by his ideas. It supported Flexner's conception of how medical education should be organised, and historians have tended to draw a direct link between Haldane's agenda for reform and the professorial units established after the First World War.[3] These new units have been described as a revolutionary departure from established modes of teaching, but there is more to the story than the traditional chronology. Flexner's evidence did influence the royal commission, but the decision to create two professorial units at St Bartholomew's reflected an interest in scientific medicine, research and increasing cooperation with the University of London that, if influenced by Flexner and the commission, pre-dated it.

New views of medical education

Before Flexner presented his evidence to the Royal Commission in 1911 interest in reforming how medicine was taught was already apparent. Flexner's *Medical Education in Europe* quickly attracted attention in Britain against a background of dissatisfaction with the nature of training.[4] From the 1870s onwards the medial curriculum had come under increasing attack. The importance of character in training and how to achieve 'fitness for practice' in an overcrowded curriculum worried contemporaries. In these late nineteenth-century debates, science was safely confined to pre-clinical study. Under pressure from the General Medical Council, most medical schools had reluctantly accepted the importance of appointing pre-clinical teachers and had established links with local universities, especially outside London.[5] However, advances in laboratory medicine in the 1890s raised questions

[2] Kenneth Ludmerer, *Learning to Heal: The Development of American Medical Education* (New York, 1985); William Rothstein, *American Medical Schools and the Practice of Medicine* (New York, 1987).

[3] George Graham, 'Formation of the Medical and Surgical Professorial Units in the London Teaching Hospitals', *Annals of Science* xxvi (1970), pp. 1–22.

[4] Abraham Flexner, *Medical Education in Europe: A Report to the Carnegie Foundation for the Advancement of Teaching* (New York, 1912).

[5] Stella V. F. Butler, 'A Transformation in Training: The Formation of University Medical Facilities in Manchester, Leeds and Liverpool, 1870–84', *Medical History* xxx (1986), pp. 115–32.

about training and the role of science in clinical practice. Concern grew that England was falling behind; that newly qualified doctors were ill-equipped for the type of scientific practice patients were thought to be demanding on the back of a growing popular faith in scientific progress. Medical schools began to be judged not just on the size of the hospital to which they were attached but also on their laboratory accommodation.

Reformers and doctors were divided over the relevance of the laboratory and an academic environment to the training of general practitioners. At Oxford, William Osler, who had arrived from Johns Hopkins University School of Medicine to fill the Regius chair of medicine in 1905, was already attacking the neglect of laboratory studies in English medical schools.[6] Osler had been an important figure in reforming Johns Hopkins. Although less successful in establishing a clinical school at Oxford, his views were widely reported. Calls for radical reforms to teaching were also being put forward in a number of London teaching hospitals. The public was not insulated from these debates: science was incorporated into discussions about Britain's education and the nation's economic and political position in the world.

At St Bartholomew's the complacency that was felt to exist about learning and the nature of medical education in the last decade of the nineteenth century was under attack by the 1900s. Here Archibald Edward Garrod and Wilmot Parker Herringham were in the forefront of discussion on the relevance of science and academic medicine to clinical training. Holburt Jacob Waring and others were equally aware of the need for reform. It was their reworking of how academic clinical units should be established that was finally implemented.

Garrod came from a medical family and, after graduating with a first-class degree in the natural sciences from Christ Church, Oxford, he followed his father into medicine rather than pursuing a purely scientific career. After training at St Bartholomew's, further study in Vienna confirmed Garrod's enthusiasm for science, which went hand-in-hand with his interest in clinical practice. After collaborating with his father in a study of rheumatoid arthritis, he started researching the chemical aspects of urine with Frederick Gowland Hopkins. Work with Hopkins (who won the Nobel Prize in 1929 for his biochemical research) encouraged in Garrod a passion for the 'rigorous application of physiological chemistry to clinical problems'. The significance of Garrod's pioneering work on 'inborn errors of metabolism' was overlooked by contemporaries, but his interest in research and chemical pathology shaped his approach to clinical training.[7] Although, like many of his contemporaries, Garrod had received an education that stressed the importance of the bedside, the 'lack of scientific spirit and atmosphere' in

---

[6] For Osler, see Michael Bliss, *William Osler: A Life in Medicine* (Oxford, 1999).
[7] Alexander G. Bearn and Elizabeth D. Miller, 'Archibald Garrod and the Development of the Concept of Inborn Errors of Metabolism', *BHM* liii (1979), pp. 315–28.

English medical schools alarmed him.[8] The *Lancet* felt that 'there are probably few who would not agree that Dr. GARROD has . . . laid bare one of the chief defects of British methods'.[9]

Garrod looked to Germany for the solution. Interest in German methods had been present in British educational discourse since the 1850s and postgraduate study in Vienna, and frequent visits to German clinics for his research made Garrod a disciple of the German system. By the 1880s, German universities had become prestigious centres for research after earlier reforms had transformed them into institutions for 'knowledge-creation'. Medicine, exemplified by the work of Virchow on cellular pathology and Koch on bacteriology, was one of the main beneficiaries. With universities providing a framework of equipment and funding, research was believed to be easier in Germany where professors exercised direct control over wards and laboratories. The large number of students who flocked to study there supported this view, while many of the leaders of the new scientific medicine in England had also studied in Germany.[10]

Like many, Garrod recognised that the German educational system under-pinned the country's scientific standing and demonstrated the importance of science to medicine. Reflecting anxiety about England's position in relation to Germany's industrial and military expansion, he worried that England's scientific output was also falling behind. The science lobby had exploited mounting fears of German economic and military power to argue for state support: in medicine, reformers used the same arguments to call for a reorientation of the English system of training. Garrod argued that England's apparent scientific lethargy could be reversed only by adopting the best of the German system so that a new culture of research and scientific study was merged with the culture of the bedside. Osler and others had intro-duced similar reforms at Johns Hopkins in the last decade of the nineteenth century. To reproduce the system in England required a revision of medical teaching and a change in the physical environment of many schools where clinical laboratories were often separate from the wards. Garrod believed that by organising medical schools into German-style clinics to include wards and a clinical laboratory, these defects could be overcome.[11] Garrod was outlining a system of academic medicine in which he believed science and research would flourish. He was not calling for the wholesale substitution of existing facilities and practices, but a series of clinical units under professorial control.

---

[8] Archibald Garrod, 'Individuality in its Medical Aspects', *St Bartholomew's Hospital Journal*, November 1908, p. 21.

[9] *Lancet* ii (1912), p. 1599.

[10] W. H. Brock, 'Science Education', in *Companion to the History of Modern Science*, R. C. Olby *et al.* (London, 1990), pp. 946–9.

[11] Archibald Garrod, 'Laboratory and the Ward', *St Bartholomew's Hospital Journal*, 1908, pp. 65, 67.

Herringham was equally enthusiastic. He and Garrod had worked together at the West London Hospital and on a handbook of medical pathology for students. They had helped Osler form the Association of Physicians for academically minded practitioners and pressed for the opening of a chemical pathology laboratory at St Bartholomew's in 1904.[12] Having studied at Keble College, Oxford, Herringham came to St Bartholomew's once he had given up law after a few months' study at Lincoln's Inn. After a period of study in Vienna, Herringham started teaching in the College as an assistant demonstrator of practical anatomy in 1884. A specialist in kidney disease, and with considerable administrative abilities, he was an idealist with a disregard for inessentials. These qualities made him appear formidable. Like Garrod, he felt 'justly proud' of the practical nature of medical education in England but was acutely aware of the need for reform. While praising the work of general practitioners, Herringham felt that in eschewing experimentation 'a spirit of content with a hand-to-mouth existence' had been fostered. This attitude had belittled the laboratory. Herringham agreed with Garrod that the solution lay in a series of clinical units under professorial control. Rather than rendering existing clinical teaching redundant, he believed these would build on established practices and 'throw a new light even upon the common problems'. Under clinical professors, Herringham argued, students would be infused with 'not only a spirit of criticism . . . but the hopeful spirit of inquiry', so that England would 'recover . . . that place in [medical science] which she has lost'.[13]

Garrod and Herringham were not alone at St Bartholomew's in advocating an academic model of medical education. The College had a tradition that stressed 'academic' performance, and Garrod and Herringham were supported by Anthony Bowlby, lecturer in surgery and close friend of Herringham's, Thomas Shore, dean from 1906, and Hoburt Waring, lecturer in surgery. Shore had originally opposed any extension of the University of London's authority, but, frustrated by the lack of time he was able to devote to his research, he gradually moderated his stance and came to support a university model as the best way of promoting science, research and the interests of the College. At a practical level, however, Waring was the most influential. He worked tirelessly for St Bartholomew's and was an avid supporter of the University of London, representing the Faculty of Medicine on the University Senate between 1911 and 1920, when he was elected dean of the faculty. Waring had strong convictions and saw the need for closer links between the London medical schools and the University. Although

[12] Wilmot Parker Herringham, Archibald Garrod and W. J. Gow, *A Handbook of Medical Pathology, for the Use of Students in the Museum of St Bartholomew's Hospital* (London, 1894).

[13] Wilmot Parker Herringham, 'On Medical Education in London', *St Bartholomew's Hospital Journal*, February 1919, pp. 47–9, 59–61.

inconsiderate, his domineering character ensured that he was able to exert a considerable influence on the College's administration, pushing it towards an academic system.

The interest Garrod and Herringham expressed in research, and their vision of creating academic clinics in existing London hospitals, was a reaction to shifts in medical practice that were encouraging optimism about the value of science. Neither was their support for the university and clinic unusual: both were endorsing a university model at a time when the university had re-emerged 'as the favoured site of medical instruction' in the search to democratise higher education and match it to the demands of industrialisation. In the university, many found the best way to bring together the laboratory and the clinic.[14] How a university would promote research was more uncertain. Johns Hopkins, where the best of the German professorial system had been combined with a British emphasis on clinical experience, provided a model for reform. By 1920, this university model had become the goal in how clinical training should be organised in Britain.

Science and the practice of medicine

At the beginning of the twentieth century the ideas outlined by Garrod and Herringham were gaining acceptance at St Bartholomew's after a series of retirements made them easier to express. Old stalwarts like Dyce Duckworth, who already feared the decline of art in medicine, were being replaced by younger men more willing to combine laboratory science and clinical work. Many had studied in Germany. A growing generational split challenged the College's traditional conservatism and faith in empiricism, promoting a climate more sympathetic to change. Yet, in many ways, the acceptance of science remained limited to diagnosis and treatment where it could be seen to have practical benefits. Although Herringham and Garrod's conception of how medical education should be advanced was not universally shared, their calls for a scientific spirit and better system of clinical instruction reflected a gradual shift in emphasis at St Bartholomew's.

Science emerged at the bedside at a slower rate than in pre-clinical teaching or in the rhetoric of practitioners who used it to assert their professional status. The laboratory was a symbol of scientific medicine that overlaid a variety of practices and attitudes. In most hospitals, however, a new spirit had started to emerge by 1900, though not without a struggle. From the 1870s, a growing number of doctors had begun to argue that the laboratory and diagnostic technology could offer a certainty in diagnosis that medicine lacked. 'From Listerian antisepsis . . . to the new serum and chemotherapeutic

[14] A. H. Halsey, *Decline of Donnish Dominion: The British Academic Professions in the Twentieth Century* (Oxford, 1992), pp. 37–8.

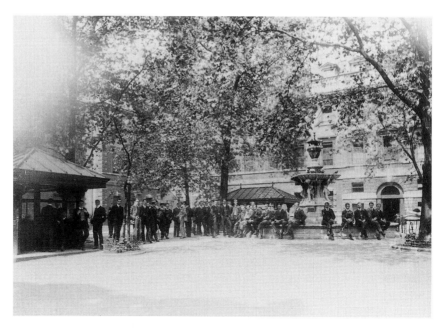

Plate 5.1 Doctors and students congregating in the Square before the start of ward rounds, 1906

regimes of the 1890s and 1900s', those working in hospitals slowly 'came to embrace a constellation of concepts and techniques' associated with the laboratory.[15] For Blume, such methods became a resource for further professionalisation and specialisation and a way of attracting patients and money.[16] Scientists' and clinicians' interest in science often diverged, but their rhetoric and enthusiasm paved the way for the development of laboratories in the diagnosis, treatment and labelling of diseases. Although few doctors were prepared to call themselves scientists, the laboratory had been assimilated into the culture of the medical elite by the 1920s. Tensions remained between the bench and the bedside, and many tried to strike a balance to produce a 'safe' science that did not threaten traditional clinical skills. It was this balance that Garrod and Herringham were calling for.

Earlier hostility to science at St Bartholomew's declined as a laboratory and bacteriological construction of disease supplanted earlier models of

---

[15] Russell C. Maulitz, '"Physician versus Bacteriologist": The Ideology of Science in Clinical Medicine', in *The Therapeutic Revolution*, ed. Morris J. Vogel and Charles E. Rosenberg (Philadelphia, 1979), p. 92. For how the laboratory began to shape the explanation of diseases, see Andrew Cunningham and Perry Williams, eds, *The Laboratory Revolution in Medicine* (Cambridge, 1992), pp. 209–47.

[16] Stuart S. Blume, *Insight and Industry: On the Dynamic of Technological Change in Medicine* (Cambridge, Mass., 1992).

explanation. By 1900, a certain fervour for bacteriology had come to exert an influence over teaching and clinical practise at St Bartholomew's where previously staff had advocated a more empirical approach. Old and new approaches existed side by side until after the First World War by which time many of the older staff had retired. This enthusiasm for pathology and bacteriology was more than just rhetorical. The number of surgeons appointed in the 1900s who had worked either in the pathological museum or as demonstrators of pathology helped the College embrace laboratory medicine. The more progressive doctors read up about new advances and pressed for their adoption in the wards. They considered scientific investigation 'an essential step towards the adequate treatment not only of the patients in general, but also of particular cases actually in the wards'.[17] This view was espoused by Thomas Horder, demonstrator of practical medicine and pathology. He warned of the dangers of 'divorcing clinical observation from pathological research' and advocated that clinicians should undertake clinical pathological procedures.[18] Horder introduced lumbar punctures and established blood cultures as a diagnostic tool for infective endocarditus despite opposition. He also celebrated the importance of the bedside and was highly critical of laboratory workers, asserting that 'to change the physician for the pathologist can but end in disaster'. While welcoming science at the bedside, Horder firmly believed that doctors should undertake all such clinical work.[19] Horder's attitudes revealed a tension that was not easily resolved. However, his enthusiasm for science, together with that of other lecturers in the College, forced new ways of thinking about disease that did not fit easily with older attitudes or the initial lack of practical pay-offs.

Although neither the hospital nor the College became major centres for bacteriological or pathological advance, staff did attempt to employ laboratory techniques in the wards. The surgeon Henry Butlin found it 'difficult to understand' in 1900 how doctors in the hospital could 'work efficiently before the institution of the pathological laboratory'.[20] It helped that laboratory diagnosis was easily constructed as an adjunct to clinical work with the clinical staff remaining in control of what was requested for testing and how the results were used. As Worboys has stressed, this made the

[17] Subcommittee, 18 June 1894, MS 34/1; ibid., 25 November 1905, MS 34/2; Statistical tables, MR 42/24, pp. 188–95.
[18] Abernethian Society, 18 November 1910, SA 1/14.
[19] Thomas Horder, *Clinical Pathology in Practice: With a Short Account of Vaccine-therapy* (London, 1910), pp. 13, 9. For Horder's approach to science and the bedside, see Christopher Lawrence, 'A Tale of Two Sciences: Bedside and Bench in Twentieth Century Britain', *Medical History* xlii (1999), pp. 421–49.
[20] Thomas Horder, 'On the Importance of Pathological Examinations', *St Bartholomew's Hospital Journal*, January 1911, p. 55; *Lancet* i (1900), p. 1859.

incursion of the laboratory less threatening for clinicians.[21] Under Alfredo Kanthack, lecturer in pathology, the pathological department worked to apply new advances to the wards at a time when clinicians at other hospitals were not so easily convinced of the value of pathology.[22] At first, applied pathology was used to verify diagnoses by 'microscopic examination', but a new technique devised by Kanthack for providing faster tissue diagnosis made it indispensable to the 'practical surgical diagnosis of tumours'. To ensure the effective application of these methods, the demonstrator of pathology was frequently asked to attend operations to help guide surgeons. Laboratory-based analysis was not limited to pathology. The preparation of vaccines and sera, with its promise of a specific cure, became part of the 'every-day work connected with vaccine-therapy'.[23] Blood, sputum and secretions were tested for anthrax, tuberculosis, anaemia or leukaemia, but the number of cases investigated was at first small in comparison to total admissions.[24] The adoption of these methods was not, as Sturdy has suggested, to enhance medical administration or to meet local public health needs, but to improve diagnosis and therapeutic efficacy.[25]

However, by 1903 it had become clear that St Bartholomew's was losing ground. Almroth Wright's laboratory at St Mary's was attracting influential support and had grown rapidly since it was opened in 1902. At University College, plans were well advanced for a new 'School of Advanced Medical Studies' to overhaul teaching and research, while The London, St Thomas's and the Middlesex could boast an expansion of their research and laboratory facilities.[26] The pathological laboratory at St Bartholomew's on the other hand was confined to a small area separated by a screen from the main physiological classroom with additional space in the science workroom. Rooms were overcrowded, and this was felt to hinder research and teaching at a time when other schools were establishing new departments. A fall in

---

[21] Michael Worboys, 'Vaccine Therapy and Laboratory Medicine in Edwardian Britain', in *Medical Innovation in Historical Perspective*, ed. John V. Pickstone (Basingstoke, 1992), p. 97.

[22] Steve Sturdy, 'Medical Chemistry and Clinical Medicine: Academics and the Scientisation of Medical Practice in Britain', in *Medicine and Change: Historical and Social Studies of Medical Innovation*, ed. Ilana Löwy (Montrouge, 1993), pp. 381–2; L. S. Jacyna, 'The Laboratory and the Clinic: The Impact of Pathology on Surgical Diagnosis in the Glasgow Western Infirmary, 1875–1910', *BHM* lxii (1988), pp. 384–406.

[23] Thomas Horder and William Girling Ball, 'Notes on the Preparation and Uses of Bacterial Vaccines', *St Bartholomew's Hospital Journal*, November 1908, p. 69.

[24] Lelland Rather, *The Genesis of Cancer: A Study in the History of Ideas* (Baltimore, 1978), p. 111.

[25] See Steve Sturdy, 'The Political Economy of Scientific Medicine: Science, Education and the Transformation of Medical Practice in Sheffield, 1890–1922', *Medical History* xxxvi (1992), pp. 125–59.

[26] *BMJ* i (1906), p. 1444.

student numbers was blamed on 'the want of accommodation'. Staff pressed for better facilities for 'a more complete bacteriological and histological investigation of every case'.[27] The need not to be seen to be falling behind in a competitive market for students, and a concern about fees, saw moves to reverse this perceived trend.

The governors were approached and the interests of the College and hospital were again linked. Temporary arrangements were made to provide additional space for pathology and bacteriology and a separate pathology block, funded by the governors, was opened in 1909. Additional laboratory accommodation and a separate library named after Kanthack (where staff had their afternoon tea) were added. The new block was designed to 'bring our Hospital thoroughly up to date'; to help staff and students 'keep pace with the increase of knowledge which is so rapidly changing the conditions of medical practice'. It expressed a robust faith in the future of pathology in the treatment of disease. Frederick Andrewes, who headed the department, believed that the building represented 'a new epoch in the history of the hospital'.[28] Pathological chemistry, haematology, bacteriology and morbid histology were seen as new tools for doctors that would amplify the ordinary observation of the patient. Separate laboratories were provided for each field of inquiry. The *BMJ* thought the new building would do 'much to promote the chances of successful treatment in the wards, and go far towards ensuring the utilisation of scientific methods among the general practitioners of the future'. In 1910, it was seen as the 'most complete pathological department in the country'.[29]

With the opening of the new block, and efforts to extend vaccine therapy in the wards, a concerted effort was made to develop the bacteriological and histological investigations carried out on patients. The variety and frequency of tests increased as doctors sought confirmation or explanation in the laboratory. Pathological investigations of tumours to determine malignancy were routine by 1910. Interest in blood chemistry and the presence of leukocytes as an indicator of infection was furthered by new methods of testing that required a smaller amount of blood, making the procedure more practical. New techniques encouraged a greater use of blood counts and cultures to aid or confirm treatment, especially for fevers.[30] Chemical and urine tests were used in differing degrees by the medical staff now that they had lost some of the unreliability that had characterised earlier procedures. Patients were also more likely to have a series of bacteriological and pathological samples taken from them during the course of their treatment.[31] 'Speaking

[27] Board of studies in pathology, 19 March 1908, MS 106/1.

[28] *St Bartholomew's Hospital Journal*, June 1909, p. 129; Frederick Andrewes, 'The Meaning of the New Pathological Block', ibid., pp. 136–7.

[29] *BMJ* i (1909), p. 1188; ibid., ii (1910), p. 690.

[30] Statistical tables, MR 42/16–21; Medical register, MR 16/57.

[31] Statistical tables, MR 42/21–4; Surgical pathological register, PATH 8/2–8; Medical and surgical registers, MR 16/67–81; Horder, *Clinical Pathology*, p. 151.

generally', explained Andrewes, 'when any patient vomits, coughs up, or passes from the bowel any unfamiliar substance, it is sent up for pathological investigation'.[32] Because they were 'beyond the powers of the clinician' these had to be conducted away from the wards in a laboratory. These procedures were the essence of Garrod's 'scientific method'. However, the complexity of these pathological and bacteriological methods made it harder for students to observe or undertake all but the simplest of tests.

Scientific teaching and research

Before 1890, students received little training in the new branches of pathology and had few opportunities to work in laboratories. Training at St Bartholomew's was equated with tradition and observers felt that in many respects students were treated like schoolboys. By the start of the twentieth century, the importance of applying science to medicine had begun to gain acceptance and teaching was beginning to be put on 'a basis of experimental science'.[33] The successes of bacteriology in diagnosing and controlling diseases gave reformers a persuasive argument for placing greater emphasis on science in the medical curriculum. Younger lecturers at St Bartholomew's shared the reformers' faith, but uncertainty was still voiced about the validity of the new methods at the expense of a gentlemanly education and clinical experience. Teaching was caught in a paradox. It remained firmly located in the clinical culture that had come to characterise English medical education, but the College also prided itself on the efforts it had made from the late 1880s to introduce experimental science. The new sciences of pathology and bacteriology were seen as an extension of this. Such an attitude, backed by a wealthy hospital, initially made the introduction of pathological and bacteriological teaching easier than elsewhere, where uncertainty and lack of funds hampered development.

Classes were introduced in practical and clinical pathology and bacteriology in 1903. Teaching across the College was divided into fifteen departments to promote systematic instruction: pathology was placed on the same footing as medicine, surgery and obstetrics. Facilities were at first primitive, but the pathology block, with its combination of accommodation for research, instruction and routine work, greatly increased the teaching facilities. The opening of the venereal department further extended the pathological work conducted in the hospital, instruction being provided in

---

[32] Frederick Andrewes, 'The Work and Needs of the Pathological Department', *St Bartholomew's Hospital Journal*, April 1904, p. 106.
[33] W. S. Feldberg, 'Henry Hallet Dale', *Biographical Memoirs of the Fellows of the Royal Society* xvi (1970), p. 90.

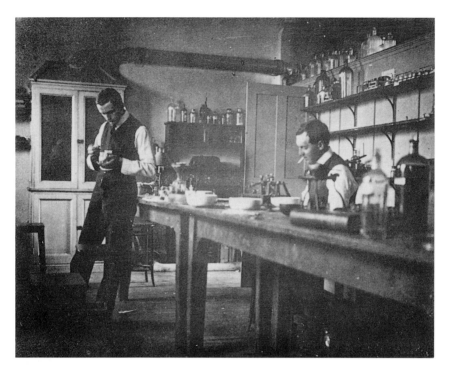

Plate 5.2 Two men at work in the 'scientific workroom', undated

taking blood for testing.[34] In 1912, a new scheme of pathological clerking was adopted, mainly at the insistence of the energetic William Girling Ball, who had been awarded the Luther Holden research scholarship for his work on surgical pathology and had recently been appointed senior demonstrator of pathology. Students working in the pathological department had been unsupervised and had carried out work 'not always considered as sufficiently reliable'. They had often been asked to identify unfamiliar micro-organisms or even to prepare vaccines without previous bacteriological training. Under the system devised by Girling Ball, pathological clerks were placed under the demonstrator on duty and encouraged to work in pairs. Additional demonstrations were organised. The hope was that better work would be produced for the department and that students would be given training in 'direct reference to individual patients'.[35] As a result, clinical teaching was reorganised and a system of practical lectures and demonstrations introduced

[34] Medical Council, 3 April 1901, MC 1/2; *St Bartholomew's Hospital Journal*, September 1917, p. 113.
[35] Board of studies in pathology, 22 May 1911, MS 106/1.

which saw all staff undertaking some teaching.[36] The aim was to promote systematic instruction within a less rigid structure, but the changes had been made with clinical practice in mind. The new system was praised as admirable, and by the 1920s it was felt that all students were being 'brought up in a bacteriological atmosphere'.[37]

An interest in bacteriology, histology and pathology at ward level did not mean a rejection of bedside medicine or a dramatic change in the style of teaching. Formal teaching was confined to lectures or demonstrations with a 'question-and-answer' style of teaching (which was to become predominant by the 1940s) only beginning to emerge. However, clinical consultations did start to form an important part of teaching. Students were invited to attend meetings of the clinical staff when doubtful or difficult cases were discussed. This served to counterbalance the instruction in the outpatient departments where students often went 'without proper supervision' and did much of the work. Despite problems, staff were clear that laboratory and clinical medicine had to go hand-in-hand, with the laboratory providing the scientific study of disease not always possible at the bedside.[38] A close dependence between the two was seen as vital. Even Flexner, who was critical of English medical education, admitted that such methods filled 'every requirement of sound and thorough teaching' because 'the student observes the patient from all sides'.[39]

A bacteriological understanding of infectious disease also improved the status of medical research. Late nineteenth-century debates over the value of science in education had included calls for a greater emphasis on research. Scientists started to colonise universities and force a research agenda to raise their professional status. Claims were made that this would make universities useful to the nation, but attitudes were slow to change.[40] Lecturers at St Bartholomew's were ambivalent. Staff working in the 'scientific workroom' in the 1890s pointed to the absence of a research culture and remembered investigations to be essentially amateur. Researchers at other medical schools faced similar problems and staff at St Bartholomew's admitted that more needed to be done to support research.[41]

In 1900, the importance of research was finally acknowledged when Thomas Lauder Brunton, lecturer in clinical medicine, appealed for a

---

[36] *St Bartholomew's Hospital Journal*, October 1912, p. 3.

[37] 'Beginnings of Bacteriology at St Bartholomew's', ibid., April 1928, p. 100.

[38] Ibid., May 1951, p. 197; 'Clinical Medicine as an Aid to Pathology', ibid., December 1909, p. 34.

[39] Flexner, *Medical Education*, p. 128.

[40] T. W. Heyck, *Transformation of Intellectual Life in Victorian England* (London, 1982), pp. 114, 173–5.

[41] *St Bartholomew's Hospital Journal*, February 1951, p. 31; Stella V. F. Butler, 'Centres and Peripheries: British Physiology, 1870–1914', *Journal of the History of Biology* xxi (1988), pp. 487–8.

research laboratory. Actively engaged in physiological and pharmacological research and having studied for three years in Germany, he had built up a pharmacological laboratory in the hospital's scullery. By 1900, this was clearly inadequate for the modern school St Bartholomew's claimed to be. Brunton argued that the presence of a research laboratory was essential to the proper functioning of the College.[42] The governors acknowledged Brunton's plea and helped to build up the College's research infrastructure. Edward Klein, as lecturer in bacteriology, had already encouraged some students to use his laboratory for bacteriological research, and when the Local Government Board withdrew support in 1904 the additional space was used for students.[43] Kanthack had been less successful in establishing a research department: in 1905 it was rejuvenated and given a commercial role as the Clinical Research Department, mirroring the public health departments established in civic universities. As part of the new treatment and teaching complex, it aimed to promote research by selling its services to those who otherwise did not have access to a laboratory.[44] However, the governors remained uncertain about using hospital funds to support research when it was not linked to patient care; nor could student fees cover expensive research or laboratory facilities. With the College unable to hold endowments, there was little possibility that new initiatives could be paid for by charity.

The creation of the Medical Research Committee (later the Medical Research Council (MRC)) in 1912 as part of the 1911 National Insurance Act dramatically increased funding for research.[45] The MRC sought to encourage a biomedical approached that did not fit easily with the research pursued in London's hospitals. Research cultures clashed in the 1920s, but the idea of making money available to support researchers had already been accepted by St Bartholomew's. In 1910, the unpopular Lawrence scholarship, awarded to clinical students for proficiency in medicine, surgery and midwifery, was converted to the Lawrence research scholarship to promote chemical pathology, largely at the insistence of Herringham.[46] Six years earlier, a scholarship had been established to facilitate research on surgical pathology. By 1919, research work of all kinds had become, if not a byword in the College, at least an acknowledged feature of clinical work. Many of the younger staff had come to recognise that a 'spirit of research' had to form part of the normal working of the College.[47] However, research continued to be sandwiched between the demands of clinical and private practice. It

---

[42] Wellcome: Lauder Brunton to College, 1900, MS 5970.

[43] Subcommittee, 22 June 1904, MS 34/2.

[44] Board of studies in pathology, 12 February 1905, MS 106/1.

[45] See Joan Austoker and Linda Bryder, eds, *Historical Perspectives on the Role of the Medical Research Council: Essays in the History of the Medical Research Council* (Oxford, 1989).

[46] Memorandum, May 1910, DF 118; Luther Holden scholarship, MS 73/10.

[47] Mervyn Gordon, 'The Spirit of Research', *St Bartholomew's Hospital Journal*, June 1920, pp. 128–9.

remained essentially a private enterprise. Scientific investigations were often 'confined to those most urgently required for the immediate treatment of patients'. With 'so much routine work ... and so many patients to deal with', lecturers at St Bartholomew's suffered the same frustrations experienced by doctors at other schools.[48]

Haldane and the clinic

Changes in the practice of medicine at St Bartholomew's and the views put forward by Garrod, Herringham and others started to shift teaching towards a more academic model. At the same time, debates over the structure of the University of London and the nature of medical education offered a context for discussion. Since 1888, efforts had been made to develop the University beyond an examining body so that it had more control over teaching and a greater role in research. From the start, medicine was seen as an important field for development, but late nineteenth-century reforms proved unsatisfactory and left a legacy of problems.[49] In 1909, a Royal Commission on university education in London was established to settle disputes between those who supported the primacy of internal degrees and those who felt that the external degree was being marginalised. The commission was also concerned with the University's administration. Various faculties had complained that the University's internal management favoured paralysis and medical schools championed the need for a more representative system that did not favour inactivity. The commission was a political solution to a difficult set of problems, part of a national policy to improve access to university education.

Haldane's appointment to chair the commission was a significant choice. Although later active in the War Office and as Lord Chancellor, Haldane 'lived in the cause of education' and wished to develop university life away from what he believed were the stultifying traditions of Oxford and Cambridge. He saw the endowment of research as crucial, but resisted plans for a second professorial university in London in favour of reforming the existing system. Working with the Fabian social reformer Sidney Webb, he had forced legislation to give the University 'a powerful teaching side', in an attempt to break a system that lent itself to cramming. However, even Haldane admitted that the 1898 London University Act was far from 'ideal' and did little more than patch up the existing system. The Act allowed the

---

[48] *Medical Education in London: Being a Guide to the Schools of the University of London in the Faculty of Medicine* (London, 1908), p. 104.

[49] *RC on a University for London*, PP (1889) xxxix; *RC to consider the draft charter for the proposed Gresham University in London*, PP (1894) xxxiv; Negley Harte, *The University of London, 1836–1986* (London, 1986), pp. 144–60.

incorporation of University College and King's College (finalised in 1905 and 1908 respectively), and united the ten London medical schools into a faculty of medicine while leaving them independent.[50]

The 1898 Act did encourage limited reforms. Attempts were made to realign the University's administration to give colleges more influence. Seven boards of studies in medicine and the related sciences were established. A decision by the government in 1901 to award a fixed grant further boosted teaching by increasing the number of endowments the University received. In medicine, grievances about the examining system, which was considered too hard and unattractive to students, were immediately addressed along with the structure of the arts and science degrees.[51] Efforts to devise a new medical curriculum had been delayed by the restructuring of the University and it was not until 1903 that a revised MB examination was finalised. Pre-clinical subjects were separated from clinical study, reflecting how these subjects were taught, and separate examinations were introduced in medicine, surgery and obstetrics.[52] Changes to teaching at St Bartholomew's were linked to this rethinking of how the different disciplines were administered. The existing pre-clinical subcommittees were converted into boards of studies, and additional boards were created for the clinical subjects to produce a departmental structure on to which professorial posts were later grafted.[53]

Efforts to instil a more homogeneous university identity were less successful. The new structure disappointed the medical schools, which in turn frustrated the University's efforts to promote greater coordination. Abortive attempts to create a University pre-clinical school encouraged criticism and the revised MB came under attack. Groups within the University saw the greater flexibility of the MB as leniency, and the matriculation examination as an unnecessary obstacle. Fears about declining standards combined with falling student numbers to raise questions about the structure of medical teaching. In 1908, the BMJ was clear that in the eight years since the revised regulations had been introduced defects had emerged that required urgent investigation.[54] Medical education was seen to be in crisis.

The Royal Commission of 1909 to 1913 was aware of the hostilities that existed between the medical schools and the University. How this relationship could be improved and how medical teaching should be organised were therefore important concerns from the start. Outside London, medical education had already undergone a major institutional restructuring

[50] 'Lord Haldane and the Prospects of Educational Reform', Contemporary Review ciii (1913), pp. 305–14; Richard B. Haldane, An Autobiography (London, 1929), p. 125.
[51] Harte, University of London, pp. 164–78.
[52] ULL: Report of the Principal on the work of the University, VP 1/1/1.
[53] Subcommittee, 17 November 1905, MS 34/2.
[54] BMJ i (1907), pp. 886–7, 960, 1005–8, 1093, 1496; ibid., i (1908), p. 946.

that had pushed medical schools into closer contact with civic universities. The move had promoted the development of pre-clinical laboratory-based departments and improved the status of provincial schools.[55] As they became more successful in attracting students, the London schools felt threatened and the general downward trend in student numbers became linked to pressure to reform the University. The 1898 Act was not the answer the London schools were looking for. A growing body of opinion argued for rationalisation, and critics of the non-university structure of medical training voiced fears about the neglect of laboratory medicine. Looking to Germany and the USA, reformers and critics agreed that the solution lay in a university medical education. Influenced by these concerns and by events outside London, the commission turned its full attention to medicine in 1911.

Flexner was already in Europe to garner an account of medical education for the Carnegie Foundation. He found the time 'one of the richest episodes of my life' and he later believed that he had personally persuaded Haldane to address the problems presented by medical education.[56] Flexner was encouraged to state his ideas clearly and, though his evidence did not entirely match the system he was describing, his support for the German-style professorial clinics adopted at Johns Hopkins influenced Haldane. Haldane was easily won over. He had studied comparative education in Berlin and favoured the German approach to science and research.[57] The other commissioners were also well aware of Flexner's ideas. In repeating criticisms made in *Medical Education in Europe*, Flexner voiced concerns that were finding expression in the London medical community and played on fears for England's scientific standing that echoed anxieties about national efficiency.

Flexner's main criticism was that 'clinical teaching . . . remains an incident in the life of a busy consultant'. Few subjects, he went on to argue, had consequently been emancipated from clinical control. This had stunted development in an environment where no rewards were given to stimulate research. The solution was a university model with closer interaction between medical science and the clinic to 'break the existing level of mediocrity'.[58] University College was identified as the most suitable starting point for reform: it had been influenced by German and Scottish university teaching, and had already appointed professors of medicine and surgery. The need to promote research had been recognised by the Faculty of Medicine in

---

[55] Butler, 'Transformation in Training', pp. 115–32.

[56] Abraham Flexner, *I Remember: The Autobiography of Abraham Flexner* (New York, 1940), p. 133.

[57] See Richard B. Haldane, *Education and Empire: Addresses on Certain Topics of the Day* (London, 1902).

[58] *RC on University Education in London, Third Report*, PP (1911) xx, q. 2–6; *Final Report*, PP (1913) xl.

1905, but Flexner's ideas reinforced existing efforts in the University to build up a professoriate.[59]

The need for a 'teaching' university in London had been asserted since 1888 and other witnesses agreed with Flexner that medical education had to be restructured to achieve this. Osler was the main proponent of these views and was considered an expert on medical education and clinical teaching. In a widely reported address to the Northumberland and Durham Medical Society in 1911, he had already asserted the primacy of the hospital unit and noted the glaring defects in provision for laboratory-based medicine. He pleaded for more funding to support hospitals' scientific work, arguing that universities were indebted to hospitals for the training they provided.[60] Addressing the Commission, he recognised that despite obvious handicaps a considerable amount of research was already being undertaken in London but felt more could be achieved and better teaching secured if the University played a greater role. This could be accomplished, he argued, only through the creation of three medical and three surgical units in London similar in style to those he had helped introduce at Johns Hopkins. Units, in his view, represented a grafting of the University on to the hospital, 'an active invasion of the hospitals by the universities'.[61]

Not all welcomed the Germanic/Hopkins model, feeling that it was the antithesis of the English system. Differences emerged over the exact nature of the units and whether the professorial staff should be full- or part-time. Most of the London schools were sympathetic, however, and suggested variations on the theme.

'A foolish way of beginning'?

Before the Royal Commission was appointed, staff at St Bartholomew's had started to discuss the structure of teaching. In 1903, the *Times* speculated that staff were pressing for a closer relationship with the University.[62] Three years later, Waring secured the appointment of a 'special committee' to investigate whether St Bartholomew's should follow University College to become an incorporated college.[63] At the time, the idea that the College should end its voluntary association with the hospital was an attractive proposition. Divisions had emerged between the medical staff and the governors over the

[59] ULL: Report of the Academic Council for transmission to the Royal Commission on university education in London, Part i, May 1910, pp. 99–100, AC 1/2; ibid., Part ii, May 1912, 7, AC 1/2.

[60] *Lancet* i (1911), pp. 211–13.

[61] *RC on University Education, Third Report*, pp. 342–5.

[62] *Times*, 11 December 1903, p. 11.

[63] Agenda book, 31 May, 28 June 1905, MS 16/2; Subcommittee, 9 March 1906, MS 34/2.

provision of a new outpatient department and suggestions that the hospital should be rebuilt on another site. In 1906, relations between the two continued to be uneasy. Links between the hospital and College ensured that the latter was affected by the dispute just at a time when it wanted money to extend its research and laboratory accommodation. The financial position of the College had been deteriorating from the 1890s onwards as the cost of medical education rose. It became difficult for the College to pay 'a living wage' to its teaching staff, while the need for an additional £20,800 for modernisation (a sum that could not be realistically met from student fees) further strained resources. The College had traditionally expected the governors to come to its aid, but with the hospital facing financial problems with rebuilding, it was no longer in a position to support the College. Endowment was believed to be the only alternative that did not commit the College to either stagnation or a level of borrowing it could not sustain. At University College, incorporation had encouraged an influx of endowments, and provincial schools had already attached themselves to the new civic universities to gain access to facilities they could not otherwise afford.[64] Other London medical schools were thinking along similar lines. Interest in incorporation was not motivated only by internal politics or financial concerns however. In 1910, the University's Academic Council recommended that incorporation should be pursued 'where possible' to promote the 'unity of higher education in London'.[65] Although the London medical schools resisted being 'pushed around by the upstart University', Waring and Herringham were able to persuade lecturers at St Bartholomew's that incorporation would solve most of the financial difficulties facing the College.[66]

From the 1840s, the College had worked to associate itself with the University of London, and James Paget's tenure as Vice-Chancellor between 1883 and 1895 had strengthened these links. By 1894, staff were prepared to support any university that gave medical schools greater representation.[67] Between 1902 and 1907 clinical staff welcomed plans to create a single centre funded by the University to provide instruction in chemistry, physics and biology. Existing accommodation for these subjects was considered outdated at St Bartholomew's and the lecturers were pressing for additional room for pathological and surgical teaching. By transferring these subjects, which were seen as of lesser importance by the clinical staff, room could be found for expansion. Cooperation with the University over the Institute for Medical Science was seen as one way of restructuring the College. The other London

[64] ULL: Report of the Academic Council, Part ii, May 1912, 34, AC 1/2; Butler, 'Transformation in Training', pp. 115–32.

[65] ULL: Report of the Academic Council, Part i, pp. 12–17, AC 1/2.

[66] Harte, *University of London*, p. 193.

[67] *RC to Consider the Proposed Gresham University*, q. 11786–815.

medical schools remained unconvinced. Jealousies between the schools encouraged resistance, many fearing that the proposed Institute for Medical Science was designed to strengthen University College and King's College. Although the Westminster and St George's, followed by Charing Cross, agreed to abandon pre-clinical teaching, the scheme collapsed and the other medical schools set about strengthening their pre-clinical departments, frustrating further attempts at coordination.[68] At St Bartholomew's, teaching was reorganised, and the space provided by the new pathological and outpatient block was reluctantly utilised to meet some of the deficiencies in pre-clinical teaching.[69]

However, efforts to work with the University did not end. During the building of the pathological block the College approached the Senate to determine if it was willing to cooperate to develop the block 'into a Centre for Higher Teaching and Research' along similar lines to the University Physiological Laboratory established under Augustus Waller. Interest was voiced in 'bringing the University into closer touch with its Colleges'. Although the Academic Council agreed to investigate, the appointment of a Royal Commission halted discussions.[70] In other respects, the College was already closely involved in the management of the University. Many of the lecturers were active in the Senate and in the Faculty of Medicine, often taking a prominent part in discussions. Pride was taken in the academic standing and university status of the College. Incorporation was therefore seen not as a radical departure but as the extension of an already close relationship.

Waring's committee reported in 1909. It confirmed that the College had 'no corporate existence' and was entirely dependent on the governors, who appointed the lecturers and owned the buildings. The situation was considered to place the College at a 'serious disadvantage in comparison with University Colleges in London and the Provinces', preventing it from holding property or endowments to support 'Lecturerships, maintain laboratories and carry on research'. The committee suggested that incorporation would remove these problems but believed that the 'active cooperation of the Governors' was vital.[71] Not every member of the teaching staff welcomed the move: some wondered if the prospect of endowment was sufficiently real to warrant an 'alteration in our present fortunate relations with the hospital'.[72] The governors had their own misgivings and feared a loss

[68] A. H. Sykes, 'A. D. Waller and the University of London Physiological Laboratory', *Medical History* xxxiii (1989), pp. 228–9.

[69] Subcommittee, 9 May, 16 June, 6 November 1905, MS 34/2.

[70] ULL: Minutes of Senate, 24 February 1909, ST 2/2/25.

[71] Report on the advisability of making the medical school a separate corporate institution, 1909, DF 7.

[72] Moore to Shore, 8 February 1909, DF 7.

of control. Waring helped soothe these concerns, but, with difficulties in agreeing to the wording of the proposed charter, frustration mounted on both sides.

During discussions over a charter, attention was given to the reorganisation of clinical teaching on a university model. St Bartholomew's was relatively unaffected by the atmosphere of uncertainty that surrounded Haldane's investigation and, as the largest medical school in London, it was less worried about falling student numbers. However, it aimed to offer something different to attract students at a time when all courses in London were considered to be fundamentally the same. To collect more information about clinical teaching Garrod visited clinics in Munich and at Guy's, and Herringham travelled to Edinburgh. Their reports confirmed a growing view that whereas 'the system of clinical teaching now in use in the College is on the whole best for the training of the undergraduates' there was room for improvement.[73] With reform being discussed, Flexner became a regular visitor to the College and Osler was invited to address the Abernethian Society.[74] A decision was made to supplement the 'ample Laboratories, Libraries or other facilities for Research' with a closer association between teaching in the inpatient and outpatient departments. Existing firms were coordinated into clinics under the control of a physician or surgeon, redistributing pedagogical authority and establishing a clear hierarchy to promote coherent and practical teaching. Lectures were made more practical, and were reorganised into medical and surgical strands with one lecture in three designated 'clinical'. Five medical outpatient clinics, each under a specialist, were created to give a greater role to teaching in the new outpatient department.[75] The proposed alterations had implications for the hospital and staffing. To solve the latter problem, and to help 'such research as the Physician or Surgeon may direct to make', a new tier of chief assistants was established. Efforts were made to fill these posts and staff discussed the possibility of appointing clinical professors to give the new clinics academic guidance in response to the University's attempts to expand its professorial staff.[76]

It was no surprise therefore that when representatives from St Bartholomew's were asked to give evidence to the Royal Commission in 1912 they presented a detailed statement that supported the need for professorial units across London. Of all the medical schools giving evidence, St Bartholomew's presented the most detailed proposals, outlining a practical way of achieving the ideals expressed by Flexner, Osler and others. Existing clinical teaching was staunchly defended and the need for more research

---

[73] Subcommittee, 11 July 1911, MS 34/2.
[74] Flexner, *I Remember*, p. 145.
[75] Subcommittee, 22 January 1912, MS 34/2.
[76] Ibid., 8 January 1912, MS 34/2.

asserted. Garrod stressed that far more could be achieved in England if those without 'original' minds were guided by a professor. Herringham dismissed Flexner's idea of strengthening teaching in a university hospital. He believed that not only were there enough competent men in London to run clinics, but that 'if you begin by creating the maximum ill will, it is a foolish way of beginning'.[77] The idea was to graft 'some of the points which are characteristic of the German methods' on to existing accommodation and bedside teaching. No revolutionary plan was suggested because those giving evidence believed that it was important to find a way of establishing units quickly without engendering too much opposition or disruption. Recognising that medical schools found it difficult to attract endowments, they recommended that any units established should be open to every medical student in London and funded by the University. It was anticipated that this would avoid adding to existing jealousies. The commissioners were not impressed. Despite the practical nature of the College's proposals, the commissioners concluded that they would not 'give the University even the beginning of a properly organised Faculty of Medicine' and that this would lead to fragmentation between competing schools.[78] This was precisely what St Bartholomew's had been trying to avoid.

The Commission's recommendations fitted with established thinking on the need to raise the level of science in the curriculum. Influenced by the evidence of Ernest Henry Starling, professor of physiology at University College, the commissioners called for the strengthening of traditional scientific departments. The same interests were continued in its recommendations for clinical teaching. 'The main features of the [report]', explained Haldane, 'are a recognition of the great strides being made in university education by the United States and Germany'. Medical education in London was described as weakly organised with subjects not taught by men 'actively . . . engaged in the advancement of knowledge in the subject they teach'. The existing system of appointments was attacked, as was the lack of cooperation between doctors and those working in laboratories. The report concluded that the only way forward was to place medicine on the same full-time and academic footing as other university subjects. This would ensure that teaching was no longer dominated by doctors teaching on a part-time basis and by men who, it was felt, often promoted their own diagnostic and therapeutic skills by focusing on difficult or spectacular cases. Hospitals, the report explained, had to be used 'to the fullest extent for medical education and the advance of medical science', so that the distinctive system of English clinical teaching be maintained. Medical schools were therefore to be brought under the control of the University and a university medical centre

---

[77] RC on Medical Education, Fifth Report, PP (1912) xxii, q. 12577–94, q. 126001–4, q. 12798–810, q. 12656–98.
[78] Ibid., Final Report, p. 117.

formed. As a transitional measure, the commissioners suggested that units be created in medicine, surgery and gynaecology at three existing schools under professors who would 'devote the greater part of their time to teaching' final year students and research.[79] Change was to be gradual.

Flexner was pleased with the outcome of the Commission and believed that 'no more incisive document on the subject has ever been written'.[80] The *BMJ* recognised that it was more than just a series of criticisms and saw the report as a 'treatise on the aims of university education'. The ideas expressed in the report became the new orthodoxy. It justified critics' assessment of the problems facing London's medical schools and endorsed their solutions.[81] Support and substantial funding from the American Rockefeller Foundation encouraged the conviction that it was essential to develop professorial units.[82] How much science should be taught, when and by whom proved harder questions to answer. The solution was not as straightforward as Haldane hoped and the aspirations outlined by the report resurfaced, finding expression in the Goodenough (1944) and Todd (1968) reports.

After Haldane

The final report of the Royal Commission had a mixed reception. Although controversy over proposals that the University should be concentrated in a 'University quarter' in Bloomsbury deflected attention from the findings on medical education, these remained a source of anxiety. Some welcomed the fusion of the basic medical science with hospital medicine, feeling that the unit system was the logical extension of existing trends.[83] Among these were Garrod and Herringham. A larger, more conservative body of opinion criticised Flexner's doctrinaire approach and attacked the Commission as 'the attempted Germanisation of London University'.[84] They feared a loss of authority and were suspicious that in adopting the Commission's recommendations the University would look no further than King's College or University College. Others worried that in moving towards a system of academic teachers, doctors 'obsessed by something they called scientific medicine' would be produced who had little contact with patients. The main

---

[79] Ibid., pp. 98–136.

[80] Thomas N. Bonner, 'Abraham Flexner as Critic of British and Continental Medical Education', *Medical History* xxxiii (1989), p. 475.

[81] *BMJ* i (1913), p. 836.

[82] See Donald Fisher, 'The Rockefeller Foundation and the Development of Scientific Medicine in Great Britain', *Minerva* xvi (1978), pp. 20–41.

[83] *BMJ* ii (1920), p. 8.

[84] 'The Attempted Germanisation of London University', *Medical Press and Circular*, 7 October 1914, pp. 368–9; *TES*, 6 May 1913, p. 79.

concern was that by bringing research and laboratory work into the hospital traditional bedside skills would be lost.[85]

The Faculty of Medicine of the University pronounced a mixed verdict that defended the nature of clinical teaching in London. It agreed that medicine should be taught 'by a community of workers devoted to the pursuit of knowledge', and that this required a close alliance between teaching and research. Concerns were expressed about the commissioners' understanding of the structure of clinical teaching. The faculty thought the Commission's notion of a 'hospital unit' was very different from the ideas expressed by Osler and others. It reasoned that if units were to be established they should not be limited to medicine, surgery and gynaecology. Convinced that Osler had a better understanding of the problems facing London, it concluded that whereas the overall tenet of the report was to be supported, in practical terms many of its proposals were either ill-suited to London or ill-thought-out. It asserted that

the University atmosphere would be best created in a medical school by the encouragement of those who seem to possess the necessary qualifications to pursue research untrammelled by the necessity for earning their daily bread, and this end could be obtained with the least disturbance of existing methods by the appointment in each medical school of one or more professors of advanced medical subjects.

These professors were to devote their time to research and 'a certain amount of teaching of the academic type'.[86] The faculty rejected the Commission's notion of a homogeneous faculty and new university hospital, preferring a modification of the existing structure by grafting 'medical teaching of a University type' on to three schools. With the faculty made up of representatives from existing medical schools, and with staff from St Bartholomew's playing a prominent role, this attitude was hardly surprising.

At St Bartholomew's the final report had a similar reception. Fears were voiced by the governors' solicitor that an effort to move towards a university model would mean a sacrifice of control and domination of scientific interests over patient care.[87] These views alarmed sections of the governing body and made it more cautious over plans for incorporation. *St Bartholomew's Hospital Journal* defended the practical nature of teaching and was anxious about recommendations that promised revolution not evolution. It interpreted the idea of placing only three schools on an academic footing as liable to ensure

---

[85] *Edinburgh Medical Journal* x (1918), p. 46.

[86] ULL: Minutes of Senate, 20 May 1914, Ac: D, ST 2/2/30; Faculty of Medicine, 1 December 1913, AC 5/5/1.

[87] A review of the position created within the hospital by the Royal Commission, August 1914, MS 7/3.

that students would be constantly moving between these schools and their own institutions. This, it was feared, would waste time and encourage many to abandon the University's degrees in favour of the less prestigious Conjoint Board. London, it was felt, was too big to mimic Cambridge.[88] The *Lancet* agreed: it worried that a two-tier system would be created and reflected a widespread opinion at St Bartholomew's that 'if the hospital unit organisation is a good one, why should the advantages of the university influence be limited to three hospital schools?'[89]

Doubts about the Commission's findings were not shared by those running the College. They aimed to coordinate teaching and improve research, and used the report to reinvigorate discussion. The ideas suggested in 1911 were revisited and the need for a system of clinical units under a director was stressed to make 'teaching more complete'. This was not seen as a departure from the existing system of clinical teaching, which was already considered to be 'of University type'. Changes in 1911 had restructured clinical departments so that they were similar to the proposed 'Hospital Units'.[90] It was felt that more control had to be sacrificed to the University through the appointment of full-time professors to promote cooperation with the University. Incorporation, many in the College argued, would achieve this, serving to revitalise discussions between the College and the governors. The financial situation had deteriorated since 1906 when discussions over incorporation had started. The rebuilding of the outpatient department and a rolling programme of internal renovation to modernise the hospital had strained resources. The governors had implied that steps should be 'taken in order to make the Medical School self-supporting and thus relieve the hospital of the heavy annual expenditure', but disagreements over the aims of incorporation prevented the charter from being finalised.[91] It was only after a further year of negotiation that Lord Sandhurst, the hospital's treasurer, was able to secure a compromise. Advising both sides that the charter would not create an administration too dissimilar from existing arrangements, he encouraged the lecturers to agree to maintain the school 'to the satisfaction of the Governors'.[92] The governors were then persuaded that in return they should render the lecturers 'any reasonable assistance and facilities for that purpose'.[93] With an agreement reached, a petition for a charter was presented to the Privy Council and then to the Board of Education.

---

[88] *St Bartholomew's Hospital Journal*, December 1913, p. 36.

[89] *Lancet* ii (1913), p. 1637.

[90] Subcommittee, 3 July 1913, MS 34/2; Statement on the views of the medical officers and lecturers, 8 December 1913, MC 5/7.

[91] Resolution, 1908, MS 6/2.

[92] Memorandum, May 1912, DF 8.

[93] Shore to Sandhurst, 6 November 1912, DF 8.

The Board of Education, already convinced that the 'scheme of the Royal Commission [was] calculated to produce a University of London worthy of the name', welcomed the proposal. The Board had been formed in 1902 to supervise the educational provision of local authorities, but a successful application for a grant-in-aid by St Mary's Hospital in 1908 gave the Board a financial interest in how medical education was organised.[94] The Board in giving money recognised that fees, civic money and philanthropy were insufficient to fund higher education. Other schools in London quickly followed St Mary's after a decision by the King Edward Hospital Fund for London in 1906 prevented any portion of its collections from being diverted to teaching or research. The Fund's decision threatened the philanthropic income of London's medical schools just as they were seeking to endow teaching and research.[95] A fall in student numbers from 650 per annum in the 1860s to some 250 in the 1900s heightened fears. The poor financial climate made it difficult for schools to meet the cost of laboratories and encouraged them to approach the Board for funding as one way of securing additional support.[96] Grants came at a price, however. In adopting a model already embraced by other government bodies, the Board used its grants to exert influence on how medical education was organised. To encourage medical schools to transfer preliminary teaching to the University of London, students undergoing preliminary training were excluded from how grants were calculated. The Board also insisted that the payment of clinical teachers had to be placed on a defined basis and that medical schools it assisted should establish a 'proper system of government and management'.[97]

St Bartholomew's was the last London medical school to secure a grant from the Board of Education, coming under the scheme in 1913. Efforts were immediately made to comply with the Board's guidelines. Student registration was improved and a salaried structure introduced for the staff. The process of allocating shares of the fees to staff, which had defined payment since the 1790s, had become overly complicated. The move to a salary structure did simplify the process, but increased financial burdens made comparisons with other medical schools possible, adding to pressure for a more uniform system. The grant also strengthened interests in incorporation.[98]

[94] W. F. Bynum, 'Sir George Newman and the American Way', in *The History of Medical Education in Britain*, ed. Vivian Nutton and Roy Porter (Amsterdam, 1995), pp. 41–2.
[95] Frank K. Prochaska, *Philanthropy and the Hospitals of London: The King's Fund, 1897–1990* (Oxford, 1992), pp. 57–8.
[96] Leslie P. Le Quesne, 'Medicine', in *The University of London and the World of Learning, 1836–1986*, ed. F. M. L. Thompson (London, 1900), p. 137.
[97] George Newman, *Some Notes on Medical Education in England: A Memorandum Addressed to the President of the Board* (London, 1918), pp. 3–4.
[98] Hetherington to Shore, 30 July 1914, DF 184; Finance Committee, 11 November 1914, MS 31/2.

In September 1913, the Board of Education appointed a departmental committee to consider the implementation of the recommendations of the Royal Commission. The committee saw its duty 'to approach the governing bodies of three hospitals of sufficient size and endeavour to make arrangements for the transfer to the University of the financial and education control of the medical schools attached to them'.[99] St Bartholomew's was the first to be approached. Delegates from St Bartholomew's stressed that while they 'were in sympathy with the aim of the Commissioners and wished to give their hearty co-operation in carrying out the principles of the support' they wanted to protect patient care. They accepted that the University should assert more control over the College, and welcomed the idea that St Bartholomew's might become a constituent college, placing it on a par with University College. After further meetings with St Bartholomew's, University College, The London and St Thomas's, the committee supported efforts to create units and went on to adopt most of the suggestions which Garrod and his colleagues had presented to the Royal Commission. It agreed with St Bartholomew's and the Faculty of Medicine that local professorial units should be established, predicting that those schools which did not become incorporated colleges would be placed in an inferior position.[100]

European and national events overtook the Board of Education. The outbreak of war with Germany in 1914 cut short debate and redirected attention from the University of London and the problem of medical education.

A Barts man at the Board of Education

According to Bonner, the First World War acted as a 'dramatic reminder' of the clinical and observational roots of medicine. A more practical balance between the laboratory and the ward did emerge after 1918, but the value of science continued to be stressed as part of concerns that future economic competition would 'call for far larger, greater, more persistent and more intelligent efforts' in science than before.[101] The end of the war saw a rush of statements on the public responsibility for science. Educationists and the government became convinced that science could be effectively encouraged by extending the state's support for universities. Government patronage through the newly formed University Grants Committee (UGC) increased and professional training was made a priority. A higher level of state support combined with predictions that there would be a flood of researchers returning from the trenches to stimulate universities to expand their

---

[99] PRO: Memorandum, UGC 5/2.
[100] PRO: Departmental committee on the University of London, 22 July 1914, UGC 5/2.
[101] *The Times*, 28 March 1919, p. 14; Thomas N. Bonner, *Becoming a Physician: Medical Education in Great Britain, France and Germany and the United States, 1750–1945* (New York, 1995), p. 307.

laboratory facilities.[102] In this new climate, the link established between medicine and science in the late nineteenth century ensured that medicine was seen as an important area for development. War had strengthened the appeal of clinical research and the 'union of laboratory studies with the close observation of disease at the bedside' became part of the MRC's eclectic funding policy.[103] War, in the *Lancet's* opinion, had also allowed for mature consideration of the issues surrounding medical education. Revolutionary change was predicted.[104]

Medical issues were high on the postwar Board of Education's agenda. Robert Morant, permanent secretary to the Board, and George Newman, late chief medical officer and the Board's principal assistant secretary, were leading figures in the campaign that led to the creation of the Ministry of Health in 1919. After 1917, the Board advocated a hierarchical structure for medicine that required a shift in how doctors were trained. With the Board awarding grants to all but four of the twenty-two medical schools in England, it had a stake in reform as part of the spirit of wholesale reconstruction. The MRC offered its support, believing that work of real value was being hampered by the lack of an effective university base.[105]

In 1918, Newman published *Some Notes on Medical Education in England*, which set out the Board's agenda on medical education. Energetic and influential but considered by some to be cautious and a poor administrator, Newman was a strange mix of educationist, clinician and medical officer of health (MOH). The press saw him as an eminent civil servant, an 'apostle of preventive medicine', and an expert on infant mortality. Friends regarded him as an enthusiast who went about his work tirelessly.[106] Born into a Quaker family, he had a short formal academic career at King's College London, where he had studied before he was appointed MOH for Bedfordshire and then for Finsbury having taken the Diploma in Public Health at Cambridge. In 1906, he accepted the post of public health lecturer at St Bartholomew's, perhaps because of the College's proximity to Finsbury and Clerkenwell where he had worked as an MOH. He arrived already well established in the field, having publishing extensively on bacteriology and child health.[107] In the following year, he was appointed lecturer in sanitary

---

[102] Robert E. Kohler, 'Walter Fletcher, F. G. Hopkins and the Dunn Institute of Biochemistry: A Case Study in the Patronage of Science', *Isis* lxix (1978), p. 348.

[103] PRO: MRC annual report 1919/20, p. 28, FD 2/6.

[104] *Lancet* ii (1918), p. 259.

[105] PRO: MRC annual report 1919/20, p. 29, FD 2/6.

[106] *The Times*, 22 July 1916, p. 6; *TES*, 27 February 1919, p. 103. For Newman's early career see Margaret A. E. Hammer, 'The Building of a National's Health: The Life and Work of George Newman to 1921' (unpublished D.Phil. diss., Cambridge, 1995).

[107] See George Newman, *Bacteria, Especially as they are Related to the Economy of Nature, to Industrial Processes, and to the Public Health* (London, 1900); George Newman and Harold Swithinbank, *Bacteriology of Milk* (London, 1903); Newman, *Infant Mortality: A Social Problem* (London, 1906).

law and then chief medical officer to the Board of Education. Although he continued to teach at St Bartholomew's, the Board of Education attracted an increasing amount of his time and was for him 'like a blooming dream'.[108] The College responded by appointing a public health tutor. Newman remained connected to St Bartholomew's in a formal capacity until 1914 and then as emeritus lecturer, keeping in contact with the staff despite his growing commitments at the Board of Education.[109]

At the Board, Newman worked hard to establish the school medical service, and after St Mary's had made a successful application for a grant-in-aid he was appointed medical assessor to the standing committee that allocated the grants. As medical assessor, Newman visited London's medical schools where he felt he discussed 'fully and frankly with the staffs difficulties and defects which they have themselves pointed out'. The Royal Commission, changes in the practice of medicine, and wider interest in the value of science and the need to train effective general practitioners, encouraged Newman to look into how medical education was organised. He met Osler and Flexner, and in 1912 made a rapid tour of medical schools in both the USA and Germany to collect information. War redirected his efforts but once the burden of his wartime administrative duties had declined, he resumed visiting medical schools in England.

Newman had 'absorbed relatively little from his tour' of America and Germany, but *Some Notes on Medical Education in England* echoed many of the ideas outlined by Flexner.[110] As a public statement, *Some Notes* was a moderate version of the views he had outlined in a memorandum to the Board of Education in December 1917. To the Board, he deplored a system of medical education where there was 'no unification; no University standard and no central control' and was dominated by 'too many "casuals" and too much "pot-boiling"'. 'Complete medical education of a university standard', with clinical lectures, bedside teaching and instruction in the laboratory and outpatient clinics within the setting of a clinical unit, presented a way of resolving these problems. Newman's support for a unit system came from his interest in training general practitioners. In the published version, he called for a holistic approach to medicine that stressed the importance of preventive medicine. The creation of clinical units was for Newman essential in achieving these aims.[111]

The system Newman was pressing for was closely allied to the practices he

---

[108] Wellcome: Newman to Hatty, 6 September 1907, MS 6206.

[109] Agenda book, MS 16/4.

[110] Bynum, 'Newman and the American Way', pp. 41–2.

[111] PRO: George Newman, 'Some notes on medical education', Memorandum to the Secretary of the Board of Education, 28 December 1917, ED 24/1961; Steve Sturdy, 'Hippocrates and State Medicine: George Newman outlines the Founding Policy of the Ministry of Health', in *Greater than the Parts: Holism in Biomedicine, 1920–1950*, ed. Christopher Lawrence and George Weisz (Oxford, 1998), pp. 112–34.

had seen at St Bartholomew's, and to the ideas that were being discussed in the College when he was there. Close contact already existed between St Bartholomew's and the University and pressure for incorporation was growing. Efforts had been made to teach students in the various outpatient departments and Newman praised the College's 'regular and numerous lectures by the whole staff, medical group consultations and clinical demonstrations in special subjects'.[112] These had all been introduced between 1905 and 1912.

Newman remained pragmatic at the Board of Education and in his public support for clinical units. He defended bedside medicine, and agreed with staff at St Bartholomew's that a wholesale adoption of the recommendations made by the Royal Commission would provoke hostility. A policy of gradual reform was therefore needed. To achieve these ends, Newman advocated further grants from the Board of Education, reflecting the state's increased financial commitment to science. Initially, money was to be used to fund units at St Bartholomew's, The London and University College because he believed they were the most likely to establish units. From this starting point, Newman anticipated that further units would be created. To prevent grants from becoming 'a system of doles for which there is no adequate reform in educational value', he recommended that they should cover only three-quarters of the costs.[113] The Board of Education accepted the ideas outlined in the memorandum and started negotiations with the Treasury for additional funds. The MRC was equally receptive and put aside plans to fund hospital beds for clinical research in favour of the unit system.[114]

The published version of 'Some Notes' was not intended as an '*ex cathedra* pronouncement' and underplayed the full force of Newman's support for clinical units. However, in endorsing a view of medicine that was both academic and practical and a more 'intimate association' between teaching and research so that the 'conquests of physiology and pathology [could] be brought into the work and applied by clinical teachers', it stressed the need to place medical schools under university control and establish full-time professorial units. This, Newman argued, would promote the necessary 'interrelationship between the study in laboratory science and the clinical practice of medicine'.[115] Newman's idea challenged not only the existing structure of medical education subsequent to the Haldane report but also the social organisation of clinical training.

When *Some Notes* was published, few were aware of the extent of the Board of Education's commitment to the unit system. Doctors, politicians and educationists, including Flexner, Haldane and Osler, wrote to Newman

---

[112] Newman, *Some Notes*, p. 76.

[113] Ibid.

[114] Christopher C. Booth, 'Clinical Research', in *Historical Perspectives on the Role of the Medical Research Council*, ed. Austoker and Bryder, pp. 208–9.

[115] Newman, *Some Notes*, pp. 18–27, 74–9.

expressing their approval, but it was his ideas on clinical units, rather than his enthusiasm for extending preventive medicine that attracted attention.[116] *The Times* wholeheartedly attacked what it felt was a system that 'prostitutes teaching appointments' and upheld Newman's call for a university medical education.[117] In his review of *Some Notes*, Clifford Allbutt, Regius professor of medicine at Cambridge, called for units to be established 'in every adequate clinical school', implying that a school would be inadequate without one. Only through units could schools be freed from Harley Street, that 'grave of the great clinical teacher'.[118] The London medical schools were, however, less certain and were reluctant to cede their independence as Haldane and Newman suggested.

Postwar reconstruction

Teaching had been carried on at St Bartholomew's with considerable difficulty during the war. Part of the hospital had been given over to the War Office and tensions had mounted between the demands of the military casualties and the needs of the civilian patients. The number of students (and therefore the income of the College) had fallen, and many of the teaching staff were either in the Services or had been stationed at other hospitals to treat returning casualties. With the collapse of the German front in 1918, St Bartholomew's and the country turned its attention to reconstruction. Imperfections in the medical curriculum and examination system were discussed with renewed vigour. Waring persuaded the University's Faculty of Medicine to establish a committee to investigate 'the changes that may be desirable in Medical Education'. At St Bartholomew's, a reconstruction committee was formed on the advice of Shore and Girling Ball. Its members were influenced by *Some Notes*, and the committee overlooked the problems facing the hospital to concentrate on 'medical education and research'.[119]

The committee's first report in 1919 returned to the ideas expressed before 1914. St Bartholomew's, unlike other medical schools in London, was no longer 'generally unsympathetic to experimental, academic medicine'.[120] A fall in student numbers added an additional incentive. With the College's income cut by one-third, closer contact with the University offered the potential of extending teaching and research without cost to the College. It also promised to set the College apart, improving its chances of competing with other teaching hospitals.[121] After considering these points, the report recommended

[116] PRO: Newman diary, August 1918, f.110, MH 139/3.
[117] *The Times*, 1 August 1918, p. 18.
[118] *BMJ* i (1919), p. 438; ibid., ii (1918), pp. 113, 118.
[119] ULL: Minutes of Senate, 20 November 1918, pp. 543–4, ST 2/2/35.
[120] Cited in Bonner, *Becoming a Physician*, p. 331.
[121] Shore to Newman, 26 April 1918, DF 23.

a compromise with suggestions made by the Royal Commission. Four years of war with Germany ensured that no reference was made to continental clinics: the more Germanic ideals of the Commission had been discredited and Haldane's pro-German leanings had consigned him to the political wilderness. The idea that the University should assume more control was sidelined partly because the Board of Education had indicated that while it favoured full incorporation, it would support the creation of professorial units in advance of the University.[122] The Board had rejected withholding grants as a means of encouraging reform, believing that it was best to organise units quickly, 'to demonstrate . . . the necessity of reforming the university system'. Lewis Amherst Selby-Brigg, Morant's successor at the Board and an opponent of Haldane's brand of liberalism, did not want university reform to obstruct a system of clinical training that Newman had convinced him was essential. This was not what Haldane had envisaged and it went against the idea of a unified, homogeneous medical faculty.[123]

Whether Newman, given the time he had spent at St Bartholomew's, had persuaded the Board of Education to offer more than it might otherwise have done is uncertain. What is clear is that the College was already moving towards a model of teaching that Haldane and Newman had pressed for and the Board of Education wished to endorse. Although the Board claimed that it did not intend to dictate any prescribed method of teaching, special grants were given to those schools 'which are doing thorough and efficient work'.[124] However, it was Newman's promise of funding that encouraged the committee to address the need for clinical units and to look further into the issue of incorporation. Thomas Hayes, clerk to the hospital, was clear that the 'Medical Staff . . . would tell you frankly that it is purely upon financial grounds' that they favoured incorporation, given that 'a medical education on modern lines' could not be provided out of fees.[125] The fall in student numbers encouraged other medical schools to come to similar conclusions. The promise of additional funding for clinical units offered medical schools in a position to establish them a way of increasing their income without compromising their independence.

Reassurances from the Board of Education that it would not interfere in the running of St Bartholomew's swayed the reconstruction committee. Confident that autonomy would be protected, it had no hesitation in recommending the creation of three professorial clinical units in medicine, surgery and gynaecology to run in tandem with existing firms, which were reorganised into non-professorial units. No attempt was made to wait for university reform, and an application was submitted to the UGC for assistance in 'maintaining the

---

[122] Medical Council, 26 February 1919, MC 1/5.
[123] PRO: Minute from Newman, 21 November 1918, ED 24/1961.
[124] *BMJ* i (1919), p. 107.
[125] Hayes to Sanhurst, 1 August 1914, HA 11/2.

reorganised [system] of teaching'.[126] Given the situation in obstetrics and gynaecology, where an emphasis on outpatient care had resulted in an acute shortage of beds, the committee felt it was best to postpone the creation of a gynaecological unit until better provision could be made.[127] However, the committee was confident that units could be established in medicine and surgery with little disruption. Mirroring suggestions in the Royal Commission, each professor (or director) was full-time and had 'a free hand to obtain material from all Departments of the Hospital for the illustration of their lectures'. To protect the interests of the clinicians, the new professors were to have no overall 'control over the treatment of patients'. The move to a salaried system at St Bartholomew's in 1914 made these ideas easier to accept, while reassurances about clinical control, and the fact that only a limited number of professors were to be grafted on to the existing structure of clinical teaching, did not threaten clinicians' authority. Each professorial unit was to have approximately fifty beds and an outpatient clinic in addition to a clinical laboratory and an operating theatre.[128] The approval of the governors was secured in March 1919 once it became clear that they would not be expected to cover the cost of converting the wards.[129]

Other changes were suggested in line with Newman's recommendations. Teaching was extended, with the creation of a new preliminary course in practical medicine, surgery and pathology to prepare students for the wards. Other courses were changed to make teaching more relevant to the postwar clinical setting, especially in therapeutics and orthopaedics. It was recommended that all departments should be improved with additional laboratory accommodation created in the pre-clinical departments to promote 'good teaching'. To solve the problem of an inadequate obstetrics department, pre- and antenatal clinics and additional beds for the 'diseases of pregnancy' were called for.[130] Part of a rising national campaign bolstered by the 1918 Maternal and Child Welfare Act, services were designed to extend antenatal work and develop teaching. However, the need for professorial units initially overshadowed these objectives.[131]

By August 1919, the Board of Education had agreed to award an additional grant to those schools seeking to establish professional units. Despite being

---

[126] Medical Council, 26 February 1919, MC 1/5.

[127] Medical Council, 26 February 1919, MC 1/5. It was not a position unique to St Bartholomew's. The failure to standardise medical teaching of obstetrics had become a scandal, and the need to provide more beds and better training in obstetrics worried the College throughout the interwar period: see Chapter 6.

[128] Medical Council, 26 February 1919, MC 1/5.

[129] Treasurer's and almoner's minute book, 28 March 1919, HA 3/40.

[130] Medical Council, 21 May, 8 July, 1 October 1919, MC 1/5.

[131] Ibid., 10 March 1920, MC 1/5; Board of studies in midwifery, 9 July 1919, MS 105/1; see Lara Marks, *Metropolitan Maternity: Maternal and Infant Welfare Services in Early-Twentieth Century London* (Amsterdam, 1996), pp. 195–226.

embroiled in discussions over the new Ministry of Health, Newman provided constant advice. The Board considered the application from St Bartholomew's first. To fulfil Newman's idea of using grants to influence teaching, the Board imposed conditions on St Bartholomew's that neither the lecturers nor the governors had anticipated. It insisted that each unit had 'appropriate accommodation' and that 'appropriate and competent persons' should be available to teach. It was also expected that St Bartholomew's would adhere to the principles outlined in *Some Notes*, with extra instruction introduced in psychiatry, orthopaedics and paediatrics.[132] The same standards were adopted by the UGC once Newman had convinced it that the need for professorial units was too urgent and that further investigation might prejudice reform. In acceding to the Board's policy, the UGC reinforced the idea that St Bartholomew's was the most likely medical school to establish a unit and awarded a grant of £6,000.[133] Room was found for both professorial units in the south wing. Wards were reorganised and the top floor of the isolation block, recently rebuilt as part of the programme of modernisation, was converted into a temporary home for the new laboratories. This took beds away from other clinical staff, storing up antagonism for the future.

Normal procedures were suspended in the appointment of directors. To reduce opposition from clinicians who had lost beds in the reorganisation, it was decided to invite applications from the existing staff.[134] Garrod and George Gask were nominated: both had travelled extensively in Europe and America and were pioneers in their fields. Gask, a specialist in thoracic surgery known as 'Uncle George' to his students, was seen as an extremely able surgeon with an imperturbable character. Moved by a deep sense of mission to improve the education of surgeons, and renowned for his clear exposition of basic principles and unhurried manner, he was considered to be the ideal man to head the surgical unit.

Garrod and Gask took office in October 1919 after approval had been gained from the UGC. Garrod had a 'very deep sense . . . of the task which I am undertaking'.[135] Bowlby and Herringham resigned to make way for the new directors. Herringham welcomed the 'new appointment for which I have long worked and which will I am sure be of greatest benefit to the Hospital, the School and Medicine in general'.[136] It was not until February 1920 that the University was approached to ratify these appointments after the UGC had decided that it was not 'an expert Educational Body in the matter'. Although problems were also encountered over professional appointments at St Thomas's and The London, the situation at St Bartholomew's was

[132] Treasurer's and almoner's minute book, 7 August 1919, HA 3/40.
[133] PRO: UGC minutes, 25 July, 9 October, 13 November 1919, UGC 1/1.
[134] Board of governors, 24 April, 27 November 1919, HA 1/29.
[135] Garrod to Hayes, 23 September 1919, HA 34/1/33/12.
[136] General court, 24 July 1919, HA 1/29.

straightforward. The College informed the University of the arrangements, and recommended that Gask be appointed professor of surgery. As Garrod had resigned to succeed Osler as Regius professor of medicine at Oxford, the assistant director Francis Fraser was nominated to take over Garrod's fledgling unit.[137]

By October 1919, the two units had started to take patients and students.[138] Unlike University College, the College did not receive £1,205,000 from the Rockefeller Foundation. The money was seen as a 'gift to British medicine' and was backed by the MRC's interest in the hospital. The aim was to make University College into the model for other schools.[139] Incorporation and the presence of dynamic clinicians committed to research made University College an attractive site for the Rockefeller. Without such funding, and with only an annual grant of £5000 from the UGC, St Bartholomew's found it harder to provide the ideal number of beds. It was only just able to match the minimum criteria formulated by the UGC, but inspectors appointed by the University in 1920 decided to overlook this and commended both the 'zeal and energy displayed on all hands', and the working environment.[140]

Aftermath

The scheme outlined by the Haldane Commission was reduced in practical terms to the creation of a series of professorial units in London and the provinces. No new university hospital was created and the foundation of units depended on the initiative of individual schools. Those medical schools that did move to a unit system received official backing (and funding) from the UGC. It insisted that 'a University Medical Education requires that the latest advances in science which affect medicine, chemistry and physics, anatomy and physiology, pathology and pharmacology should be continually brought into the teaching of clinical subjects and applied to the observation and treatment of disease'.[141] Science and a freedom from grinding were now the desired aims, and the UGC saw in professorial units the perfect medium through which this could be achieved.

The ideas behind the units remained controversial, raising questions about how to reconcile the work of clinicians with that of university academics. Doubts were expressed about their validity and contribution to research, but by 1921 five other professorial units besides the two at St Bartholomew's had

---

[137] ULL: Minutes of Senate, 25 February 1920, pp. 1971, 3690–4, ST 2/2/36; Graham, 'Professorial Units', pp. 13–20.
[138] Medical Council, 15 October, 20 August 1919, MC 1/5.
[139] Fisher, 'Rockefeller Foundation', pp. 30–1.
[140] ULL: Minutes of Senate, 21 July 1920, p. 4348; 20 October 1920, p. 237, ST 2/2/36.
[141] BMJ i (1920), p. 776.

been established at The London, St Mary's, St Thomas's and University College. Outside London, the colonisation of civic universities by Oxbridge academics and a move away from science ensured that units were slower to emerge. In those schools where units were established, an immediate improvement was seen in teaching and treatment. More systematic lectures and clinical demonstrations in a wider variety of subjects were offered, and links with the University of London were strengthened.[142]

Although units had been established in four other schools, it was felt that the two at St Bartholomew's were 'probably beyond question' the most successful. They remained the only units where full-time directors were appointed, and were regarded in the University as 'pattern units' despite the funding University College was able to attract.[143] Student admissions rose and teaching was reorganised, but the units had another effect, forcing the issue of incorporation. Discussions deferred in 1914 with the outbreak of war were resumed and a dramatic slump in the economy in 1920 made the governors more inclined to reduce their financial responsibility. An agreement was reached over the wording of the Charter, and a new lease between the lecturers and the hospital was negotiated.[144] By 1921, the charter had been granted and 'the Medical College of St Bartholomew's Hospital in the City of London' given legal form with the right to hold investments and 'provide opportunity for research so as to advance knowledge of medicine and surgery and the allied sciences, and to promote the investigation of disease by lectures and demonstrations'. A board of governors was created and two admin-istrative bodies (the College council and the College committee) were formed, with elected representatives from the governors and lecturers. Waring was appointed vice-president; Herringham and Bowlby were made governors, and Shore, as dean, became the 'executive officer'.[145] Hospital and College were officially separated, although strong links remained. The effect was to reduce tension. St Bartholomew's became the incorporated college Waring had called for in 1906, with close links to the University assured through the professorial units.

The creation of the medical and surgical professorial units quickly revealed deficiencies in the College. The units did not bring about the immediate fusion of medicine with science that Garrod and Herringham had foreseen. An academic style of medicine had been accepted, but financial problems in the early 1920s ensured that the optimistic schemes for reconstruction were never fully implemented. With the UGC and MRC unable to fund capital projects or to endow research, additional support was difficult to obtain. Changes in the medical curriculum also prevented staff working in the units

[142] Ibid., ii (1960), p. 1823.
[143] Memorandum, 1942, DF 192.
[144] Draft lease, MS 9/10/1–4.
[145] Charter of incorporation, MS 26/1.

from undertaking the level of research originally envisaged. Although the problem was recognised in 1924 by George Adami, he concluded that professorial units had made such a significant contribution to teaching that no changes should be made.[146] Staff at St Bartholomew's were not so certain. Within four years of Garrod's appointment as director, disquiet was being expressed about the poor quality of laboratory accommodation. Particular difficulties were seen in the pre-clinical departments. It was these concerns and the question of how teaching should be developed that dominated the College from the 1920s to the outbreak of war in 1939, committing St Bartholomew's to a further period of building and expansion.

[146] *BMJ* i (1939), p. 797.

6

Deficiencies revealed

Teaching in the interwar period

Higher education expanded immediately after the First World War as demand rose and the number of students engaged in research increased. The formation of the University Grants Committee (UGC), the Committee of Vice-chancellors and Principals, the Association of University Teachers, and the National Union of Students in the early 1920s established a definable system of higher education within which contemporaries agreed medicine should be located. Prewar debates on the value of science to medical education persisted however, and became more intense. Abraham Flexner's report and the Haldane Commission were, according to the *Lancet*, revelations that had resulted in a 'troubling of the waters ever since'.[1] The academic construction of medicine outlined by the two reports vied with a view that wanted a return to traditional notions of clinical medicine – albeit modified by the findings of contemporary science. This highlighted different approaches on how medical knowledge should be constructed.

Tensions over the nature of medicine in the interwar period were worked out in discussions about the form and content of the medical curriculum, as reformers struggled to rethink the social organisation of clinical training. Familiar arguments on the value of a liberal education and the autonomy of the bedside were repeated. Dissatisfaction increased throughout the interwar period to shape the structure of teaching at St Bartholomew's, as efforts were made to promote greater cooperation with the University of London. Although a fragile consensus on the shape of reform had emerged by the late 1930s, action was pre-empted by war in 1939.

The creation of the clinical professorial units at St Bartholomew's in 1919 had resulted from a partial shift from the culture of empiricism that had dominated the school. By the end of the First World War, earlier doubts about the effect of the laboratory on the art of medicine had resurfaced among the senior staff. These men, who formed part of Lawrence's 'patrician' class, invoked a language that stressed the importance of the generalist and an English medical tradition rooted in the art of medicine.[2] Their view

---

[1] *Lancet* i (1925), p. 667.
[2] Christopher Lawrence, 'A Tale of Two Sciences: Bedside and Bench in Twentieth-Century Britain', *Medical History* xlii (1999), pp. 421–49.

diverged from that embodied in the professorial units. Although the difference was not enough to split the College – largely because the patricians' influence was in decline – St Bartholomew's remained, in effect, several institutions throughout the interwar period. It had a pre-clinical side separate from the clinical school, which was itself divided between the non-professorial and professorial units, and between full-time and part-time staff. Laboratory medicine remained contested, but facilities for laboratory teaching and research were expanded. Tension also existed between those who saw St Bartholomew's as a teaching institution, and those who wanted to encourage research. A focus on academic and clinical medicine restricted the pre-clinical departments and it was not until 1930 that agreement was reached over the need to rethink pre-clinical teaching. In moving the 'science' departments to Charterhouse, teaching was revitalised but the result proved a mixed blessing.

Deficiencies resolved!

Postwar debates in medical education returned to familiar territory as concerns about the value of specialist training were reasserted. Although St Bartholomew's had six specialist outpatient clinics by 1900, those running the College and hospital remained reluctant to appoint specialists, preferring instead to employ generalists with specialist interests. This situation was seen as symptomatic. Contemporaries keen to advance their area of expertise felt that teaching hospitals erected 'idealogical [sic] barricades' that maintained an educational framework geared to the generalist.[3] However, growing specialisation in medicine, fuelled by the expansion of university-centred training and the laboratory, patient demand, and by doctors returning from war who used it to rebuild lost private practices, gave specialists a greater role. As pressure grew to develop specialist clinics and diagnostic services in the 1920s and 1930s, London's medical schools established departments with specialists in control in areas that did not immediately threaten the incomes or intellectual traditions of the dominant generalist culture.

Following a nineteenth-century pattern, most of the specialist clinics were created to extend outpatient care. An outpatient department was less controversial than inpatient beds, and teaching was used to justify the existence of these new departments. For example, in 1926 an outpatient fracture clinic was discussed at St Bartholomew's for 'improving the teaching of the Treatment of Fractures'. No mention was made of patient care for fear of threatening the interests of the general surgeons.[4] Clinics often followed

---

[3] Cited in Roger Cooter, *Surgery and Society in Peace and War: Orthopaedics and the Organisation of Modern Medicine, 1880–1948* (Basingstoke, 1993), p. 184.
[4] Medical Council, 24 February 1926, MC 1/7.

the appointment of a lecturer, as teaching (which could be limited to lectures) responded faster than institutions. Although a delay existed between the codification of specialist fields and their institutionalisation, the pace at which they were included in training increased in the interwar period. The result was a further overburdening of the curriculum, so that the type of training geared to the needs of the majority of students who entered general practice was often neglected. This alarmed many clinicians who felt that the 'bewildering haste' to add new disciplines was not matched by a willingness to 'sweep away much that has slowly fallen into discredit'.[5] The British Medication Association (BMA) feared that the curriculum was becoming needlessly specialised and failed to meet the needs of a majority of future practitioners.[6] These views were voiced as part of an ongoing debate on the content of the curriculum but reflected anxiety about specialisation in the interwar years.

Tension remained at St Bartholomew's between support for a holistic approach that defended the role of the generalist and the inclusion of specialist fields into teaching. Attempts to employ Harold Gillies as a plastic surgeon in the 1920s were initially frustrated on the grounds of 'unnecessary' specialisation. Gillies, who had developed a leading plastic surgery unit at Sidcup during the war, was appointed to the ear and throat department as a general surgeon. It did not help that his ideas on cosmetic surgery were seen as unethical. Patients were often referred to him as a last resort and, although Gillies used them to build up the status of plastic surgery in the hospital, a plastic surgery clinic was not formed until 1933, a year after lectures in the field began.[7] Demands made on training by the General Medical Council (GMC) and by the Board of Education, which made its funding conditional on the provision of additional instruction in psychiatry, orthopaedics and paediatrics, modified this opposition to specialisation.[8] The result was a further compartmentalisation of the curriculum and an increase in the number of clinical subjects which students studied, a process that led the College to rethink clinical training.

As new specialist fields were institutionalised and examining bodies acknowledged the need to extend clinical training to incorporate them, pressure mounted on outpatient services. Between 1900 and 1939 the College encouraged the formation of a number of specialist outpatient clinics at St Bartholomew's. In 1904, a children's outpatient department was created, which under Herbert Morely Fletcher and James Thursfield quickly established a leading reputation. Two years later, the throat and nose department was consolidated; a dermatology clinic followed in 1908. More beds were called for and greater attention was paid to providing students with

---

[5] *BMJ* i (1932), p. 485.
[6] Ibid., i (1936), p. 1212.
[7] Medical Council, 31 May 1933, MC 1/9.
[8] Treasurer's and almoner's minute book, 7 August 1919, HA 3/40.

experience in specialist clinics. Other specialist clinics (for fractures, cardiology, plastic surgery and neurosurgery) took longer to emerge. On the overcrowded island site in West Smithfield the creation of specialist services was problematic. Action was limited by the interests of the general surgical and medical staff who resisted having beds taken away from them. They felt that most patients could be treated in the medical or surgical wards, ensuring that clinical instruction was given within the existing ward structure. Even with growing waiting lists and mounting concern about admissions, the hospital's governors found it hard to fund additional beds. In an effort to circumvent these problems and provide patients for teaching, the College, following initiatives elsewhere, established links with other institutions to create a patchwork of services that could be used for teaching. In 1914, a tuberculosis dispensary was opened in cooperation with the City of London; three years later another joint scheme saw the creation of the special treatment centre for venereal disease. However, it was efforts to provide clinical training in midwifery, which did not fit the ward structure, that attracted most attention. Revived from the burgeoning discourse on preventive medicine, the drive to establish maternity services reflected efforts to reconceptualise public health and strengthen hospital-centred medicine. The holistic and curative emphasis this encouraged merged with the growing professional status of obstetrics to produce a series of schemes designed to extend teaching. This brought St Bartholomew's into cooperation with other hospitals, and with the London County Council (LCC).

If the creation of specialist outpatient clinics presented a dilemma, obstetric teaching created serious problems. Although obstetrics was the cornerstone of many general practices, standards of training nationally were poor.[9] Attempts to extend practical training met with little success. Although teaching in midwifery had been offered at St Bartholomew's since the 1790s, instruction was restricted largely to lectures; limited use was made of the small number of obstetrics patients admitted.[10] The appointment of James Matthews Duncan in 1877 as midwifery lecturer to reorganise teaching did raise the moral tone and extend instruction. Duncan had been a dedicated lecturer in Edinburgh, and at St Bartholomew's he set about transforming midwifery teaching. Standards were raised and students started doing better in examinations. Although he advocated a medical model and secured the appointment of a midwifery tutor, obstetrics was still viewed as a secondary subject and Duncan's plans for a maternity department to improve training were dismissed.[11] Only in 1886 did the second Medical Act draw

[9] See Ornella Moscucci, *The Science of Woman: Gynaecology and Gender in England, 1800–1929* (Cambridge, 1990) for debates over obstetric training in the nineteenth century.
[10] *Lancet* ii (1868), pp. 708–9.
[11] Subcommittee, 11 February 1882, MS 34/1; James Matthews Duncan, Miscellaneous Letters, p. 40.

specific attention to midwifery as a necessary subject for qualification. In response, the GMC required students either to spend three months in a lying-in ward or to be present at twelve deliveries; yet midwifery continued to be neglected.[12] It was mounting concern for infant and maternal mortality in the 1900s that finally forced the College to rethink its obstetrics teaching. As childbirth moved out of the domestic sphere into the hospital, St Bartholomew's fell behind. The need for students to attend a lying-in hospital or ward was recognised in 1909 as an important area for development, but the district and inpatient services available in neighbouring hospitals and local boroughs were only gradually emulated at St Bartholomew's.[13] For the College, the need to meet deficiencies in teaching outweighed consideration of the needs of the local population.

When plans were outlined for the medical and surgical professorial units in 1919, they were viewed as two parts of a triumvirate and it was anticipated that a third unit for obstetrics and gynaecology would follow.[14] The GMC had stressed the importance of better teaching in obstetrics, and a committee of the Royal Society of Medicine had just concluded that instruction in obstetrics 'merits [in some cases] emphatic condemnation'.[15] However, when the units were finalised at St Bartholomew's a shortage of maternity beds prevented an obstetrics unit from being created.[16] The governors had traditionally seen midwifery as 'indirectly – if indeed at all – a department of the Hospital'. Maternity cases were officially excluded until 1911 after the lecturers had spent two years arguing that increased lying-in provision was vital for training. The governors agreed only because students required instruction in midwifery 'to enable them to qualify'.[17] Although the College wished to see beds added 'as soon as practicable', neither the surgical nor the medical staff were willing to give up room for them. As a short-term measure, it was decided to press for an expansion of outpatient services. Child welfare and maternity care were identified as two areas through which this could be achieved at a time when both had become important social and political concerns.[18]

---

[12] *Interim Report of the Departmental Committee on Maternal Mortality and Morbidity* (London, 1930), pp. 31–2.

[13] Finance subcommittee, 1 February 1909, MS 31/2. See Lara Marks, 'Mothers, Babies and Hospitals: "The London" and the Provision of Maternity Care in East London 1870–1939', in *Women and Children First: International Maternal and Infant Welfare, 1870–1945*, ed. Valerie Fildes, Lara Marks and Hilary Marland (London, 1992), pp. 48–73.

[14] Medical Council, 26 February 1919, MC 1/5.

[15] *Proceedings of the Royal Society of Medicine* xii (1919), pp. 108–34.

[16] Medical Council, 21 May, 8 July, 1 October 1919, MC 1/5.

[17] Lawrence to the College, 28 January 1902, MS 6/3/4; *League News*, 1911, pp. 214–15.

[18] Medical Council, 13 February 1918, MC, 1/5.

War revived fears about future generations.[19] Doctors were redefining their attitudes to pregnancy and had begun to shift attention from the infant to the mother. The result was greater emphasis on antenatal care and hospitalisation. The newly formed Ministry of Health made money available to voluntary and local bodies under the 1918 Maternity and Child Welfare Act, which encouraged local authorities to extend maternity services, and the City of London approached St Bartholomew's with the idea of establishing a maternity clinic. Adopting the language of the maternal and child welfare movement, the College anticipated that the hospital could become a centre to coordinate 'present charitable work' and 'raise the national standard of physical health' by reducing infant mortality. With obstetrics becoming a branch of public health, lecturers argued that child welfare and maternity services created an 'additional means of education both of students and nurses' so that they became 'acquainted with these branches of preventive medicine'.[20] An infant welfare centre and antenatal clinic followed in 1920, adding to the maternal and infant welfare services encouraged by the 1918 Act. By 1926, the clinic treated over 1000 women a year and sought to provide 'opportunities both for the teacher and the student of investigation for the early evidence of pathological conditions'.[21] Although the clinic was seen as an important part of any future professorial unit, students had to fit in attendance while visiting other specialist clinics. Until the appointment of Wilfred Shaw in 1925 emphasis continued to be placed on observation, intervention and anaesthesia, and the clinics remained underutilised for teaching.[22]

Although support for a professorial unit was reaffirmed in 1925 after University College Hospital opened an obstetrics unit, attempts to create one at St Bartholomew's were temporarily abandoned. The governors had failed to add to the existing thirty-two maternity beds (twelve of which were used for antenatal cases), or to set aside laboratory accommodation necessary for an obstetric unit.[23] Doubts were voiced about whether the UGC would support 'another Professorial Unit'. However, with the UGC willing to fund a laboratory and a resident physician-accoucheur to provide clinical instruction, teaching was extended at a rudimentary level.[24] The move was

[19] See Deborah Dwork, *War is Good for Babies and Other Young Children: A History of the Infant and Child Welfare Movement in England, 1898–1918* (London, 1987); Jane Lewis, *Politics of Motherhood: Child and Maternal Welfare in England, 1900–1939* (London, 1980); Lara Marks, *Metropolitan Maternity: Maternal and Infant Welfare Services in Early-Twentieth Century London* (Amsterdam, 1996).

[20] Medical Council, 10 March 1920, MC 1/5.

[21] *St Bartholomew's Hospital Journal*, January 1920, p. 56.

[22] Lewis, *Politics of Motherhood*, pp. 124–5; Board of Studies in Midwifery, 2 February 1923, MS 105/1.

[23] AGM, 10 March 1926, MS 27/1.

[24] Joint committee, 16 February, 17 June 1925, MC 1/7.

seen as an interim measure that offered some of the advantages of a unit. Shaw was appointed because of his skill 'in teaching midwifery and evidence of research', and set about developing the obstetrics research laboratory.[25]

Shaw's appointment and the creation of outpatient maternity services did not remove pressure for a professorial unit. When the hospital started to discuss plans for the redevelopment of the Smithfield site in the mid-1920s, the College pressed for a maternity department 'comparable to that provided for patients suffering from medical and surgical diseases'.[26] Studies by the Ministry of Health revealed that efforts to combat maternal mortality had not been successful, while the formation of the National Birthday Trust Fund for Maternity Services in 1928 and campaigns by women's organisations were raising the profile of maternity care. Lack of skill or knowledge on the part of doctors, who increasingly relinquished care in ordinary cases to midwives, was blamed for the rising maternal mortality. Practical training was widely seen as insufficient, fuelling demands for medical schools to provide better obstetric services and training. Guidelines drawn up by the 1932 departmental committee on maternal mortality stressed the importance of attendance over 'mere observation', insisting that all students should spend six months on obstetrics with two-thirds of the time allotted to midwifery. It also recommended that students should spend two months working in a maternity hospital. The committee hoped that by providing better training maternal mortality would be reduced.[27] The British College of Obstetricians and Gynaecologists outlined a similar programme in 1932, further emphasising the need for doctors to be trained in antenatal care, management of normal labours, postnatal care, recognition of abnormalities and minor obstetrical procedures.[28]

Changing views on how doctors should be taught was only one aspect of the drive to create more maternity beds. Doctors were also under pressure from the Ministry of Health to ensure that all abnormal cases were hospitalised. Medical opinion was beginning to favour hospital births as an answer to high maternal mortality. For obstetricians, this offered the additional advantage of advancing their speciality. At the same time, more women were demanding hospital confinement as it became safer and cheaper. Some London medical schools had already realised that if they failed to expand their obstetric departments they would be unable to maintain their quota of maternity patients for teaching, as women would go elsewhere.[29]

[25] Medical Council, 28 October 1925, MC 1/7.
[26] College Council, 19 March 1931, MS 28/1.
[27] *Interim Report*, pp. 83–4.
[28] See *Memorandum on the Training of Medical Students in Midwifery and Gynaecology* (London, 1932).
[29] Jean Donnison, *Midwives and Medical Men: A History of the Struggle for the Control of Childbirth* (London, 1988), p. 184; *University College Hospital Magazine*, August 1930.

The College was under pressure from all sides to extend the number of maternity beds and develop teaching.

Existing training, however, had focused on a different model. Until 1911, students at St Bartholomew's had been sent to 'Mackenzie's' to learn midwifery. Mackenzie's was a shop in Cloth Fair where butcher's clothing was sold to the Smithfield meat-porters, and in the three ramshackle storeys above rooms were rented for the District Midwifery Team. Eight to ten students were in the Team, which confined its work to the mothers of the adjoining slums.[30] Every student had to spend a month in the bug-infested, 'dirty and neglected' Mackenzie's, but they received little formal instruction in midwifery before this other than a few demonstrations with a pelvis and a rubber dummy. For students, it was often their first real clinical responsibility. Duties were therefore taken seriously. Much of their work dealt with 'treating' poverty as much as it did with assisting at births. The newly qualified Extern Midwifery Assistant would take students to their first few deliveries, after which they were expected to cope on their own.[31] Students noticed a considerable improvement when Mackenzie's was closed in 1911 and accommodation provided in the hospital. Students now spent more time in the labour ward where they were taught the value of asepsis before attending births.[32]

Improvements in training could not solve the problem of access to patients. Students were seldom able to attend more than eight deliveries where the GMC and University of London required a minimum of twenty. The 1902 Midwives Act had encouraged trained midwives to send for doctors in difficult births, making it essential that doctors become familiar with home births and surgical complications. Facing a fall in the number of midwifery cases to which students had access in the districts surrounding the hospital, the College approached the Borough of Finsbury about its midwifery arrangements.[33] Recommendations from the Ministry of Health that all emergency cases should be admitted to a hospital worried the College. It also feared that Finsbury was planning to send its emergency maternity cases to the City of London Maternity Hospital since St Bartholomew's was unable to offer emergency beds. Plans to divide Finsbury into catchment areas raised further questions. The College felt that these proposals threatened to reduce the number of midwifery cases available for teaching.[34] To offset this, an arrangement was reached with the borough. The essential role midwives played in local maternity services was recognised given the shortfall in

[30] Andrewes to Lawrence, 3 July 1901, MS 6/3/1.

[31] St Bartholomew's Hospital Journal, February 1947, 3; 'The Changing Face of Bart's', ibid., December 1945, pp. 149–51.

[32] Marks, 'Mothers, Babies and Hospitals', p. 56.

[33] College Council, 31 March 1931, MS 28/1.

[34] Medical Council, 27 February 1929, 25 May 1932, MC 1/8.

obstetric beds at St Bartholomew's.[35] The College agreed to fund two midwives in return for responsibility for midwifery care in the borough. All pregnant women were asked if they were willing to be attended by a midwifery extern, and those who agreed came under the care of the hospital's antenatal clinic. Cases of antenatal abnormality were referred to the clinic, and all complications were admitted to the hospital. Postnatal care was divided between St Bartholomew's and the municipal clinic. The service survived with few modifications until 1959. For Finsbury, the arrangement removed the need to pay for midwives in an area where obstetric beds were limited; for the College it allowed students to obtain practical experience and ensured that all cases 'useful for teaching' were sent to St Bartholomew's.[36] Similar agreements with other boroughs were made by other teaching hospitals.[37] To reassure Finsbury, which worried about the standard of supervision, midwifery training was placed 'at the end of [the] curriculum'. In 1939, an additional chief assistant was appointed to improve 'practical teaching in obstetrics during actual deliveries', when it was realised that with students attending births in the district most of the teaching had to be done 'out of hours' or at night.[38]

A continuing fall in the number of home deliveries as more and more pregnancies were hospitalised forced a different approach in 1933. Attempts had been made in 1930 to reach an agreement with the City of London Maternity Hospital, which was at 'the centre of the district from which the cases are drawn for the teaching of our students'.[39] The Maternity Hospital had extensive in- and outpatient facilities, admitting an average of 1581 patients each year.[40] Staff felt that amalgamation would attract students and solve the College's problems. Although staff at St Bartholomew's and at the Maternity Hospital were enthusiastic, negotiations broke down. Discouraged, the College rejected developing links with a voluntary hospital in favour of establishing an association with the LCC's St Giles Hospital, Camberwell and St Andrew's Hospital, Bow. The move built on attempts to promote cooperation between voluntary and municipal hospitals encouraged by the Ministry of Health, which wanted to develop a more unified London hospital system. St Bartholomew's and other voluntary hospitals had already agreed to a policy of cooperation with the LCC when the Council took over the Poor

---

[35] Donnison, *Midwives and Medical Men*, p. 184.

[36] College Council, 8 July 1931, MS 28/1; *Maternal Mortality Report* (London, 1934), pp. 4–12.

[37] LMA: Central public health committee staff subcommittee, 18 November 1932, LCC/MIN/2180.

[38] College Committee, 3 May 1939, MS 29/1.

[39] Medical Council, 31 December 1930, MC 1/8.

[40] Lara Marks, 'Irish and Jewish Women's Experience of Childbirth and Infant Care in East London, 1870–1939' (unpublished D.Phil. diss., Oxford, 1990), pp. 184.

Law medical services under the 1929 Local Government Act. Elements in the voluntary hospital community remained suspicious of municipalisation, but with the 1929 Act supporting the need for 'cordial relationships' between voluntary and municipal hospitals joint consultative committees were established.[41] If the relationship was not always as envisaged, the most successful efforts to develop cooperation in London were made between the teaching hospitals and the LCC. Several teaching hospitals had already started to send their students to local infirmaries, and the LCC, under the guidance of its chief medical officer Frederick Menzies, was keen to work with individual medical schools rather than with the arrogant Voluntary Hospitals Committee.[42] An agreement between the LCC and the deans of the London schools in 1933 allowed a maximum of twelve to fifteen students to attend certain LCC hospitals on a weekly basis for demonstrations. Access to obstetric beds took longer to arrange because it was seen as a more complicated issue.[43]

The College's decision in 1933 was part of this growing cooperation and a recognition that had been increasing since the 1890s that municipal hospitals offered useful clinical facilities for teachings. Links with the LCC were made easier by its division of hospital services into treatment and residential care.[44] A rise in the number of institutional confinements helped the LCC to extend its maternity services, and local authorities became 'disinclined to allow the patients in their districts to be dealt with in their houses by students'.[45] Under the agreement, students from St Bartholomew's were sent to St Giles' and St Andrew's for two weeks for their midwifery training. It was felt that the arrangement, if not ideal, at least 'obviated the difficulties previously experienced in the teaching of midwifery'.[46] Staff from St Bartholomew's were required to select patients from a list and undertook not to intervene in diagnosis or treatment. Similar agreements were reached between other medical schools and nineteen LCC hospitals.[47] The relationship was not always harmonious.

The decisions to cooperate with the Borough of Finsbury and the LCC was a short-term solution to deficiencies in the College's teaching resources imposed by the need to extend training into specialties that had previously

[41] PRO: Cooperation between local authorities and voluntary hospitals, 1933–4, MH 58/209.
[42] Geoffrey Rivett, *The Development of the London Hospital System, 1823–1982* (London, 1986), pp. 198–9, 113–14.
[43] LMA: LCC minutes, 31 January 1933, 21 February 1933; LCC central public health committee, 26 January 1933, LCC/MIN/2181.
[44] *Annual Report of the Ministry of Health 1934–5*, p. 56.
[45] Medical Council, 10 April 1929, MC 1/8; ibid., 27 November 1935, MC 1/10.
[46] AGM, 13 February 1933, MS 27/1.
[47] *Hospital*, August 1933, p. 210.

received little attention. The model of developing teaching links and sending students to other hospitals became increasingly prominent after 1945, as the pattern of medical education and healthcare changed in postwar Britain.

Impact of the units

The opening of the medical and surgical professorial units was hailed as a great advance in medical education. The units were a result of a combination of forces that hoped to place medicine on an academic footing and fuse the laboratory with the ward. Those who advocated the units anticipated that they would impose a new intellectual order on teaching and promote research. In 1923, George Newman, in his role as chief medical officer at the Ministry of Health, reaffirmed their importance. He saw the professorial unit as embodying 'the University spirit' and the 'University standard of learning' and providing a corrective to the 'old empirical approach'. In them he felt laboratory and clinic were combined 'to train the student and extend the frontiers of knowledge'.[48] To what extent did the units at St Bartholomew's achieve these aims?

The professorial units established a full-time academic element in the College without challenging the existing structure of clinical teaching. In aligning the College with a system of training that was seen to be in the vanguard of reform, the units attracted students and staff, breaking with tradition by encouraging outside lecturers to visit and by making it easier for those not trained at St Bartholomew's to secure a post. George Gask, head of the surgical unit, shared the view of the Haldane Commission that units should be resources for the University of London and not just for the individual school. As a way of furthering his aim, he invited speakers to the College to give university lectures. Outside formal teaching, the Abernethian Society (see Chapter 7) was used to attract prominent speakers to discuss clinical and political issues keeping staff and students abreast of the latest intellectual and scientific developments.[49] The idea was to create an intellectually stimulating environment. Particular attention was given to developments in America and junior staff were encouraged to visit the USA (aided by grants from the Rockefeller Foundation). A more ambitious scheme was to invite visiting academics and surgeons to run the professorial units for a short period. Gask had hit upon the idea after his visit to the Peter Brigham Bent Hospital in Boston, where he had been invited in 1921 as temporary chief. The first to be invited to St Bartholomew's therefore was Harvey Cushing from Peter Brigham Bent. Gask wanted to develop neurosurgery and

---

[48] George Newman, *Recent Advances in Medical Education in England* (London, 1923), pp. 89, 90, 91.
[49] Abernethian Society, attendance at meetings, SA 10/4.

hoped to use Cushing's interest in cerebral surgery to encourage staff at St Bartholomew's. Cushing found the experience 'illuminating'.[50] When Gask left for the British Postgraduate Medical School in 1935 the practice declined.

Efforts to offer systematic lectures and integrate medical and surgical teaching had already been introduced before 1914, but the units were seen to bring a new enthusiasm to the College. Teaching was rethought and 'the whole Staff put its back into bringing to Bart's . . . high standards'. Work in the units was compared to 'a rocket that goes off with a bang about 9.30 am every day and sinks expiring to the ground at 6 o'clock'. Lectures became less stuffy and the previous habit of delivering them in academic dress was symbolically abandoned in favour of the laboratory coat.[51] However, divisions emerged between the academic and clinical staff, creating friction that threatened to split the College. Clinical staff with their private practices often resented the units, and kept them in a subordinate position, so that their impact on teaching was not as great as initially desired.

After the initial enthusiasm for science and the laboratory that surrounded the creation of the units had faded, some staff in the College started to worry that too much stress on science could damage clinical practice. Nationally, controversy developed over the merits of the bedside in the advancement of medical knowledge. However, as Thomas Horder explained in his retirement speech, the College resisted 'the divorce of clinical from laboratory methods' common in other schools.[52] Here the professorial units were seen to provide the science, and the non-professorial units the bedside instruction and clinical medicine that had come to typify medical education in Britain. Through the professorial units, students were introduced to laboratory medicine early in their training. George Gask and Francis Fraser, head of the professorial medical unit, tried to adapt teaching to 'the practice of medicine in its march to the goal of applied science'.[53] In the short time they spent in the units, students were trained in how to perform a variety of bacteriological and pathological examinations and were given an 'intimate acquaintance with . . . what is *not*, just as much as what *is*, possible with them'. Students were also advised to carry out practical scientific work, but it was recognised that this was not always possible. Teaching strove 'to cultivate the power of accurate observation, and to insist upon clear thinking' whether in the wards or in the laboratory.[54] New courses, centred on the units, were added, increasing the number of clinical teachers. Many adopted a therapeutic approach that by merging science and art in treatment did not challenge

[50] *St Bartholomew's Hospital Journal*, June 1922, p. 138; ibid., February 1923, p. 66.

[51] William Girling Ball, 'Autobiography' (typescript), p. 66; *St Bartholomew's Hospital Journal*, May 1938, p. 176.

[52] *Lancet* ii (1928), pp. 136–9; *St Bartholomew's Hospital Journal*, July 1920, p. 144.

[53] *St Bartholomew's Hospital Journal*, April 1929, p. 101.

[54] Ibid., January 1936, p. 76; ibid., February 1923, p. 66.

clinical autonomy, and met Fraser's interest in a functional and physiological approach to medicine.

The provision of new courses, and the need to develop the units as research departments, quickly raised questions about their accommodation. While the units aimed to institutionalise science into medicine, the makeshift arrangements required to house them were not what had been envisaged. Within two years of the units opening, serious deficiencies in the laboratory accommodation had become clear.

The opportunity to redevelop the units' laboratory facilities was presented by Walter Morley Fletcher, secretary of the MRC and principal architect of the interwar biomedical science policy. He had clear ideas about MRC patronage. Fletcher wanted to sponsor fundamental research under the guidance and direction of those with a rigorous scientific training and accepted the idea of academic units as a way of achieving this. He therefore welcomed the units at St Bartholomew's. For him they were a challenge to the poor state of academic medicine in London, and he encouraged the MRC to support research in the College. Initially the College, unlike other medical schools, made little attempt to seek funding from the MRC, much to Fletcher's concern. Fletcher had more success in directing charitable funding to the College. Under his guidance, philanthropic interest in medical science was exploited and he came to see the endowment of university departments and laboratories as essential.[55] Fletcher's position as the authority on biomedical science policy attracted the Dunn Trustees, who wanted to shift their philanthropic support to favour permanent schemes. The Trustees had started to take an active interest in postwar debates on national reconstruction in an effort to stop the 'aimless dispersal' of their funds. Growing philanthropic enthusiasm for science, and the prominence of science and education in the discussions on national regeneration, led them to approach Fletcher.[56] Guided by Fletcher, the units at St Bartholomew's and The London (along with Oxford and Cambridge) were identified as requiring the Trustees' support. Fletcher hoped to use this to promote scientific rather than practical medicine, upholding the MRC's assessment of the value of academic units and providing the College with much needed funds.

Shortly after speaking at the hospital's octocentenary celebrations in 1922, Fletcher informed the College that the Dunn Trustees had agreed to award £10,000 'for the provision of new laboratories for the scientific work of your Medical and Surgical Units'. They had already given money to the hospital

---

[55] Joan Austoker, 'Walter Morley Fletcher and the Origins of a Basic Biomedical Research Policy', in *Historical Perspectives on the Role of the Medical Research Council: Essays in the History of the Medical Research Council*, ed. Joan Austoker and Linda Bryder (Oxford, 1989), p. 26.
[56] Robert E. Kohler, 'Walter Fletcher, F. G. Hopkins and the Dunn Institute of Biochemistry', *Isis* lxix (1978), pp. 340–1.

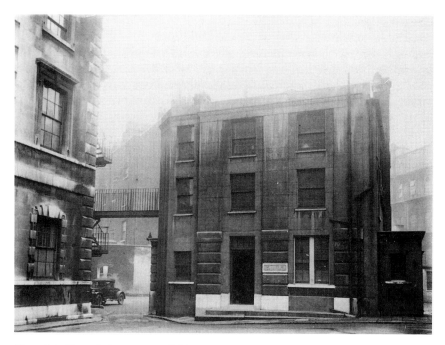

Plate 6.1 Dunn Laboratory, *c.*1924

to endow two beds, and Fletcher had no trouble convincing the Trustees that St Bartholomew's and medical science would benefit from their support.[57] Within a month, plans were made to convert the isolation block into a suite of laboratories to be called the 'Sir William Dunn Laboratories'. The idea of building a new block had been rejected as too expensive and it was hoped that the money saved could be used to support the laboratories. It was anticipated that the laboratories would form part of the existing pathological complex and conduct routine work, but that the main emphasis would be on research.[58]

The Dunn Laboratories became a focus for organising and monitoring clinical trials. It attracted MRC funding, and St Bartholomew's became one of the largest centres for MRC-sponsored research after University College and the Lister Institute. As a result, the College established a reputation for research into viruses and streptococcal infection.[59] In funding the Dunn Laboratories, the MRC's enthusiasm for moving research away from the London hospitals to universities was contradicted by the desire to develop academic medicine through the professorial units. Fletcher anticipated using

[57] PRO: Fletcher to Hayes, 19 June 1922, FD 1/1839.
[58] PRO: Hayes to Fletcher, 13 July 1922, FD 1/1839.
[59] PRO: MRC annual reports, 1924–9, FD 2/11–15.

the Dunn bequest to establish at St Bartholomew's an independent academic base favourable to experimental research which would counter the existing culture of clinical studies.[60] The laboratories certainly represented vital academic and research space. However, research in the College was often conducted outside the units and owed more to clinical studies than the style of research that Fletcher was keen to encourage.

Interest in clinical research and the value of clinical observation grew in the 1920s and found strong support in London's medical schools. Senior staff continued to articulate a model of medicine that owed much to the empirical methods of the nineteenth century and what was perceived as an English tradition of clinical medicine.[61] Experimental research was remote from the experiences of most clinicians. As they dominated the London teaching hospitals, professorial units were often marginal, ensuring that clinical research continued to dominate. Specialists also used clinical research to improve their status, helping to reinforce the clinical ethos in hospital research. At St Bartholomew's, the creation of the follow-up department in 1922, the relative weakness of the professorial units and concentration on cancer research ensured that clinical research held strong.[62] This emphasis left little room for the type of experimental and scientific studies Fletcher strove to promote and ensured that research was seldom focused on the academic model embodied in the units. Although the follow-up department was designed to improve teaching, it was used by the surgical staff to evaluate their procedures as part of what Thomas Lewis at University College saw as 'a fertile science that deals primarily with patients'.[63] Power remained with those clinicians who emphasised the value of the follow-up department rather than the laboratory as a site for research. Although this did not constitute a concerted attack on the laboratory or academic medicine, the MRC was forced to adapt. By the 1930s, the MRC, now under Lewis's influence, was directing a greater part of its funding to clinical research. At one level it remained 'disdainful of clinical activities', at another it awarded substantial grants to non-professorial and professorial departments at St Bartholomew's and other London schools to fund clinical studies.[64] While the MRC hoped this might 'produce many men [sic] able and willing to devote themselves to a life of clinical research in experimental medicine', by 1930 it had recognised that this had not yet happened.[65]

---

[60] PRO: Fletcher to Mann, 9 August 1923, FD 1/1839.

[61] See Christopher Lawrence, 'Still Incommunicable: Clinical Holists and Medical Knowledge in Interwar Britain', in *Greater than the Parts: Holism in Biomedicine, 1920–1950*, ed. Christopher Lawrence and George Weisz (Oxford, 1998), pp. 94–112.

[62] Medical Council, 31 December 1924, 24 June 1925, MC 1/7.

[63] BMJ i (1930), pp. 479–83.

[64] PRO: MRC annual reports, 1928/9, p. 60, FD 2/13; ibid., 1931/2, p. 105, FD 2/18; Green to Rootham, 17 November 1939, FD 1/3131.

[65] PRO: MRC annual report, 1928/9, p. 29.

Although multidisciplinary research and the selection of patients for study became easier, few staff in the professorial units had time for large-scale studies. Research opportunities remained fragmented outside university science departments, and medical research was only beginning to emerge as part of a career structure. Research at St Bartholomew's was not always compatible with the demands of teaching, clinical work or private practice. Fraser did attempt to develop an atmosphere in which staff could work on problems for which they were specially trained. However, despite a rise in grants from the MRC and other bodies, many working in the units were forced from financial necessity to spend most of their non-hospital time in private practice. Frank Green, chief assistant in the medical unit, noted in 1927 that he had only 'the evenings and Sundays to devote to my research'.[66] 'Serious original research' was often prevented by a lack of adequate facilities and makeshift accommodation outside the Dunn Laboratories.[67] Leslie Witts, Fraser's successor, was more successful given his interest in clinical medicine, which met with approval from the medical staff. Witts had come from Guy's where he had played a leading part in modernising teaching and research. He had a firm faith in academic medicine, and as secretary of the Association of Physicians he actively encouraged research into haematology and gastroenterology. The College was not alone in the problems (even under Witts) it encountered. Fletcher recognised that the heavy demands upon units 'necessarily limit the volume of . . . successful research work coming from them'.[68] Criticisms were made that the units in London had failed because of their limited contribution to medical knowledge, but as Witts noted in 1938, staff were often too busy teaching and caring for patients for anything else.[69]

Building work in the hospital in the 1930s threw teaching into confusion as wards and special departments were rearranged or used for temporary accommodation. Departments vied for beds and clinical teaching was constantly disrupted. An investigation into student clinical appointments in 1931 revealed that the creation of the academic units had not been a uniform success. The demands of working in the units and the time allocated to clinical appointments made it impossible for students to visit all the special departments especially as many clinics were held at the same time. To ensure that they gained the widest possible clinical experience, students tended to overlook pathology. Staff were alarmed. Since 1927 it had been recognised that pathology had been poorly organised and 'inadequately taught', with new classes added 'here and there whenever necessity arose'. To resolve this,

[66] PRO: Green to MRC, 22 April 1927, FD 1/2234.
[67] Board of Studies in Pathology, 7 March 1938, MS 106/2.
[68] PRO: MRC annual report 1928/9, p. 27.
[69] St Bartholomew's Hospital Journal, May 1938, p. 176.

pathology teaching was restructured, the teaching staff enlarged, and more demonstrations organised.[70]

By 1931, it was clear that the new arrangements had not worked. The removal of responsibility for pathology from the professorial units proved detrimental to 'the proper training of men for the clinical staff' and caused tension between the pathology department and the chief assistants in the units who wanted to carry their own pathological work.[71] The development of laboratory facilities for blood grouping, pushed by Geoffrey Keynes and Ronald Canti as part of the London Blood Transfusion Service, had also increased pressure on the pathology department.[72] Although St Bartholomew's became the power-base of the transfusion service, its presence highlighted deficiencies in the units. Clinical appointments were rethought and a new plan was devised whereby students spent nine months in general clinical work, followed by nine months in the special departments. They then spent six months in outpatients before attending a three-month pathology course, so preventing pathology from being spread throughout the year. The final period consisted of five months for obstetrics and gynaecology and a month for anaesthetics. An extra three months' clerking was made available for students wishing to take the University of London's MB. The new scheme was seen as a solution to students completing their 'appointments in an extremely rushed manner in considerably less time than this'.[73]

Changes to the structure of clinical appointments had a limited impact on the effectiveness of the units, especially when students spent only a short time in them. Ronald Christie, Witts' successor, felt that some in the College saw the units as little more than a 'scientific or pseudo-scientific excrescence'.[74] Routine administration and too many students sapped both units' strength, while the academic climate they were designed to create was not reflected in examination results. Teaching in the professorial units was varied and remained uncoordinated, and initial efforts to give them a greater role in training and moves to coordinate teaching with the eight non-professorial units were only partially successful. This was more effective on the surgical side. Gask, who had been at St Bartholomew's since 1893 and pioneered thoracic surgery in the hospital, was able to overcome some of the resentment the formation of the units had created. A devolutionist, Gask believed in giving his staff plenty of responsibility, which fitted with the ethos of the College, and he sought to encourage rather than guide his staff and helped them find time for research. The surgical staff, dominated by

---

[70] Board of Studies in Pathology, 17 January 1927, MS 106/1.
[71] Medical Council, 31 May 1922, MC 1/6; ibid., 2 February 1927, MC 1/7; Memorandum, 1942, DF 192.
[72] See Geoffrey Keynes, *Blood Transfusion* (London, 1922).
[73] College Council, 29 April 1931, MS 28/1.
[74] *St Bartholomew's Hospital Journal*, July 1938, p. 249.

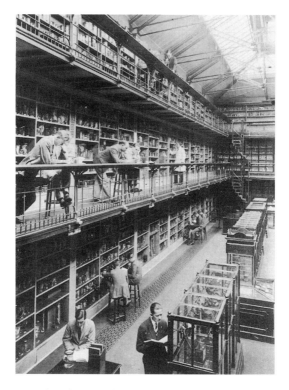

Plate 6.2 Doctors and students in the pathology museum, *c.*1929

abdominal surgeons, welcomed his practical approach and surgical ability. Both factors made it easier for him to promote his ideas.

Fraser as director of the medical unit was less fortunate. Unlike Gask, he had not trained at St Bartholomew's and had joined the College in 1920 as assistant director of the medical professorial unit before being promoted to director. Committed to an academic model, he adopted a different style to that found at St Bartholomew's. Fraser saw his role as directing a unit that would have few clinical duties. Although Fraser's rounds were considered to be 'the highlight of medical life at Barts', he found it difficult to impose his ideas on his staunchly individualistic colleagues.[75] With senior colleagues upholding the individuality of each case and the healing power of nature, Fraser's experimental approach created friction; he initially compared St Bartholomew's to a 'technical shop'. The retirement of the caustic John Drysdale in 1924 did reduce feuding, but the medical consultations continued to provide an opportunity for conflict. The situation improved marginally

[75] Cited in Booth, 'Clinical Research', n.69.

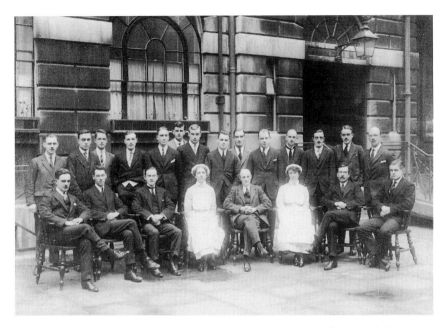

Plate 6.3 Francis Fraser and the staff of the medical professorial unit, *c*.1922

after the appointment of William Girling Ball as dean in 1930. Girling Ball was able to break down 'parochial standards' and encourage 'academic methods', but the muted antagonism between doctors engaged in private practice and the academic staff remained.[76] Junior doctors became trapped in assistant posts. While it was hoped that staff should be selected 'in such a way that each Unit should train men to fill future Professorial appointments', this was not always possible.[77] The need to make a 'medical living' and the demands of private practice curtailed the academic initiative behind the units. Fraser was only able to build up a full-time academic staff and encourage the research programme he had envisaged before coming to St Bartholomew's after leaving the College in 1935 for the British Post-graduate Medical School. Here, as the first professor of medicine, he developed the type of academic environment he had only partly succeeded in establishing at the College.

The units had not brought the full reorganisation of medical education envisaged. The process of grafting units on to existing medical schools along the lines put forward by Herringham and Garrod, though the most practical, was not the most successful. Work in the professorial units was diluted by routine clinical duties, funding problems, and the culture of private practice

[76] Fraser to Girling Ball, 11 December 1934, Girling Ball Scrapbook 3.
[77] Medical Council, 28 February 1923, MC 1/6; ibid., 28 October 1925, MC 1/7.

that made working in a voluntary hospital and medical school possible. When compared to the other units in London, however, those at St Bartholomew's had a better record. They were able to promote greater coordination and systematic teaching at ward and laboratory level, but, with few full-time appointments and endowments, the units struggled to offer the academic teaching and research expected of them in 1919.

A 'captive of research'?

Although research in the professorial units was curtailed by private practice and teaching, the surgical unit did stimulate study in one area. The formation of the Radiotherapeutic Research Committee (later the Cancer Research Committee) in 1923, partly on the initiative of Gask and Neville Finzi, lecturer in radiotherapeutics, followed a wave of public interest in cancer mortality. Cancer had become more 'visible' during the nineteenth century and the understanding of the structure of tumours (if not their nature) had grown. Work at the Middlesex Hospital led the field and the establishment of the Cancer Research Fund (later the Imperial Cancer Research Fund (ICRF)) in 1902 'heralded a new era in experimental cancer studies'. The Fund stimulated research and encompassed changing perceptions of the role of science in medicine.

At St Bartholomew's, some attempt was made to outline a scheme for 'systematic investigation' shortly after the creation of the ICRF, but the move proved stillborn and, when established, the radiotherapeutic research committee embodied an agenda different from that adopted by the ICRF. After the First World War, the identification of a rise in cancer mortality and enthusiasm for radium treatment combined to encourage a number of institutional initiatives. The foundation of the British Empire Cancer Campaign (BECC) in 1923 by leading clinicians (including Horder, Charles Gordon-Watson and Bernard Spilsbury from St Bartholomew's) aimed to encourage treatment over the style of laboratory research favoured by the ICRF. Contemporaries were clear that the BECC represented a challenge to scientific authority and laboratory medicine.[78] The radiotherapeutic research committee at St Bartholomew's was a response to these interests. As an attempt by staff outside the professorial units to reassert their role in research, it helped develop an informal research school in the College.

Research into cancer had come to represent a growing field of inquiry at the College by 1914. Under Finzi, the X-ray department had been expanded to provide an important focus for early work on radium therapy, which aroused less patient anxiety than surgery. Finzi's work with filtered gamma

---

[78] David Cantor, 'Cancer', in *Companion Encyclopaedia of the History of Medicine*, ed. W. F. Bynum and Roy Porter, 2 vols (London, 1997), Vol. 1, p. 537; Joan Austoker, *A History of the Imperial Cancer Research Fund, 1902–1986* (Oxford, 1988), pp. 69–90.

rays suggested that they could be used to destroy malignant cells. This encouraged him to use radium instead of X-rays in treatment and, supported by Gask, he pressed for the use of higher voltages. Work with radium was not limited to Finzi's studies. Keynes, already making a name for himself over his advocacy of blood transfusion, developed his controversial ideas on the treatment of breast cancer. He advocated radium and conservative surgery as opposed to the radical approach espoused by William Halsted and worked closely with Frank Hopwood, physicist to the hospital, who used radium for research when it was not required for treatment.[79] At the same time, Canti was conducting experiments into X-ray treatment in the pathology department and advising the BECC. However, Malcolm Donaldson led the field. With Finzi, he experimented on the use of radium needles in the treatment of ovarian cancer, and tried to use the MRC to encourage research into radiotherapy. With his efforts resisted, he switched to promoting the type of cancer research centre at St Bartholomew's that he wanted to see established elsewhere. Working with Finzi, he raised enough money to buy the hospital's first deep X-ray machine, which formed the nucleus for the radiotherapeutic research committee. Donaldson, like Finzi and Gask, hoped that the committee might go some way towards preventing clinical material from being wasted and provide a means of facilitating research in an environment where private practice was the norm.[80] Although staff at St Bartholomew's were far from unique in their interest in radium therapy, the committee institutionalised existing clinical work and established a structure for research often lacking in other schools.

The radiotherapeutic research committee, although linked to the professorial units and follow-up department, developed its own research infrastructure using funds from the BECC and National Radium Trust. Success in securing external funding – made easier by the fact that several surgeons from the College sat on the BECC – provided the committee with a way around residual opposition from those who felt that 'money should not be spent on cancer'.[81] In doing so, the committee allied itself to the BECC's model of clinical research. Although Fletcher secured considerable influence for the MRC in the BECC, and helped shape its early interest in radiology, the BECC continued to promote clinical study.[82] At St Bartholomew's

[79] Reginald Murley, 'Breast Cancer: Keynes and Conservatism', *British Journal of Clinical Practice* xl (1986), pp. 49–58.

[80] For Donaldson's national role, see David Cantor, 'MRC's Support for Experimental Radiology during the Interwar Years', in *Medical Research Council*, ed. Austoker and Bryder, pp. 181–204.

[81] Donaldson to Aylwen, 27 June 1939, HA 14/39.

[82] Austoker, 'Walter Morley Fletcher', pp. 29–30; Cantor, 'MRC's Support for Experimental Radiology', pp. 201–2. For tensions between BECC and MRC, see Joan Austoker, 'The Politics of Cancer Research', *Bulletin of the Society for the Social History of Medicine* xxxvii (1985), pp. 63–7.

the two approaches represented by the MRC and BECC were combined, suggesting an inherent contradiction overlooked by those who have stressed the discord between scientific and clinical approaches to medicine in the interwar period.

Privileged access to the BECC concentrated research on irradiation and X-ray treatment, while money from the National Radium Trust promoted a separation of X-ray therapy from diagnosis.[83] Comparative studies were undertaken between surgical results and those obtained from deep X-ray therapy and the use of radium puncture. Private gifts of radium gave the College more freedom than many other institutions, and rooms in the Harvey Laboratories (see below) were converted to provide laboratory and treatment accommodation. The nature of studies gradually changed. In the 1930s, more attention was given to the influence of radium on cells *in vitro*, individual cancers and the effects of radiation, after the deaths of several prominent radiologists aroused concern about its harmful effects.[84] Much of this work was multidisciplinary. The committee also stimulated the creation of several subsidiary research departments, including a special department for animal experiments. In 1934, a new cancer department, with a full-time registrar post, was created to coordinate experimental work. Two years later, through the benefaction of Mrs Meyer Sassoon who had been convinced by Finzi of the need for work in this field, a 1000kv machine was installed to aid research into high-voltage X-rays. The department was seen as one of the most advanced in the world.[85]

By the mid-1930s, interest in cancer research had become firmly established at St Bartholomew's. Although the Middlesex remained the leading centre for cancer, the College was able to acquire an international reputation for its work while the support of cancer research promoted the growth of a research infrastructure. Teaching and treatment benefited and emphasis was placed on early diagnosis and care. In 1932, a 'progressive' course on radiological anatomy was started: at the time, only three other schools in London had incorporated radiological findings into their anatomy courses.[86] Teaching, however, was not limited to lectures and demonstrations. Canti's frustration with the tedium of watching change in cancerous cells through a microscope led him to film the process. The use of film in training was only just beginning to be appreciated, and although films were seen as adjuncts to reading rather than to lectures, Canti's work attracted considerable attention and came to play an important part in teaching in the College.[87]

---

[83] Medical Council, 29 November 1928, 30 January 1929, MC 1/8; ibid., 30 January 1935, MC 1/10.

[84] Ibid., 8 October 1929, MC 1/8; T. S. P. Strangeways and Frank Hopwood, 'Effects of X-rays upon Mitotic Cell Division', *Proceedings of the Royal Society* c (1926), p. 283.

[85] *St Bartholomew's Hospital Journal*, November 1964, p. 469.

[86] *Lancet* i (1936), p. 1027.

[87] Ibid., p. 461.

The formation of the Radiotherapeutic Research Committee stressed the clinical dimension to research at St Bartholomew's. The work it encouraged contrasted with the more experimental studies of causation and tumour growth undertaken elsewhere. However, the committee was not universally successful in promoting new treatments: when Donaldson left for Mount Vernon Hospital, his parting shot was 'Wake up, Barts'.

Deficiencies revealed

The presence of the professorial units and the work of the radiotherapeutic research committee poorly concealed deficiencies in the College. In 1918, the reconstruction committee concluded that the existing buildings were only adequate 'for the immediate necessity'. Suggestions that the hospital be moved to a new site or rebuilt were rejected in favour of buying a neighbouring site for the College. The hospital already ran a special treatment centre for 'parturient Women suffering from Venereal diseases' as part of the venereal department in Golden Lane, and it was felt that pre-clinical teaching and special departments could also be moved. This would create room for new laboratory accommodation and operating theatres, which were seen as essential.[88] The second report of the reconstruction committee shared the assessment reached by the Haldane Commission and Board of Education, that there was an urgent need to develop pre-clinical teaching and equipment.[89] Full-time academics had been quietly ushered into the College through the pre-clinical departments in the 1910s as part of the University's policy of professorial appointments, but they were given little influence and presided over outdated departments. The committee highlighted the need for more accommodation in anatomy and chemistry and recommended that a physics workroom was essential given the growing importance of radiology and the pioneering work that Hopwood and his team were undertaking. In the physiology department the laboratory, which had not been re-equipped since 1899, was 'whole[ly] inadequate, even to deal with teaching of comparatively small classes of recent years'. It was considered 'the worst' in London.[90]

In these inadequately housed departments, one student felt he was plunged 'into a set of three incomprehensible, immiscible and highly abstract sciences'. Students were 'rushed from the development of the nervous system in the chick to the laws of mass action in chemistry, and thence to the theories of light waves in physics' to give them the 'smattering' of science that critics felt medical students lacked. The GMC and Ministry of Health,

---

[88] Medical Council, 29 March 1918, 10 March 1919, 21 July 1920, MC 1/5.
[89] See Chapter 5.
[90] Medical Council, 21 May 1919, 8 July 1919, MC 1/5.

convinced by the arguments expressed by the Royal Commission on Scientific Instruction (1871–75), wanted these subjects to be given greater emphasis in secondary education to relieve pressure on the medical curriculum. However, although over 250 secondary schools offered advanced classes in biology, chemistry and physics, the standard of training was often superficial. Most medical students lacked an 'adequate groundwork for the study of medicine' when they started, and many felt they had considerable ground to catch up when they entered medical school. Pre-clinical teachers at St Bartholomew's, as in other schools, felt constrained by the need to supplement such deficiencies as more than an elementary knowledge was required by the University of London.[91]

Students were constantly reminded of the importance of 'scientific truth' in medicine, and told how physics, chemistry and biology were vital to an understanding of physiology, anatomy and pharmacology. It was a view widely adopted in advice to medical students by the mid-1920s.[92] While biology, physics, chemistry and histology were covered in a year, anatomy, physiology and pharmacology (labelled the intermediary subjects) were taught over eighteen months; pathology was left to the fourth year. In these latter subjects, which were seen as the foundations for clinical practice, teaching was designed to be of 'direct importance to the future practitioner'.[93] To achieve this, emphasis was placed on practical classes, which ran in tandem with systematic lectures. However, deficiencies in accommodation ensured that this was not always possible.

Students felt the aim of making these subjects relevant to clinical medicine was seldom achieved outside the physics department, where Hopwood, the most feared and popular pre-clinical teacher, presided. Many pointed to a divorce between the pure science approach embodied in pre-clinical teaching and the realities of their first days on the wards. However, with staff in the pre-clinical departments having little time for research, most of their teaching was shaped by clinical rather than experimental interests. An effort was made to avoid the dilemma faced at other London schools of turning students into physiologists or biochemists. Physiology was illustrated in relation to clinical cases, especially after the appointment of Hamilton Hartridge as professor of physiology in 1927. Hartridge favoured practical instruction and disliked the vagueness of physiological concepts, developing a visual style of teaching using a specially designed projector.[94] A similar practical approach was favoured in the other pre-clinical departments. Biology, for example, was taught in terms of comparative anatomy and not as a pure science. The pre-clinical staff defended the scientific merit of their

[91] *BMJ* ii (1930), p. 617.
[92] See Alexander Miles, *A Guide to the Study of Medicine* (London, 1925).
[93] *St Bartholomew's Hospital Journal*, October 1924, pp. 11–13.
[94] W. A. Rushton, 'Hamilton Hartridge', *Biographical Memoirs of Fellows of the Royal Society* xxii (1977), p. 205.

subjects and stressed how laboratory practice was 'the art of making correct observations, and . . . of recording them neatly and accurately'. This rhetoric aimed to bolster the value of their subjects to doubtful students, who considered many of their classes tedious or unnecessary.

Little support was gained from the clinical staff who remained sceptical of the value of pre-clinical and experimental sciences. With no service role, the pre-clinical departments were seen to be peripheral to the main work of the College. Junior doctors and the newly qualified wanted to become chief assistants, not serve an apprenticeship in the pre-clinical departments where teaching was seen as 'drudgery'. This had made it 'very difficult for the College to obtain demonstrators for the scientific teaching departments'.[95] Those who joined the pre-clinical departments tended to view them as a stepping stone to better posts, and took demonstrator positions to secure a 'means of living while he completes the primary and the final fellowship'. Charles Lovatt Evans, professor of physiology, complained that 'by the time a man is beginning to be of real use, he finds that the post has served his purpose and goes to another subject in which his experience is not of great value to him'.[96] The tendency for demonstrators to be preoccupied with examinations or higher appointments, and the relatively short time they spent in the pre-clinical departments, made it 'impossible to raise the standard of instruction above an elementary level'.[97] It was a common problem: 'too frequently' students studied the pre-clinical subjects 'not as a preparation for the after-study of diseases but as a means of passing a certain examination'.[98] The willingness of one of the College porters to sign students in to preliminary and pre-clinical lectures when they were absent for a small fee helped many skip lectures. Others hid at the back of the dimly lit lecture theatre and relied on the laboratory attendant for unofficial information on examinations to pass.[99] Students' tendency to dismiss or avoid pre-clinical teaching became part of the ongoing debate on the need to balance clinical experience with demands for more science that clouded interwar discussions on the curriculum.

The pre-clinical lecturers struggled to offer the best possible training under poor and cramped conditions. The collapse of the postwar restocking boom in 1921 prevented any immediate improvement. Unemployment rose as industrial production fell during one of the worst depressions in British history.[100] A fall in income shifted attention at St Bartholomew's from

---

[95] Memorandum, DF 192.

[96] Board of Studies in Anatomy, 25 November 1935, MS 100/1; Board of Studies in Physiology, 19 June 1923, MS 109/1.

[97] Board of Studies in Anatomy, 25 November 1935, MS 100/1.

[98] W. D. Halliburton, ed., *Physiology and National Needs* (London, 1919), p. 80.

[99] *St Bartholomew's Hospital Journal*, December 1933, p. 52.

[100] See Derek H. Aldcroft, *From Versailles to Wall Street, 1919–1929* (London, 1977), pp. 67–77, 111.

reconstruction to retrenchment. It was only when the economy started to recover in 1922 that Lovatt Evans, recently appointed as professor of physiology, joined forces with dean Thomas Shore to press for a new physiology department. Lovatt Evans was committed to research and had come to St Bartholomew's from the MRC's National Institute for Medical Research in Hampstead. He felt constrained by the existing department and, with Guy's investing £45,000 in laboratory accommodation, he worried that the College was falling behind. The GMC had also just put forward a revised curriculum, which outlined the need for more physiology, anatomy and pathology as part of its efforts to approach training in clinical medicine in a more systematic manner. Physiology's status had been bolstered by wartime discoveries in nutrition, respiration and fatigue, while a move in surgery towards a more physiological approach was an additional factor. With the development of further specialised instruments, the breadth of research had increased.[101] New textbooks raised the profile of physiology and support was readily gained from physicians who had become convinced of the value of physiology. Even the old guard at St Bartholomew's subscribed to a view of medicine as applied physiology because it gave them status as a learned profession.[102] Plans in 1919 for a physiology lecture theatre and laboratory were revived and a small demonstration theatre, two research laboratories and rooms for preparation were added. An additional year of fund-raising was required before a warehouse in Giltspur Street was purchased as the 'ideal site'.[103]

Estimates for rebuilding alarmed some of the surgical staff who saw the new department as 'needless' at a time when they felt new '*operating theatres* [were] *essential* and *urgent*'.[104] Although an upturn in the economy was beginning, they doubted that money could be found for rebuilding. Lovatt Evans immediately defended the need for new accommodation. Using arguments familiar to the clinical staff, who had employed them to press for the professorial units, he suggested that the laboratory had become an essential part of a doctor's training and that existing accommodation was obsolete. Lovatt Evans believed that the new building would bring St Bartholomew's in line with other schools. The surgeons were further reassured by plans for the old physiology block: requests from the pre-clinical departments to use the accommodation were rejected and space was allocated for tutorials in medicine, practical surgery and midwifery. A laboratory for practical surgery was established and the remaining room was used to house a 'small collection of typical teaching specimens and microscope slides'. With

---

[101] See Steve Sturdy, 'From the Trenches to the Hospitals at Home: Physiologists, Clinicians and Oxygen Therapy, 1914–1930', in *Medical Innovations in Historical Perspective*, ed. John V. Pickstone (Basingstoke, 1992), pp. 104–23.

[102] *St Bartholomew's Hospital Journal*, October 1924, p. 9.

[103] General purposes committee, 13 February 1922, 6 March 1923, MS 35.

[104] Ibid., 6 March, 5 November 1923; Medical Council, 21 December 1922, MC 1/6.

room found for clinical teaching it was agreed that the new building should be named the 'Harvey Laboratories'. Most of the converted building was designed for laboratory teaching but some space was found for a physics lecture theatre.[105]

The opening of the Harvey Laboratories in 1924 encouraged the other pre-clinical departments to press for new accommodation, but tensions between pre-clinical and clinical staff and the poor financial position of the College delayed further development. Several proposals were put forward in the mid-1920s, and land in Cock Lane adjoining the Harvey Laboratories was acquired for development. However, it was not until 1929, when the governors of the hospital announced their plans to redevelop the West Smithfield site, that serious attention was turned to the College's needs.[106]

An investigation into teaching and research revealed problems. Although staff continued to believe that the College had 'been able to keep up-to-date and to rise into the highest position', they were aware that professorial posts in medicine and surgery had been funded through 'rigid economies' in other departments. The lecturers felt it 'quite impossible' to support chairs they felt were needed in obstetrics, biochemistry, clinical pathology and bacteriology, or adequately to fund the 'services of the highest type of Trained teachings'. Salaries remained largely dependent on funding from the UGC, and most of the junior staff were unpaid. Research had also suffered. Without an endowment fund, the College had been incapable of awarding 'monetary grants to those qualified to undertake research'. Although the Dunn bequest made it possible to provide laboratory accommodation for the professorial units, and an appeal helped fund the Harvey Laboratories, the College was unable to raise enough to endow posts or 'for new laboratories and modern scientific equipment'.[107] Research and teaching in the pre-clinical departments was hardest hit, suffering from the concentration on clinical medicine that had dominated the College since the mid-Victorian period.

Since the First World War, teaching in the pre-clinical department had 'entailed the provision of a large teaching staff'. At the same time, student numbers had grown by one-third. Clinical services had been expanded to cope with this increase, but the pre-clinical departments had lagged behind. As a result, rooms were overcrowded. Existing accommodation for the chemistry department was inadequate and students had had to share desks since 1918. A similar situation existed in anatomy, which was seen as an 'awful'.[108] Although senior surgical staff had resisted demands by their

---

[105] General purposes committee, 6 March 1923, 5 November 1923, MS 35; *St Bartholomew's Hospital Journal*, February 1924, p. 68.

[106] Appeal, MS 6/13.

[107] Statement of objects and needs of the College, c.1929, MS 6/8.

[108] General purpose committee, 5 November 1923, MS 35; Woollard to Girling Ball, 25 September 1936, Girling Ball Scrapbook 3.

pre-clinical colleagues for more room, all were agreed by 1929 that anatomy 'must be expanded and rebuilt on another site if the work of medical education is to be carried on with efficiency in accordance with modern ideas'. Changes had occurred in the structure of anatomy as a subject since 1920 which problems with space had made difficult to incorporate. The clinicians supported anatomy's claims because it was seen as essential to practice, and this gave the pre-clinical staff an opportunity to press their case. The transfer of College Hall to the hospital in 1923 to provide rooms for nurses while a new nursing home was built created an additional need to redevelop the College. It was estimated that £40,000 was required for research and £70,000 for a new anatomy department.[109]

The decision to rebuild the anatomy department raised questions about the other pre-clinical accommodation. Improvements to the physiology department, and the creation of the Harvey Laboratories, revealed a backlog of problems. In addition, the departments were scattered over several sites and it was deemed important to concentrate them in one place. Clinical attitudes to pre-clinical teaching had also started to shift. Doctors were coming to accept that the basic sciences also had a role to play in providing a theoretical framework for practice and had gradually learned not to 'scoff at the early scientific teaching to students'.[110] The pre-clinical sciences had expanded rapidly, and although there was room for modification in how they were taught, the role of pure science in medicine was accepted as an 'essential foundation'.[111] The same process may be seen at St Bartholomew's. By the late 1920s a consensus had emerged that facilities were needed 'to instil into the mind of the student from his earliest days such scientific knowledge as will enable him to understand the chemical, physical, and biological problems which are bound to confront him during the clinical period of his training'. The growing importance of radiology raised the profile of the physics department where Hopwood was carrying out groundbreaking research. In anatomy Herbert Woollard, the newly appointed professor, rapidly set about introducing an experimental environment into the department and strengthening the 'scientific spirit in the oncoming men'.[112] His interest in the sympathetic nervous and lymphatic systems saw him working closely with the clinical staff. At the same time, Fraser's support for more links between physiology and clinical medicine was beginning to find expression.[113] The clinically related work undertaken in these departments strengthened their claims.

By 1930, College Council was persuaded to accept that 'in any recon-struction of the Anatomical and Chemical Departments, the whole of the

---

[109] General purpose committee, 13 February 1922, MS 35.
[110] BMJ ii (1931), p. 409.
[111] Lancet ii (1936), p. 938.
[112] Woollard to Girling Ball, 25 September 1936, DF.
[113] BMJ ii (1929), p. 308.

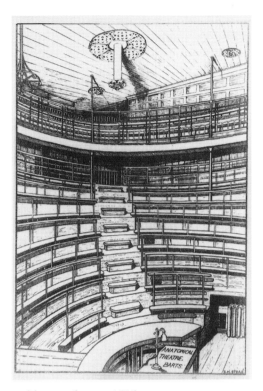

Plate 6.4 Anatomical lecture theatre, 1935

accommodation for the Pre-Clinical Subjects should be found outside the Hospital site'.[114] The College was not alone in its decision to rebuild: St Mary's had started on new buildings in 1930 in an effort to extend laboratory and student accommodation. Under pressure from the hospital's governors, who wanted to use the anatomy department for a radiological institute, the College had bought a site in Cock Lane in 1927.[115] However, with the proposed site considered too small, an impasse was reached. Girling Ball pressed for a review of the situation.

Girling Ball had recently been appointed dean, despite attempts to dissuade him by some of the surgeons who felt he lacked vision. He had already held a series of administrative posts including warden and sub-dean, but despite being a passionate administrator, he was nervous about the prospect. Familiar with the problems facing the College, Girling Ball immediately set about reforming its administrative structure and promoting closer links with the University in an attempt to encourage an academic

---

[114] College Council, 12 February, 10 December 1930, MS 28/1.
[115] General purpose committee, 17 March 1930, 3 December 1930, MS 35.

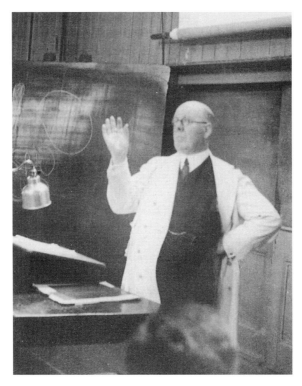

Plate 6.5 Sir William Girling Ball lecturing, *Candid Camera*, *c*.1930

environment. On the pre-clinical side, Girling Ball recognised the deficiencies facing the departments. He pressed for new accommodation to improve 'scientific education' and for the creation of more academic posts to foster an environment similar 'to one in the older universities'. At the 1930 Christmas dinner, he promised to rebuild the College within ten years. The College Council accepted his assessment and called for an investigation of other suitable sites.[116]

Move to Charterhouse

Girling Ball's intervention resulted in further deliberations over the pre-clinical departments. By 1932, two possible sites had emerged: one in Little Britain, the other in Charterhouse. The latter had been suggested by the hospital, and was owned by Merchant Taylors' School. The school, founded in 1561, had bought the five-acre site in 1872 from Charterhouse in a bid to

---

[116] Girling Ball, 'Autobiography', p. 4; College Council, 10 December 1930, MS 28/1.

extend teaching. Fitful discussions were started in the 1910s about the need to move outside London to boost admissions, and the debate was resumed after a Board of Education report in 1928 recommended a move to North London to reflect the changing pattern of residence of the City. In the light of the Board's views, a firm decision to was made to move to Rickmansworth. Negotiations were started with the Corporation of London over the Charterhouse site, but when the Corporation backed out a new purchaser was sought.[117] Charterhouse, with its existing buildings and a new science block (opened in 1926), was seen as large and quiet. It had an 'admirable refectory and kitchens' and room to build the proposed anatomy department and the residential college Girling Ball wanted. In comparison, Little Britain was cramped and pungent with the smell of meat from the vans going to Smithfield Market. Charterhouse promised a lower cost for redevelopment and pressure was exerted by the governors, who wanted to use Little Britain to extend the hospital. This, and the romantic idea that the College would be returning to a site recorded as once belonging to St Bartholomew's, swung the College Council despite initial anxieties about the distance of Charterhouse from the clinical departments.

Girling Ball had himself been uncertain. He had wanted to bring the pre-clinical and clinical departments closer together, but was swung by Woollard's enthusiasm for the potential of the site.[118] Once convinced of the possibility of using Chaterhouse to develop 'a real University Medical College' where residential and teaching accommodation were integrated, Girling Ball became committed to the scheme. With the University sceptical and unwilling to provide funding, and with the College unable to pay for Charterhouse from student fees, Girling Ball persuaded the lecturers to launch an appeal for £135,000.[119] Girling Ball already had experience of fund-raising with the City of London Truss Society (where he was a surgeon) and hoped to use the same methods at St Bartholomew's. The appeal, aimed initially at former students and staff, was a departure from previous schemes to extend the College. Lecturers had traditionally relied on the governors to pay for rebuilding, but St Bartholomew's was no longer in a position to help. In 1920, the King's Fund had threatened to withhold grants if any money donated to a teaching hospital was used to fund medical education. In addition, the hospital was itself forced to launch an appeal for £1 million in 1929 for a new surgical block and operating theatre.[120] With no money

---

[117] Guildhall: Special general court, 4 April 1866; Court minutes, 31 October 1930, 11 March 1932; F. W. Draper, *Four Centuries of Merchant Taylors' School, 1561–1961* (London, 1962), pp. 213–17.

[118] *St Bartholomew's Hospital Reports* (1936), pp. 45, 47.

[119] Report of the subcommittee on the suitability of Merchant Taylors' School for the medical college, MS 6/7; College Council, 20 January 1932, 19 October 1932, MS 28/1.

[120] *The Times*, 5 December 1929, p. 16.

available from the state, the lecturers capitalised on the fund-raising strategies employed by voluntary hospitals since the eighteenth century. A subtle shift had occurred in the nature of philanthropy to favour 'preventive' charity, encouraging more support for science within a vocabulary that linked fundamental research to prosperity.[121] The lecturers tried to use this. After support from former staff and students failed to raise the amount required, the appeal was made public. Jumble sales were organised by the Women's Guild and a 'Fiver Scheme' was established, to encourage 'Bart's men . . . to collect money from their friends'.[122] Aware that many, 'though willing to give money to a Hospital for the treatment of the sick, will not so readily come to the help of a teaching institution', an attempt was made to link the College's fund-raising to the hospital's appeal and to stress the benefits of securing better trained doctors.[123]

The metropolitan benevolent economy was highly competitive and, even with influential backing, the College could not hope to raise the money needed. A series of major appeals by hospitals and colleges in the 1920s had jaded the public, and the Wall Street crash further tightened purse strings. The Gresford mine disaster placed a further strain on resources, redirecting philanthropy away from London. To meet the shortfall, a financial package was carefully constructed that dominated the work of the College to such an extent that the organisation of teaching was neglected. Merchant Taylors' drove a hard bargain: in addition to a down payment of £35,000, the lease of the Harvey Laboratories was transferred to the Company, with the remaining amount borrowed from them at a competitive rate of interest.[124] Girling Ball accepted because he wanted to 'get on with this building at whatever the cost'. Fees to part-time staff were subsequently reduced and departments were told to cut spending. Estimates were higher than anticipated and the original aim of building a new anatomy department was delayed so that work could concentrate on altering existing buildings for physiology, chemistry and physics. The situation had become desperate by December 1934. Efforts to raise a loan faltered until Sir George Wilkinson, a close friend of Girling Ball, intervened and offered to lend the College £20,000. Girling Ball considered accepting the Wilkinson loan a 'very bold move', but admitted that without it plans for Charterhouse would have collapsed.[125]

The architects, who were responsible for numerous university and laboratory buildings and had already worked on the hospital, showed 'very

[121] Roy Macleod, 'Support for Victorian Science: The Endowment of Science Movement in Great Britain', *Minerva* iv (1971), pp. 197–230.

[122] *St Bartholomew's Hospital Journal*, June 1933, p. 158.

[123] Appeal, MS 6/13.

[124] College Council, 1 February 1933, 28 February 1933, MS 28/1.

[125] Ibid., 21 June 1933, 20 June 1934, 21 November 1934, 6 December 1934, 19 December 1934, 17 April 1935, MS 28/1.

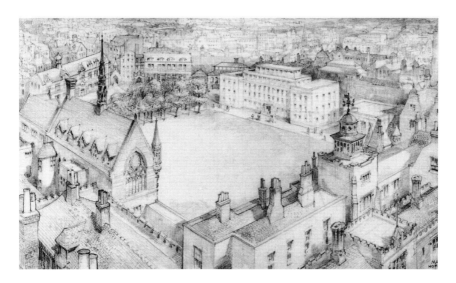

Plate 6.6 Proposed development of medical college site, Charterhouse

considerable ingenuity and patience with the great number of Teachers with whom they have had to consult'.[126] This optimistic assessment concealed problems in the planning process. William Hurtley, reader in chemistry, and Hartridge could not agree on the 'size of the new laborator[ies]'. Changes were constantly made. Despite difficulties with modifying existing buildings, the chemistry, physics, physiology and pharmacology departments and the new biochemistry building were completed in October 1935 against a background of mounting debate on the structure of the medical curriculum. Anatomy and biology followed in April 1936.[127] The whole redevelopment was considered to be along 'very modern lines'.[128] The green in the centre was handed over to the Students' Union for tennis courts and a cricket pitch, and the oak-panelled old School Hall (built in 1876) was used for cloakrooms, common rooms, a library and dinning-hall.[129] Girling Ball, as the driving force behind Charterhouse, was widely congratulated on his efforts. Woollard was praised for his work on the anatomy department which, in its combination of biology, anatomy and comparative anatomy, was seen as a physical embodiment of the desired proximity of these subjects.[130] However, cutbacks and the need to concentrate funding on the pre-clinical depart-ments ensured that a new residential college could not be built. Rooms were

---

[126] Ball to College, 11 June 1934, DF 1.
[127] Ball to Lodge, 13 July 1933, 17 January 1934, 8 March 1934, DF 1.
[128] College Handbook (1937/8), p.19.
[129] *St Bartholomew's Hospital Journal*, November 1935, p. 29.
[130] *BMJ* ii (1936), p. 36.

found in the University of London's newly opened Connaught Hall and staff worried that students from Oxford and Cambridge would avoid St Bartholomew's because it lacked 'a hostel'.[131]

The move to Charterhouse marked a change in conditions and attitudes. Students welcomed the move, seeing the new buildings as a vast improvement. For staff, Charterhouse was considered to offer better facilities for teaching and research. To promote this a Research Committee was formed to allocate laboratory accommodation. The pre-clinical staff were more impressed with the quality of the light in the new buildings, having become accustomed to gloomy or basement rooms. Those who previously had been critical of a materialistic approach to science and medicine started to defend the role of science in medicine. The editor of the *St Bartholomew's Hospital Journal* explained that the new buildings helped repair the gap between clinical and pre-clinical subjects; for Kingsley Wood, Minister of Health, they made the College a 'pioneer of modern medical education'.[132]

'Before the deluge'

No consensus had emerged by 1935 about the desired structure of the medical curriculum. A series of reports by the University of London, BMA and Ministry of Health pointed to conflicting views. Early supporters of full-time academic clinicians became uneasy. The merits of the British system were recognised, but it was left to the GMC, which was reluctant to implement substantial reforms, to secure change and revise the examination system. Although the GMC continued to support the importance of laboratory teaching, the deepening climate of economic depression and political retrenchment brought a change in emphasis. It came to believe that the best way to improve the curriculum was 'by developing and advancing the existing system' and suggested change might be better initiated by individual schools.[133] This response produced consternation: reformers were frustrated by the slow pace of change, and traditionalists continued to worry about the role of science versus bedside medicine. Individual schools were more optimistic.

Charterhouse and the professorial units gave St Bartholomew's an ideal opportunity for rethinking its curriculum. New classes on haematology, applied bacteriology and parasitology were started. In anatomy, Woollard attempted to move away from descriptive teaching and implement ideas that students should learn by handling the material. As at University College,

---

[131] AGM, 27 January 1937, MS 27/1.
[132] *St Bartholomew's Hospital Journal*, November 1935, p. 23; *The Times*, 2 October 1936, p. 11.
[133] *BMJ* i (1935), pp. 1222–3.

anatomy teaching embraced histology and neurology, breaking with traditional subject boundaries that had prevented the development of anatomy as an academic discipline. Woollard encouraged students to undertake research and introduced a new climate of experimental discipline.[134] In chemistry, the curriculum was reorganised, so that closer links were established between organic chemistry, physiological chemistry and chemical pathology. Although Hurtley had encouraged these changes because of his interest in biochemistry, the task of organising teaching passed to Arthur Wormall after Hurtley died of pneumonia in 1936.[135] Wormall was a pioneer in the use of isotopic tracers and his appointment recognised the changes that were occurring in chemistry. Under him the teaching of inorganic, organic and physiological chemistry were united.[136] Preliminary clinical teaching was transferred to Charterhouse and placed under the control of the professorial staff. It was hoped that this would answer some of the complaints made by students that their pre-clinical teaching had little clinical relevance. However, although changes were made in line with the new ideas of what students should be taught, the financial burden left by Charterhouse prevented the inauguration of more ambitious schemes. Other teaching hospitals faced similar difficulties, leading to understaffing and haphazard modernisation.

Hospitals and medical schools seemed to stagger through the 1930s from one financial crisis to another. Although the College was in a better position than many, and was able to avoid some of the financial difficulties that frustrated development at King's, Guy's, St Thomas's and the Middlesex, a deterioration in the international situation started to impose other concerns in the late 1930s. Germany's expansionist policies had started to go beyond a reversal of the Treaty of Versailles, threatening the balance of power in Europe. By 1938, concern about how the curriculum should be organised began to be replaced by anxieties about how medical education might be carried on during wartime. A communication from the University of London in September 1938 seemed to herald the future when it advised the postponement of the new term in the hope that the international situation might improve. St Bartholomew's started planning for war.

---

[134] Ibid., p. 39.
[135] Wormall was promoted to hold the first chair of biochemistry in a London medical school.
[136] AGM, 8 March 1933, 27 January 1937, MS 27/1.

7

'Bould and sawcye carryadge'

Mayhem and medical students, 1662–1939

When students were first reported at St Bartholomew's in 1664 it was because of their 'bould and sawcye carryadge'. Over the centuries, their role and behaviour changed as they came to play an important part in shaping the institutional structure of medical training and the culture of the hospital. However, despite the importance of students to the educational process, little is known about their lives. As Anderson has recognised, 'the historian's conception of "student life" inevitably concentrates on politics, clubs and societies, and the more visible forms of social life'.[1] The more picturesque aspects of student life captivated contemporaries and contributed to the myth that came to surround medical students' behaviour. By exploring the nature of student life at St Bartholomew's some of these gaps may be filled.

The 'sawcye carryadge' of seventeenth-century medical apprentices would have been familiar to Victorian commentators. By the early nineteenth century, the presence of students on the wards had become an essential feature of the medical environment at St Bartholomew's; over the next 150 years students were to have an important impact on the clinical services of the hospital. A memorandum to the Board of Education in 1914 explained that students 'render valuable services in assisting the Staff in the treatment of the patients', a point asserted by Abernethy over a hundred years earlier.[2] As clerks and dressers, students carried out routine clinical work (and paid for the privilege), relieving the honorary staff from constant attendance. Their perceived role in maintaining good practice and assisting in care became part of the rhetoric used to defend the presence of students in London's hospitals. By the mid-nineteenth century some observers had begun to worry that this trend had gone too far, that hospitals had turned into appendages of medical schools. For Victorians, the consequences could be stark: critics of the London hospital system worried that teaching demands not medical criteria determined which patients were admitted – with preference given to 'interesting and novel cases' – and how they were treated.[3] Lecturers were

---

[1] R. D. Anderson, *The Student Community at Aberdeen, 1860–1939* (Aberdeen, 1988), p. 2.
[2] Memorandum 1914, DF 184.
[3] *Charity Organisation Review*, September 1885, p. 397.

keen to refute these accusations, but by the 1940s it was clear that patient needs and teaching needs were inseparable.

The impact of medical schools on students and the corporate identity of the profession are less well defined. Sociologists have suggested that training has an important socialising role, transmitting the culture of medicine and moulding students into a professional body.[4] Studies tend to assume that students formed a homogeneous group undergoing the same experiences and ordeals. Historically the role of teaching hospitals in socialisation is less clear. Medical schools, despite their efforts to develop a disciplinary framework, were not Goffman's total institutions, but they did embody a set of values that were absorbed by students. In the process, they helped foster a professional identity that was confirmed by the General Medical Council (GMC) and the licensing bodies. At St Bartholomew's this was first achieved around the common experiences of institutional study, the evolution of a defined curriculum and the influence of the staff. Only with the development of a corporate life created through sport, clubs and the activities of the Students' Union (SU) was this identity given further shape. Bart's men did not appear suddenly formed, but their increasing number created a growing cadre of students immersed in the same values and traditions. Looking back, Geoffrey Evans, a former student, noted that St Bartholomew's 'with its tradition, atmosphere, teachers, nurses, porters and students . . . strengthened character and will' and '*made the man*'.[5]

Bart's men

Between 1788, when a medical school might be said to have come into existence, and 1939, a growing number of students could claim to be Bart's men. Admissions to the College reflected its status and the training it offered. Admissions also pointed to a degree of self-interest among those teaching: as the Charity Commission recognised in 1837, students 'form a very considerable source of profit' for staff.[6] This created internal financial pressure to maintain a healthy balance of students, pressure that frequently led to overcrowding.

London, as the cultural, economic and political centre of English life, attracted young men keen to distinguish themselves. For medical apprentices seeking to extend their experience and acquire polish, London offered

---

[4] See R. K. Merton *et al.*, *The Student-Physician. Introductory Studies in the Sociology of Medical Education* (Cambridge: Mass., 1957); Howard S. Becker *et al.*, *Boys in White. Student Culture in Medical School* (Chicago, 1961).

[5] *BMJ* ii (1950), p. 622.

[6] John Wrottesley and Samuel Smith, 'St Bartholomew's Hospital', *32nd Report of the Charity Commissions*, Part vi (London, 1840), p. 51.

something more to an essentially mobile student body. A rise in the number of lectures and new hospitals in the mid-eighteenth century increased opportunities for study, adding to the capital's attraction and enhancing London's reputation for practical medicine. Susan Lawrence estimates that 11,059 students walked the wards of London's hospitals between 1725 and 1815, the main rise occurring between the 1780s and 1815.[7] Most were surgical pupils, and a growing number came to study at St Bartholomew's after Abernethy started teaching there in 1788. The end of the Napoleonic and revolutionary wars saw a temporary reduction in numbers as demand for doctors fell, but the stimulus given to hospital-based training by the Royal College of Surgeons and the 1815 Apothecaries' Act boosted numbers. Under Abernethy, St Bartholomew's grew in prestige and size. In 1810, the number of surgical students exceeded those at the Middlesex, St Thomas's and The London, and throughout the 1810s represented approximately a quarter of the hospital students in London.[8] By 1831, St Bartholomew's was sending more students to be examined by the Royal College of Surgeons than any other medical school, and had firmly established itself as one of London's leading teaching hospitals. The governors neither encouraged nor impeded this and appeared willing to ignore students provided they did not upset the normal running of the hospital.

Abernethy's death in 1830 heralded a period of infighting. The College's position declined and student numbers fell. Advertisements were placed in the press to enhance the College's profile, but in 1842 a low point was reached (see figure 7.1). A series of reforms in the 1840s, guided by James Paget, lecturer in general and morbid anatomy and warden, encouraged a reversal of this trend and laid the foundation for the College's growth over the next fifty years. The surgeon-general Anthony Home, looking back on his time at the Middlesex Hospital, felt that 'St Bartholomew's claimed a sort of primacy amongst the schools' in the mid-nineteenth century. Students were attracted to College by 'a long succession of great men'.[9] At a practical level, the College promised relatively unrestricted access to patients in comparison to other schools, boasted a large number of beds and, if the medical press were to be believed, possessed first-class facilities. These factors were important in contributing to growth, although large numbers of students continued to attend St Bartholomew's on the advice of friends and relations. A national rise in student numbers and fears that 'everywhere medical men are jostling each other for the merest crumbs of practice' underlay this expansion. Professional anxiety about low status, underemployment, and 'significant

---

[7] Susan C. Lawrence, *Charitable Knowledge: Hospital Pupils and Practitioners in Eighteenth-Century London* (Cambridge, 1996), pp. 135–6.

[8] Ibid., pp. 357–60.

[9] Cited in H. Campbell Thomson, *The Story of the Middlesex Medical School* (London, 1935), p. 45.

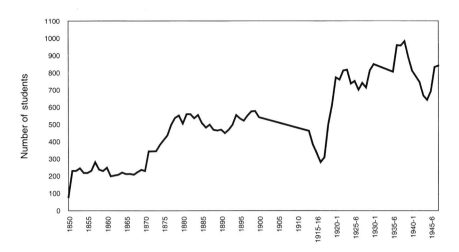

Figure 7.1 Number of students admitted, 1850–1948

downward pressure on medical incomes', resulting from acute competition, did not appear to discourage aspiring doctors.[10] Neither did antivivisectionists' attacks on medicine, or popular prejudices against studying in London, deter students from coming to St Bartholomew's. The College benefited from the inability of the medical profession to restrict its own numbers. Overcrowding increased, leading the College to press for new buildings, a move that reflected the secure and self-confident attitude that had come to permeate St Bartholomew's.[11] Although growth concealed deficiencies, by 1879 the College was once more firmly established as the largest medical school in London.

From this high point, student numbers fell. The trend in medical education towards a growing dispersion of students over a greater number of institutions (many of them civic universities) from the 1880s shifted the geography of training to favour cheaper provincial colleges. The 'Great Depression', which characterised the years between 1873 and 1896, hurt large sections of the population and increased the relative cost of medical education and studying in London. Admissions to the College only partially reflected the downward trend in recruitment. It helped that London was still acknowledged 'to be the most important centre of medical education in the world'.[12] How much the decline was due to provincial competition or

[10] *Lancet* ii (1852), pp. 268–9; Anne Digby, *Making a Medical Living: Doctors and Patients in the English Market of Medicine, 1720–1911* (Cambridge, 1994), p. 43.
[11] Butlin and Macready to Moore, 26 June 1879, MS 14/1.
[12] 'A Review of the position created within the hospital by the report of the royal commission on university education', MS 7/3.

economic circumstances is uncertain. However, the impression of falling numbers had an important impact, increasing anxiety in the London medical schools. Those teaching at St Bartholomew's were worried about admissions, prompting a series of reforms to bring the College in line with other institutions. Fear of competition rather than the level of competition was an important force in shaping services.

Uncertainties about the future of the University of London and the nature of medical education, combined with the precarious nature of medical employment, ensured a continued reduction in student numbers in the early twentieth century. Although numbers entering full-time higher education in London virtually doubled between 1900 and 1911, 1913 marked a low point in admissions to medical schools.[13] Entrants were dissuaded by the problem of competition, which was seen to be depressing medical incomes. With many young men leaving to serve in the Forces, student intake stood at its lowest by 1915/16 since 1870. After the war a backlog of applicants generated by wartime conditions and a limit on places (part of St Bartholomew's had been converted into a military hospital reducing the number of beds for teaching) saw a national and local boom in admissions, encouraged by the University Grants Committee (UGC). The national postwar boom quickly faltered, however, and student numbers fell dramatically between 1919 and 1923 in response to the collapse of the postwar restocking boom. The College was insulated from these national trends by the opening of the professorial units in 1919. It was seen to offer the professorial and academic style of education outlined by the Haldane Commission, which at first kept admissions artificially high. It was only in 1923 that the number of entrants began to slow down in spite of a recovery at other schools.[14] The addition of new laboratories and clinics solved some of the deficiencies in clinical training and the under-resourced and cramped pre-clinical departments, encouraging more students to attend as the economic situation improved.

The economic slump between 1832 and 1935 depressed the employment market for graduates of all kinds. Science and technology were hardest hit. In medicine, student numbers rose (see Table 7.1). The 1911 National Insurance Act, which created panel practice, made medicine more financially secure. An improvement in medical incomes and status continued during the interwar period, consolidating medicine's position as an attractive career for 'a better class of men'.[15] Changes in the structure of healthcare after the 1929 Local Government Act expanded the number of opportunities for practitioners. Interwar interest in malnutrition, tuberculosis and degeneration also raised the profile of medicine, while a greater emphasis on biology in secondary schools helped channel students into medicine.

[13] PRO: UGC Returns, UGC 3.
[14] Student attendance, MS 54/5; BMJ ii (1937), p. 444.
[15] BMJ ii (1935), p. 445.

Table 7.1   Student numbers in the
United Kingdom, 1929–36

Year	Number
1929	1502
1930	1792
1931	1643
1932	1947
1933	2287
1934	2350
1935	2603
1936	2544

Source: BMJ ii (1937), p. 444

Medicine proved a stable occupation and a profession with an aura of gentle-manly respectability.[16] At St Bartholomew's the opening of the widely applauded pre-clinical departments at Charterhouse set the seal for a further rise in admissions only interrupted by the war in 1939.

What did students choose to study? Medical education was dominated throughout the nineteenth and twentieth centuries by the pluralistic system of licensing upheld by the 1858 Medical Act. This left it to the student to decide which set of examinations to sit, and where. The system encouraged flexibility and allowed students to travel to London to gain clinical experience without tying them to a particular examination. Students could shop around in an open market for qualifications, matching the licence to their requirements, levels of attainment and professional norms.[17] Yet, despite the continued survival of a multitude of licensing bodies, most students at St Bartholomew's followed a similar educational path.

Before 1858, there was no formal compulsion to take a degree or obtain a licence to practice. Students at St Bartholomew's in this period were therefore not necessarily seeking a qualification. With most coming to London to walk the wards or to hear anatomy or surgery lectures, the College initially had a predominantly surgical emphasis shaped in part by demand and by the interests and strengths of the staff. Even by the early 1820s there were still few medical pupils, and the medical wards remained underused until the following decade when the teaching of physic was reformed.[18] Although the number preparing for the LSA (established by the 1815 Apothecaries' Act and practically compulsory for practitioners who dispensed) came to

---

[16] Anne Digby and Nick Bosanquet, 'Doctors and Patients in an Era of National Health Insurance and Private Practice, 1913–1938', *EcHR* xli (1988), pp. 74–94.

[17] See James Bradley, Anne Crowther and Margaret Dupree, 'Mobility and Selection in Scottish University Medical Education, 1858–1886', *Medical History* xl (1996), pp. 1–24.

[18] Robert Christison, *Life of Sir Robert Christison* ii (London, 1886), pp. 190–2.

dictate teaching in the 1820s, the College retained its surgical character. After dissatisfaction with the LSA set-in in the 1830s, a greater number of students returned to taking the MRCS. By the 1850s the MRCS had come to dominate, with approximately 60 per cent of students sitting the licence. The 1858 Medical Act, by making a diploma, degree or licence a prerequisite for an 'orthodox' practitioner, merely formalised what had already become an established trend. While the University of London's MB had a considerable impact on the structure of teaching at St Bartholomew's in the 1850s and 1860s, most students continued to favour the combination of the MRCS/LSA. High standards and a poor general education discouraged students who preferred the easier dual qualification of the MRCS and LSA, which became the accepted route into the profession.

The actual qualifications students sought did change however (see Table 7.2). In the early 1860s, students at St Bartholomew's started to reject 'College and Hall' in favour of the MRCS and LRCP. By 1882, Paget was clear that the LSA was 'too easy' and students were discouraged from sitting the examination.[19] Marland's work on Huddersfield and Wakefield, and Bradley, Crowther and Dupree's research on Scotland suggest that this was part of an overall trend.[20] Doctors moved from holding a single qualification to seeking a dual licence, with practitioners rejecting the LSA, which was associated with trade, in favour of the more prestigious qualifications offered by the royal colleges. The formation of the Conjoint Diploma in 1884 formalised this process by merging the MRCS and LRCP, without creating the single portal of entry campaigned for by reformers. Critics and staff at St Bartholomew's took a dim view of the examination, seeing it as inferior to the MB. Although the Conjoint Diploma proved popular with students, professional enthusiasm waned and the examination came under attack for poor standards.[21] At St Bartholomew's students were discouraged from taking it unless they were considered to be of a poor standard, or had repeatedly failed the MB. Numbers taking the Conjoint consequently declined, although not as dramatically as the lecturers hoped. With the opening of the professorial units, an increasing number of students opted for the MB. The College came to see itself as a school of the University, and by 1948 was 'unwilling to accept students who are not engaged on a University course'.[22]

---

[19] RC on Grant of Medical Degrees, PP (1882) xxix, p. 16.
[20] Hilary Marland, Medicine and Society in Wakefield and Huddersfield, 1780–1870 (Cambridge, 1987), p. 268; Bradley, Crowther and Dupree, 'Mobility and Selection', pp. 11–13.
[21] Minutes of the GMC xl (1903), Appendix xi.
[22] College Calendar (1949–50).

Table 7.2 Qualifications of students leaving St Bartholomew's, 1877–86

Year	MRCS	MRCS and LSA	MRCS and LRCP	MRCS, LRCP and LSA	LRCS	FRCS	LRCP	LSA	MD	MB	Other Bachelors	Other
1877	20	10	5	2	–	–	9	12	–	–	–	–
1878	42	13	11	3	–	1	14	19	–	1	2	1
1879	32	8	6	5	2	–	15	17	2	5	4	1
1880	14	2	2	2	–	–	4	5	–	2	1	–
1881	33	2	5	4	2	3	10	6	1	6	4	–
1882	53	4	17	3	2	1	23	8	2	5	1	1
1883	51	17	19	2	1	5	27	20	–	10	6	2
1884	73	15	23	1	5	1	38	26	2	6	10	2
1885	51	20	16	3	1	–	19	24	3	11	1	3
1886	68	14	27	4	1	1	34	21	2	2	2	–

Source: List of students, DF 208

Students and the 'mother hospital of the empire'

Given the absence of information on students' social backgrounds, it is hard to generalise about the type of men who came to study at St Bartholomew's, but it is possible to plot the College's geographical recruitment. While impressionistic evidence and Paget's survey suggest that most students came from medical, professional and commercial backgrounds, evidence from the student signature book provides a detailed picture of the College's appeal and how this altered over time.[23] Glynn has suggested that the University of London did not serve the metropolis but saw its role as national and imperial.[24] London's medical schools shared this attitude. In the late eighteenth century they matched the type of education they offered to student demand; in the nineteenth century they increasingly offered a curriculum that reflected the requirements of the GMC. The central role which London's hospitals came to play in medical education ensured that the capital's medical schools recruited nationally. Even with the growth of provincial medical schools, London's appeal and standing had a certain irresistible quality for those wanting to enter medicine.

By the 1920s it had become St Bartholomew's policy to admit 'all classes of students and all nationalities', a move that compromised the College's bid to maintain standards.[25] With over 3800 St Bartholomew's-trained doctors practising in England and the Empire by 1929, the College's ability to attract students nationally and internationally should not be surprising. Networks of recruitment and support existed, and strong family and local ties developed, but the pattern of recruitment gradually shifted to take account of the changing geography of medical education, population movements and regional economic development (see Figure 7.2, pp. 228–9). Students from Scotland and the Northwest were always in a minority, given the strength of the Scottish medical schools. Traditional areas of recruitment in the South and East Anglia declined as the number of students from the Home Counties increased. Students from the Midlands and the North gradually moved away from St Bartholomew's in favour of provincial schools attached to civic universities. The same process may be seen in the Southwest with the growth

[23] See James Paget, 'What Becomes of Medical Students', *St Bartholomew's Hospital Journal* (1869); M. Jeanne Peterson, 'Gentlemen and Medical Men: The Problem of Professional Recruitment', *BHM* lviii (1984), pp. 460–2. The College reflected a similar pattern of recruitment to Zwanenberg's findings for Suffolk apothecaries' apprentices, and to Rosner's work on Edinburgh: David Van Zwanenberg, 'The Training and Careers of those Apprenticed to Apothecaries in Suffolk, 1815–58', *Medical History* xxvii (1983), pp. 139–50; Lisa Rosner, *Medical Education in the Age of Improvement: Edinburgh Students and Apprentices, 1760–1826* (Edinburgh, 1991), pp. 27–8.

[24] S. Glynn, 'The Establishment of Higher Education in London', in *London Higher*, ed. Roderick Floud and Sean Glynn (London, 1998), p. 31.

[25] Memorandum, 1942, DF 192; 'Statement of objects and needs', MS 6/8.

of the Bristol medical school and depopulation. Recruitment in London declined in the twentieth century from a high point at the end of the nineteenth century, when St Bartholomew's had acquired a greater share of the educational market, as students were attracted to provincial schools.

The one group of students that consistently grew was those from overseas, rising from 1.8 per cent in 1840 to 1845 to 26.1 per cent in 1930 to 1935. This was considerably higher than in many of the smaller London medical schools.[26] As elsewhere, overt and covert quotas for foreign students were established: in the 1920s these were set at approximately 5–10 per cent of applicants. Despite protests from students about the 'number of "coloured" students', these quotas were repeatedly ignored. By 1926, St Bartholomew's was felt to cater 'for the whole world'.[27] The rising number of overseas students reflected in part the structure of Britain's imperial expansion and the reputation of St Bartholomew's as the 'mother hospital of the Empire'. Overseas applications were further encouraged in 1902 following a metropolitan decision to place joint advertisements in colonial papers to boost recruitment. As students from St Bartholomew's joined the Indian and Colonial Medical Service, so the College's links were extended and a new network of recruitment created. Students from India, South Africa and America dominated, followed by those from the West Indies, Australia and New Zealand. Most, in fact, were colonials: native students were a minority.[28]

Until the 1930s, Europe contributed a relatively small number of overseas students. Given the prestige and established position of many European universities, they formed only 6.9 per cent of the student body between 1930 and 1937. With the rise of Hitler, the College reluctantly admitted more students fleeing the Nazi regime and by 1937 the majority of European students were Nazi refugees. By 1939, the College felt 'overburdened with students from foreign countries' and throughout the Second World War resisted admitting further overseas students.[29]

Paying for medicine

Until the 1960s, no matter where students came from or what qualifications they sought, the majority had to pay for their training. State and local authority intervention did start to play a part in the finance of medical education from the 1900s but this was directed at an institutional level to

[26] See Claire L. J. Cassar, '"Of Mary's and Men": Admissions to the St Mary's Hospital Medical School "Experience", 1883–1916' (unpublished B.Sc. diss., University College London, 1999), pp. 37–41.

[27] SU minutes, 15 June 1926, SU 11/1.

[28] Overseas students, DF 85–6.

[29] Ibid.; College Council, 21 June 1939, MS 28/1.

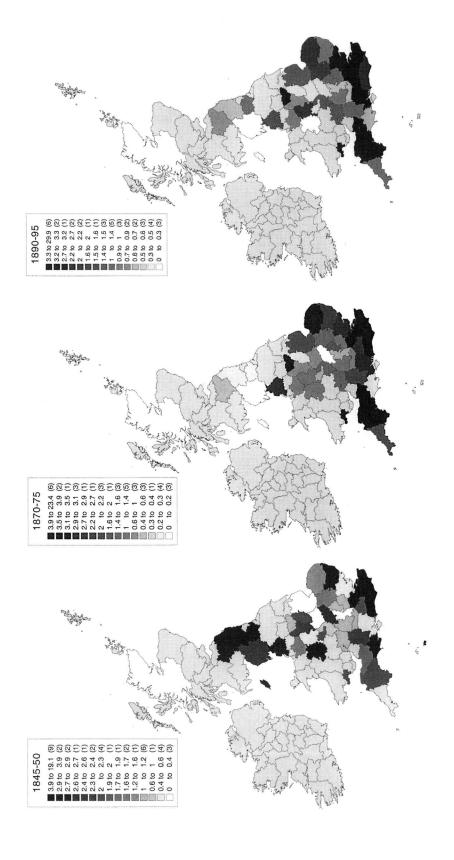

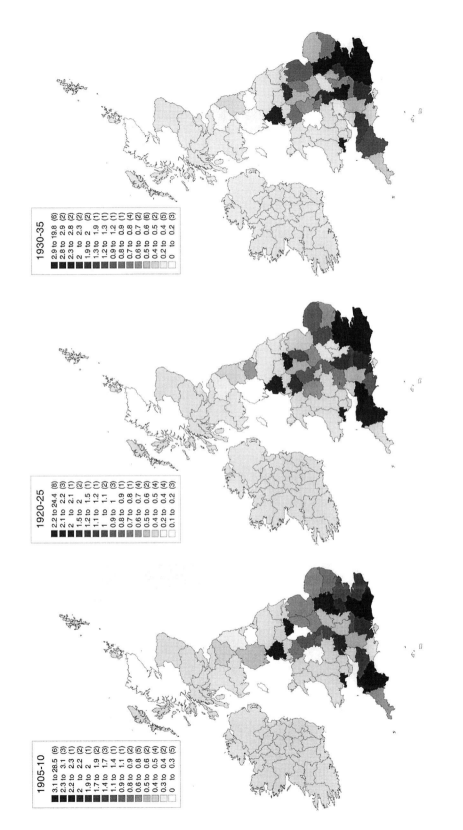

Figure 7.2 Place of residence while at St Bartholomew's, 1845–1935

cover services, not at individual students. London stood at the apex of this free market system of medical education in which students and their families were expected to shoulder the cost of training.

In the late eighteenth century, the professional advantages offered by study in London outweighed the costs, so that it was not 'only those from professional or relatively wealthy families could afford . . . [the] high expense' who entered medicine or sought an education in London.[30] Not every student opted for this route, but 'for young men seeking to enhance their professional and social status . . . a stay in the metropolis was likely to be worth the expense'.[31] Walking the wards of a London hospital put them at an advantage, while the short period of attendance initially required cut down the actual cost. However, the gradual institutionalisation of the medical curriculum required longer periods of training at a medical school, forcing up the relative cost of studying in London. In the early nineteenth century, study at a London school cost between £100 and £200 per annum depending on the institution, a figure the *Lancet* already felt to be extortionate. This rivalled the average amount spent on a public school education and the minimum deemed necessary to study at Oxford.[32] By the mid-nineteenth century the cost of studying in London had risen further. Peterson estimates that the minimum budget was £250 at a time when most clergymen earned approximately £100.[33] The average was more likely to be between £500 and £1000.[34] As the curriculum expanded and greater emphasis was placed on laboratory training, so the cost of studying rose. Medical schools raised their fees in an attempt to keep pace with rising costs, skewing recruitment and leading to fears that medicine was becoming too exclusive.

London remained the most expensive place to study medicine in Europe throughout the nineteenth and twentieth centuries, and St Bartholomew's was one of the most expensive medical schools in London. The College charged £52 10s for 'entrance to all the Lectures necessary for admission to the Members' examination at the Royal College of Physicians and Surgeons and the Society of Apothecary' in 1845.[35] Unlimited admission to lectures cost more. By the 1860s, the minimum a student could expect to pay was £73

---

[30] Cited in Thomas N. Bonner, *Becoming a Physician: Medical Education in Britain, France, Germany and the United States, 1750–1945* (New York, 1995), p. 65.

[31] Susan C. Lawrence, 'Private Enterprise and Public Interest: Medical Education and the Apothecaries' Act, 1770–1825', in *British Medicine in the Age of Reform*, ed. Roger French and Andrew Wear (London, 1991), p. 49.

[32] Sheldon Rothblatt, *The Revolution of the Dons: Cambridge and Society in Victorian England* (London, 1968), p. 56; *RC on Oxford*, PP (1852) xxii, p. 32.

[33] M. Jeanne Peterson, *The Medical Profession in Mid-Victorian London* (Berkeley, 1978), p. 74.

[34] *Westminster Review* lxx (1858), pp. 141–2.

[35] College Calendar (1845/6).

10s; at St Bartholomew's it was £97 7s.[36] The cost of board and lodging, estimated at between 25s and 37s a week in 1885, along with books and equipment, also had to be found.[37] Attempts were made to encourage other London schools to fix their fees at the level charged by the College to moderate competition, but while some success was achieved in negotiating increases, St Bartholomew's remained an expensive institution. Fees reached £150 by 1892, rising a further 25 per cent in 1920.[38] In addition, students had to pay for the privilege of becoming dressers or clerks, for special courses, for compulsory attendance at a lying-in or mental hospital, and to use the library (at least until 1880 when library charges were abolished). Only a limited number of free posts were available: preference was given to those 'who are recommended by their limited means or other special circumstances'.[39] Money was also collected for cadavers for dissection and for the hire of microscopes. With a mounting number of students unable to pay their fees on time, it was decided in 1905 not to allow defaulting students to attend classes. This provision was extended in the following year: any student who owed money to the College was prevented from starting courses or taking up a post until their account had been settled.[40]

How to pay fees and make ends meet proved a constant worry for many students, and was the main reason for failure to complete study. Surviving letters and diaries reveal the time spent at medical school as a period of financial anxiety made harder by the erosion of mid-Victorian prosperity. Initially the fee-based system that had emerged in the eighteenth century allowed flexibility. Students paid for attendance on the wards or for the courses they attended, making it possible to construct a training that matched their educational needs and purses. By the 1840s the requirement to pay for individual courses had been largely abandoned in favour of a composite fee that entitled students to attend a set course of study. To ease the financial burden, Paget introduced an instalment system in 1861 and in 1902 it was decided that the composite fee entitled students to attend lectures over a seven-year period. This allowed students to take time off from their studies to spread the cost, without incurring additional expense.[41] Students and their families took full advantage of the composite fee, but a large number still found the cost of sending their sons to St Bartholomew's

---

[36] Peterson, *Medical Profession*, p. 72.

[37] Charles Bell Keetley, *The Student's and Junior Practitioner's Guide to the Medical Profession* (London, 1885), pp. 116–17.

[38] Medical officers' and lecturers' minutes, 26 June 1858, MS 12/1; ibid., 25 May 1878, MS 12/2; meeting, June 1878, MS 14/1; Finance committee, 20 February 1920, MS 31/2.

[39] Medical officers' and lecturers' minutes, 20 July 1872, MS 12/2.

[40] Finance committee, 2 February 1905, 8 February 1906, MS 31/2.

[41] Medical officers' and lecturers' minutes, 1 July 1859, MS 12/1; Finance committee, 7 February 1902, MS 31/2.

too much. Frank Fouke, for example, summoned his son away in 1890, explaining 'he has now the opportunity of employment which will enable him at once to begin keeping himself'. Fouke had found the fees too high, and with a 'young family dependent on me' felt unable to continue paying for his son's education.[42] Regular requests were made for the refund of fees and the College did occasionally offer free places to able students, and those from impoverished medical families sponsored by the Royal Medical Benevolent Fund.

Students adopted a number of strategies for meeting the cost of attending St Bartholomew's. Many from London live at home 'for economy', although this was believed to disrupt study.[43] Others relied on sources outside their families. George Burrows saved money from his Tancred scholarship at Cambridge before continuing his medical studies at St Bartholomew's.[44] A greater number worked as unqualified assistants out of term time, although progressively restrictive practices by the GMC made this less possible until the Council all but prohibited the practice from 1888 onwards.[45] If the chance of working as an unqualified assistant became increasingly limited, it did remain possible to work for the College. Donald Macalister, a student in the late 1870s, used his post as demonstrator of physics to supplement his income. He found the '£40 or so' the appointment paid 'uncommonly welcome, *when it comes*, for the expenses are very heavy at first'.[46] For Macalister and others, teaching and other appointments (including writing for the popular and medical press) were essential in helping them through their studies. By the 1930s the College was prepared to offer some students a free education in return for service as pre-clinical demonstrators, formalising an established practice.[47]

Money from friends, family or work could be supplemented by competition for prizes and scholarships. The orthodox view has seen scholarships as established to allow the talented and respectful poor to be educated before evolving into a way of recognising academic merit.[48] London's medical schools adopted a different rationale. For the College, scholarships and prizes were designed to encourage achievement and reward success, to attract students and raise standards. Only indirectly were they promoted as a way of recruiting the sons of gentlemen into the profession. To advance the best candidates, staff rejected the 'nomination' style adopted at The London

---

[42] Fouke to Moore, 3 November 1890, MS 14/4.

[43] W. S. Feldberg, 'Henry Hallet Dale', *Biographical Memoirs of the Fellows of the Royal Society* xvi (1970), p. 89.

[44] *St Bartholomew's Hospital Reports* xxii (1887), p. xxxiv.

[45] R. G. Smith, 'Development of Guidance for Medical Practitioners by the General Medical Council', *Medical History* xxxiii (1993), p. 60.

[46] Edith F. Macalister, *Sir Donald Macalister of Tarbert* (London, 1935), p. 55.

[47] College Committee, 5 December 1938, MS 29/1.

[48] Brian Simon, *Studies in the History of Education, 1780–1870* (London, 1960), p. 299.

Hospital in favour of examinations, with money offered not with a view to helping students financially, but as a way of encouraging them to compete. This was scholarship via examination, not means-testing, and it was only in the 1960s that this attitude began to change.

Students viewed prizes and scholarships differently. Although they were regularly reminded that medicine was not about money, making ends meet was an important concern for most. Scholarships formed a potentially large reservoir of additional funding. Success in a number of competitions could prove, if not profitable, then a valuable means of offsetting the high cost of study. At St Bartholomew's scholarships ranged from £15 to £130 by the 1890s, with the Combined Hospital University Entrance Scholarship, established between the College, Guy's and St Thomas's in 1933, providing a free education for three years.[49] The addition of new scholarships enlarged the scope of potential support, and competition for them became a major part of student life: 'all the year round, and in every class of academic, institutional and professional training, men are winning prizes, losing prizes, competing for prizes or scratching for those competitions'.[50] Competition was seen as healthy and a useful preparation for practice, but for students scholarships both rewarded ability and helped ease the high cost of training. This function was highlighted during the depression of the 1930s when a fall in incomes increased the financial burden of studying at a London school. The number competing for scholarships rose: in response, both the University and the College founded new scholarships. Scholarships also presented other long-term advantages that added to their material value. Charles Bell Keetley, a former student and assistant demonstrator of anatomy, urged students in 1885 to compete, believing that a good medal worth £5 'led to an income of a thousand a year'.[51] Scholarships and prizes brought the student to the attention of the teaching staff and the medical press. Each medical school religiously advertised its prize-winners, hoping to attract new students. Whether the scholarship was announced or not it remained a useful form of self-advertisement and could help guide appointments. Paget felt that winning a series of scholarships had added greatly to his position and encouraged a belief 'that I might become connected with the Hospital and be prosperous in London'.[52] By the twentieth century, whether a student had won a scholarship or not was regarded as important as 'previous experience' in determining appointments.[53] A scholarship did not become a prerequisite for a post at St Bartholomew's, but with the decline of apprenticeships they gave staff a chance to identify the talented and industrious.

---

[49] College Calendar (1891/2); ibid. (1897/8).
[50] Cited in Peterson, *Medical Profession*, p. 83.
[51] Keetley, *Practitioner's Guide*, p. 28.
[52] Stephen Paget, ed., *Memoirs and Letters of Sir James Paget* (London, 1901), pp. 54–5.
[53] House appointment nominations, DF 239.

The onset of the Depression in the 1930s forced the College to modify its attitudes towards fees and student hardship. The amount paid in scholarship money was increased, and a more direct approach was adopted to help students meet the cost of studying. With lecturers concerned about levels of debt and the effects of the Depression, a fund was established to assist 'deserving students'. Loans rather than donations were central to the fund's efforts. To limit the number of applications, the fund was not advertised: deserving cases were recommended by the lecturers.[54] However, for most students the immediate family was still the main means of support. Although the state and local authorities stepped up their financial assistance for education, offering a handful of scholarships and grants, attention was principally directed at grammar schools. Medical students received little if any financial assistance given the professional nature of their studies.[55] By the 1940s pressure was growing for 'free university education', on the grounds that entry into medicine had been 'restricted by the cost of university fees and by maintenance for at least five years after leaving school'.[56] The need for grants was put forward by a number of bodies including the Royal College of Physicians and National Union of Students (NUS), but it was not until 1958 that the idea of mandatory grants was accepted by the Ministry of Education.[57] Mandatory grants took time to be implemented, but by the 1950s a greater number of students at St Bartholomew's were already receiving financial support from local authorities. The fee-based system that had characterised medical education, and the financial basis of the College from the late eighteenth century, was gradually being eroded.

'Riotous behaviour'

Because students paid for their training did not mean that they were always conscientious consumers. The image that has come to surround the medical student suggests an entirely different picture; one represented by the 'mildewy' Allen and 'slovenly' Sawyer, two 'sawbones . . . [in] "trainin"' from Charles Dickens' *The Pickwick Papers*. Dickens' portraits were more than crude parodies. Other contemporary writers saw medical students in a similar vein, so that the stereotypical medical student became potentially irreligious, coarse, ignorant, greedy for drink, tobacco and food.[58] Rules introduced

[54] Finance committee, 17 March 1930, MS 31/3.
[55] Harold Perkin, *The Rise of Professional Society: England since 1880* (London, 1996), p. 230.
[56] Wellcome: Royal College of Physician, planning committee report, GC/186/3.
[57] Nicholas Timmins, *The Five Giants: A Biography of the Welfare State* (London, 1995), p. 202.
[58] Charles Dickens, *The Pickwick Papers* (Oxford, 1988), pp. 363–7.

by hospital governors in the eighteenth century in a bid to regulate conduct conjured up 'images of unruly, swearing, noisy students' disrupting the wards.[59] Although student antics infuriated indignant middle-class Victorians already worried about levels of intemperance and crime, medical students did have a poor reputation. Medical schools were attacked as 'hot-beds of Bohemianism', lacking in discipline and providing an environment that turned the 'new man' from serious study to dissipation.[60]

Fears of urban life, and London in particular, made such caricatures all the more believable. London was viewed as a city of 'imprudence and depravity'. Although it was admitted that students were warned against 'the solicitations to evils' that would beset them, it was suggested that most succumbed to the metropolis's corrupting influence.[61] Reports of medical students appearing in court reinforced popular beliefs that most could not resist temptation. Stereotypes fed on a rich vein of anxiety about moral decay, intemperance and dissection. Worries about bodysnatching and fears of callous treatment at the hands of doctors flourished in a climate where lecturers advised students to cultivate a 'necessary inhumanity' to cope with dissection.[62] Here the 'terra incognita' of the city, and the associated dread of anarchy, unrest and the decay of family life, fused with general apprehensions about lawlessness and drunkenness.

Most students at St Bartholomew's worked hard and took their studies seriously, but in many respects they managed to fulfil stereotypes. A tension existed between the demands of study and life in London. Outside lectures it was felt that students made 'frequent visits to the amusement gardens in Highbury Barn', a popular place of entertainment and drinking with a large, lamplit, open-air dance floor. Here it was believed 'rioty and general disorderliness became rampant at night'. Visits were also made to the Argyle Rooms, a fashionable concert hall in Regent Street, and the Pavilion, a song and supper room in Whitechapel, and there were trips to the numerous music-halls and theatres hugely popular in Victorian London.[63] More attention was directed at regular student visits to the taverns and beershops of Smithfield and the surrounding neighbourhood. Here students ate and socialised. Beer and other alcoholic drinks were an important part of any

---

[59] Lawrence, *Charitable Knowledge*, p. 123.

[60] Samuel Squire Sprigge, *Life and Times of Thomas Wakley* (London, 1897), pp. 18–19; cited in W. H. McMenemey, 'Education and the Medical Reform Movement', in *Evolution of Medical Education in Britain*, ed. F. N. L. Poynter (London, 1966), p. 145.

[61] Cited in John H. Warner, 'American Doctors in London during the Age of Paris Medicine', in *The History of Medical Education in Britain*, ed. Vivian Nutton and Roy Porter (Amsterdam, 1995), p. 344.

[62] Cited in Ruth Richardson and Brian Hurwitz, 'Celebrating New Year in Bart's Dissecting Room', *Clinical Anatomy* ix (1996), p. 413.

[63] William Girling Ball, 'History of the Medical College of St Bartholomew's Hospital' (1941), p. 29.

meal. Drinking places also served an important social and community function providing a location for sports like boxing and for popular entertainments. When students returned from local inns and taverns, lecturers complained of 'riotous behaviour' and regularly pointed to 'wilful damage done' throughout the hospital.[64]

'Riotous behaviour' could serve a function as students asserted their role as 'rational economic actors' and consumers.[65] Students used direct confrontation to assert what they believed were their rights. The focus might be on unpopular lecturers or the school authorities over restriction of access to facilities or patients. In 1834, for example, students at St Bartholomew's carried out a campaign against John Ashburner, the lecturer in midwifery. They protested against his poor lecturing and threatened a 'flare up' if he did not resign. Eventually Ashburner did resign, 'unwilling to protract a state of disorder which is alike prejudiced to the interests of your Hospital and painful to my own feelings'.[66] However, riotous conduct often had far less to do with protest. It was part of a wider student culture, but where students in London were compared to 'irregulated schoolboys', medical students were considered to display behaviour that was far more odious.[67] According to Paget, who entered the College in 1834,

> cursing and swearing were common in ordinary talk, frequently for emphasis, and nasty stories were very often told and deemed of the same worth as witty ones. Impurity of life and conversation were scarcely thought disgraceful or worth concealing.[68]

With nowhere to go after lectures until the 1840s, many of these students were forced on to the streets and into the local taverns. It did not help that Smithfield was seen as a coarse place. The annual Cloth Fair, established in 1133 and held on the eve of St Bartholomew's Day, occasionally lasted for two weeks and was suppressed in 1855 because of debauchery. The press regularly emphasised that the meat market was a place of danger and cruelty. Although the market was moved in 1852 (after which the covered central meat market was built), Smithfield continued to be seen as 'a sink of cruelty' where 'every other building was either a slaughterhouse, a gin-palace, or a pawn-broker's shop'. Street improvements and rebuilding helped transform Smithfield from 'one of the meanest to one of the handsomest parts of London', but in the 1910s the area was still thought a 'massive melange

[64] College minutes, 9 March 1843, MS 3.

[65] Lisa Rosner, 'Student Culture at the Turn of the Century: Edinburgh and Philadelphia', *Caduceus* x (1994), p. 68.

[66] House committee, 10 February 1835, HA 1/18; Medical college, 15 February 1836, MS 15.

[67] Cited in Sheldon Rothblatt, 'London: A Metropolitan University?', in *The University and the City*, ed. T. Bender (New York, 1988), p. 126.

[68] Paget, ed., *Memoirs*, p. 40.

of beer, blood, and blasphemy'.[69] As a result, contemporaries feared that students were driven into theatres, saloons, and the company of harlots and drunkards to escape.[70]

How much truth there is in these accusations is uncertain. It seems unlikely that medical students differed from other middle-class youths and failed to seek sexual experience. At least one student, according to Paget when he was warden, married a prostitute.[71] Others no doubt benefited from the hospital's proximity to rough bars and brothels. Many of the song and supper rooms, taverns and pleasure gardens were also the haunt of prostitutes and 'street women'. Students from St Bartholomew's were known to throw 'themselves into the amusement of the Town', and to visit the 'music halls and billiard rooms' that replaced pleasure gardens as a source of popular entertainment. When students 'indulged rather too freely in wine', they were frequently called before the magistrates to be accused of theft or disorderly conduct.[72] More minor misdemeanours were also reported and the College authorities received complaints about students skipping lodgings without paying rent.[73] Such 'highly reprehensible' conduct and high spirits brought the student body into conflict with the police.[74] At times, this went beyond the usual bounds of drunkenness and disorder, heightened by the police's heavy-handed treatment of the young. Pitched battles erupted when it was felt that the police had overstepped their authority, reflecting the strong sense of hostility that existed towards the police.[75] One student recalled how 'a great crowd of people and about a dozen policemen' had collected outside the hospital's gates one day.

> The young men had been snowballing one another in the hospital grounds, and some snowballs had accidentally been hurled through the gate and landed among the gazers on the outside. A policeman entered the grounds and, laying hold of the wrong man, proceeded to take him to the lock-up. However, the student wriggled out of his ulster and took refuge in the dissecting room
>
> By now numerous policemen were in the grounds. They had collared several rebels, and as there was too great a crowd of students around the gate at which they entered, they decided to go through the surgery. . . . But by accident (doubtless) all the house surgeons and house physicians had gathered here, and found it

---

[69] Cited in Francis Sheppard, *London 1808–1870: The Infernal Wen* (London, 1971), p. 189; Geoffrey Bourne, *We Met at Bart's: The Autobiography of a Physician* (London, 1963), p. 17.

[70] William Barrett Marshall, *An Essay on Medical Education* (London, 1827).

[71] Medical students, f.44, X5/19.

[72] Medical Council, 28 May 1846, MC 1/1.

[73] Cross to Moore, 19 September 1890, MS 14/5.

[74] Ibid., 30 November 1875, MS 14/1.

[75] See David Taylor, 'Policing the Community', in *Social Conditions, Status and Community, 1860-c.1920*, ed. Keith Laybourne (Stroud, 1997), pp. 104–22.

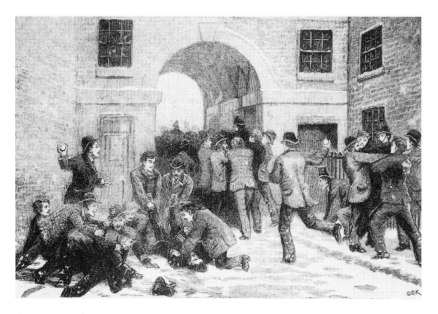

Plate 7.1 'Police and students of St Bartholomew's: A fracas during the recent snowstorms', from a contemporary print, December 1875

inconvenient just to stand aside and let the police through. Not far off a porter (who can generally understand a wink, but this time probably mistook the meaning intended to be conveyed to him) ran round and locked the door on the other side, preventing the police from doing their duty. A group of students now bundled willy-nilly into a very narrow passage, and taking the constabulary one by one, liberated the prisoners and carried the captors by heels and heads and laid them gently down on the footpath outside the hospital gates.[76]

If conflict of this nature was sporadic, student activities in the hospital and during lectures were a regular source of disturbance. Theft was common and lectures repeatedly disrupted.[77] Staff were regularly assailed by 'absurd and ridiculous performances' and lecturers were 'frequently obliged to stop'.[78] In the wards, competition between families keen for burial and students keen to acquire the recently dead for dissection resulted in 'indecent, sometimes dangerous haste'.[79] Angry letters were received from the governors implying sexual relations between students and female patients. For example, in November 1875, the Clerk reported that

[76] Girling Ball, 'History of the Medical College'.
[77] *St Bartholomew's Hospital Journal* xii (1904–5), p. 41.
[78] *BMJ* (1857), p. 1015.
[79] Christison, *Christison*, p. 192.

on Friday afternoon last, two students, Mr Farrer and Mr Young, were in the Surgery laughing and joking with two young women, who had come for admission into Magdalen Ward, and who were waiting to see the House Surgeon, and that, upon the Curator remonstrating with them on their unseemly behaviour they left the Surgery taking the women with them.

Such reported incidents were rare, but more evidence exists of students visiting nurses in the wards late at night, much to the governors' alarm.[80]

Students at other metropolitan hospitals were little better, nor were such activities limited to London. Students across Britain readily created 'their own student subculture'.[81] Such behaviour may be seen as part of an adolescent culture accentuated by the male club atmosphere strong in London's hospitals. However, by the late nineteenth century apologists for London's medical students had begun to concentrate on a different type of man. Change was already underway in the 1860s, when the medical press started to condemn attacks on students as malicious. By the 1880s, while it was reluctantly conceded that a few remained who were 'irreclaimably idle, foolish or vicious', most medical students were now shown to be industrious and gentlemanly, if full of youthful vigour.[82] The medical student was being reinvented as a respectable part of a profession, adding to a set of images that emphasised doctors' improving social status.

At St Bartholomew's the same change had apparently occurred in the student body. In 1890, Sydney Waterlow, treasurer of the hospital, could confidently tell the House of Lords that students at the College were 'better educated, and, therefore, I suppose so very much better socially than they used to be'.[83] A 'coarser stratum of society' lingered, but by the 1920s only a few 'hardy perennials' were felt to remain.[84] Petitions replaced placards and threats of riots when students felt their rights frustrated. Few incidences of drunkenness or assault were reported from the 1880s. If inexperienced lecturers still found it hard to keep their classes under control, the most common disciplinary issue was too much noise in the library.[85] Riding bicycles in the wards or sliding on the highly polished ward floors (leading one sister to impose a rule that only senior staff were allowed to do this) presented further disciplinary problems. By the Edwardian period, the

---

[80] Cross to Moore, 13 May 1884, MS 14/3; ibid., 30 November 1875, MS 14/1.

[81] M. E. Fissell, *Patients, Power and the Poor in Eighteenth Century Bristol* (Cambridge, 1991), p. 128.

[82] R. Blundell Carter, 'The London Medical Colleges', *Contemporary Review* xxxiv (1878/9), p. 585.

[83] *SC of the House of Lords on Metropolitan Hospitals, First Report*, PP (1890) xvi, p. 177.

[84] *St Bartholomew's Hospital Journal*, April 1898, p. 111; Ronald Ross, *Memoirs: With a Full Account of the Great Malaria Problem and its Solution* (London, 1923), p. 30.

[85] Bourne, *We Met at Bart's*, pp. 18–19.

difficult were characterised as the 'habitués of the local bars and dives, and cognoscenti of Leicester Square and the music halls' rather than the main student body.[86] Further changes occurred in the interwar period. The growth of cinema, dance-halls, amusement arcades and restaurants, and a rallying of the London stage, introduced new trends that were less rooted in drinking. However, it may be assumed that students also benefited from the relaxation of social protocols and sampled the more exotic world of Soho's nightclubs, in a climate where 'the example of the flapper and the "bright young thing" encouraged younger Londoners to enjoy themselves'.[87]

The events surrounding the 1926 General Strike suggests that London's medical students had firmly allied themselves with the state and become a force for conservatism. Medical students were used as strike breakers, and 170 students from St Bartholomew's joined the Special Constabulary, working in the docks and sleeping in the hospital's Great Hall. By the mid-1940s, although students at the College were certainly seen as wary of using a razor, it was asserted that they had 'a large capacity for accepting responsibility and using [their] own initiative'.[88]

Two forces may be seen at work here. The first was social. Humphries argues that by the 1890s middle-class parents had successfully inculcated their children with an 'ideology of adolescence' that was less troublesome and more restrained as Victorian society became less violent and more self-disciplined.[89] Attitudes to drinking and drunkenness were modified under the weight of the temperance movement. Fines for drunkenness, along with restrictions on opening hours, made it harder to drink throughout the day. Legal intervention combined with changing attitudes to break down the public house tradition, so that by the late Victorian period 'no respectable urban Englishman entered an ordinary public house'. Healthy recreation, sport and alternative places to eat and meet were encouraged to fill the gap.[90] Medical students, predominantly drawn from the middle classes, absorbed these values. Ironically as their numbers rose, medical students became less visible, less of a problem, as attention shifted from their carousing to the working-class 'hooligan'. Bourgeois self-doubt, firmly rooted in the dark and seductive landscape of London, fears of crime, poverty and sexual danger, presented more pressing problems for social order than drunken, essentially middle-class medical students.

The second force encouraging a modification of students' behaviour was connected with changes in the structure and nature of medical education.

---

[86] *St Bartholomew's Hospital Journal*, March 1951, p. 56.
[87] Roy Porter, *London: A Social History* (London, 1994), p. 324.
[88] Girling Ball, 'History of the Medical College' p. 348.
[89] Stephen Humphries, *Hooligans or Rebels? An Oral History of Working-class Childhood and Youth, 1889–1939* (Oxford, 1995), pp. 18–19.
[90] Brian Harrison, *Drink and the Victorians: The Temperance Question in England, 1815–1872* (Pittsburgh, 1971), pp. 309–18.

The GMC fostered a transition to a more proscriptive and longer curriculum. This had a clear impact on students' lives. Since the late eighteenth century, students had followed a broad training in preparation for a career in general practice, but with the inclusion of more subjects, lectures and demonstrations, and regular examinations, the control of learning was removed from the student. The result was less time for high living and a more disciplined and socialised student body.

The same processes may be seen at St Bartholomew's. By the mid-nineteenth century lectures were scheduled from 9 a.m. to 7 p.m., dissections from 7 a.m. to 5 p.m. In the 1880s, classes were held on a Saturday to take account of the number of new subjects students were expected to study. However, it was not just changes to the structure of education that had an impact. From the 1850s, medical schools made a concerted effort to weed out the idle or unsuitable. A move from apprenticeship and attendance at a flexible course of lectures to the corporate structure of the medical school established different routines. By the late 1880s, according to William Savory, the lecturer in clinical surgery, 'students are as carefully looked after as they can be without absolute residence within the school walls'.[91] Students did not always see it like this and complained of being treated like schoolboys. The creation of the discipline committee in 1862, along with closer monitoring through regular examinations and registers, gave students less freedom as the College, like other teaching hospitals, sought to reduce the level of 'supposed delinquents'.[92] After a flurry of activity as it asserted its authority, the committee could afford to meet less frequently by the mid-1880s, having made a series of 'purges'. Playing pitch and toss in the library was no longer acceptable. Drunkenness in the hospital or 'making noises' in lectures could result in suspension. Disturbances outside the hospital were taken more seriously.[93] In its concern with performance and attendance, the committee fostered a structure that kept students in lectures and demonstrations. In 1904, an attempt was made to check the growing custom of students absenting 'themselves from lectures and from demonstrations for indefinite periods of time without giving notice either to the warden or to their tutors'. All students who claimed to be sick now had to notify the 'Warden in writing' or face disciplinary procedures.[94] Efforts to control attendance enforced the College's patterns of study.

The general improvement in students' conduct and appearance encouraged by the College's efforts to improve study did not mean that

---

[91] *RC on a University for London*, PP (1889) xxxix, p. 79.

[92] Meeting of the medical officers and lecturers, 18 October 1873, 28 October 1876, 7 December 1878, 7 February 1874, MS 12/2.

[93] Discipline committee, 21 July 1882, 3 July 1882, MS 32/1; ibid., 13 October 1910, MS 32/2.

[94] Ibid., 30 May 1904, 20 February 1905, MS 32/2.

students were transformed from pariahs into angels. A system of education that was arduous and regimented prompted students to rebel. Nor could staff afford to be too strict. A concern about academic standards was tempered with a certain degree of leeway to prevent students from leaving. Although practical jokes remained common, 'riotous behaviour' did become more sporadic. William Girling Ball, warden between 1913 and 1921, remembered having to deal with drunken pranks but little behaviour that could be considered riotous.[95] Often these activities were channelled into inter-hospital rivalry and rag weeks, which had their heyday between 1900 and 1953. Armistice Day, 1919, saw a pitched battle between St Bartholomew's and University College when students from University College marched on West Smithfield as part of their rag week to capture the gun presented to the hospital by the War Office.[96] A further incident in 1948 suggested that students had not been entirely subdued. During the Lord Mayor's procession, four students from St Bartholomew's were arrested for 'resisting Police Officers in the execution of their duty', one being charged with 'assaulting a Chief Inspector'. As part of rag week, the four students and 100 others from the College had attempted to force their way on to the route of the Lord Mayor's procession, producing a melée when they attempted to break through police lines. However, such 'untimely incidents' had become uncommon and were now more notable for their unusual nature.[97]

'Dreary discomfort': student lives

Although students' conduct was often sufficient to justify popular prejudices, the routine of study at St Bartholomew's, and measures to improve discipline and performance, imposed a regime of lectures, ward rounds, demonstrations and examinations. Most students took their work seriously and complained that they had too much to learn. Already by 1797, Owen Evans could write to his father: 'we have a great deal too much to attend to.' Moves towards a more defined curriculum gave structure to students' learning but at the same time led to protest that work was dull and monotonous. Although the environment at St Bartholomew's was not as rigid as in some of the provincial schools, Savory reflected a common grievance in the 1840s when he noted that between lectures, dissections and the wards 'I was never at leisure'.[98] Another student, writing to his father in 1830, described how he spent his time:

[95] William Girling Ball, 'Autobiography', pp. 31–6.
[96] St Bartholomew's Hospital Journal, December 1919, pp. 38–9.
[97] Lucas to College, 12 November 1948, 1 November 1949, DF 77.
[98] John M. T. Ford, ed., A Medical Student at St Thomas's Hospital 1801–2: The Weekes Family Letters, Medical History, Supplement No. 7 (1987), pp. 35, 27.

I get my breakfast or coffee at eight or nine o'clock depending on my eight or nine o'clock lecture; read, or attend lecture at the hospital; at three I go over to a chop house in Aldersgate Street and get my dinner, and read a paper, and get a glass of porter; for this meal I pay about a shilling or thirteen pence; return to my reading again till seven, when I get coffee, and then read till bed-time.[99]

His experiences were not unusual. It was believed that only with careful planning could the student hope to condense the twelve to fourteen hours needed to study a day into something more manageable. Accounts from the 1860s amplify the mundane experience of medical school where 'every theatre except the lecture-theatre is generally forbidden fruit to a reading man'. By the 1880s the timetable had become so complex that practical physiology and practical gynaecology had to be held on Saturdays along with attendance at operations.[100] Looking back on the period, Thomas Horder suggests that the only way for most students to cope with the work was by adopting a spartan life and by working hard, even if hard-working students were often the target of ragging.[101] Not all were this studious. Ronald Ross, famous for his work on malaria, remembered his time at St Bartholomew's as occupied more by writing poetry and studying music than by being a 'good student'.[102] Such students gave colour to the medical world and their reminiscences served an important function in emphasising their progress. Most students, however, 'bore the weariness of their sordid life and worked on in dreary discomfort'. Howard Marsh remembered that the conditions under which students lived were dirty, with 'food badly cooked', and there was 'a complete absence of anything in the way of pleasant surroundings or healthy recreation'.[103]

It would be unwise to suggest that students were too impoverished by their experiences. In a survey of student living standards at St Bartholomew's in 1842, it was found that most students paid between 9s and 16s per week in rent. In the mid-nineteenth century, Mayhew estimated that a whole floor of three or four rooms cost 5s to 7s per week.[104] Medical students aimed for better accommodation even when breakfast was included. The survey showed that students would take breakfast in their rooms, with a 'great many' lunching 'at the neighbouring Bakers and the remainder at the Public houses'. In the evenings, students ate in the Clerkenwell chophouses where the food was well cooked and cheap, if not of a high standard. There were few

[99] *St Bartholomew's Hospital Journal* xii (1904/5), p. 25; Rosner, 'Student Culture', p. 73.
[100] Cited in Bonner, *Becoming a Physician*, p. 226.
[101] Mervyn Horder, *The Little Genius: A Memoir of the First Lord Horder* (London, 1966), p. 10.
[102] Ross, *Memoirs*, pp. 30–1.
[103] 'Changing Face of Bart's', p. 147.
[104] E. P. Thompson and E. Yeo, ed., *The Unknown Mayhew: Selections from the Morning Chronicle, 1849–50* (London, 1973), pp. 406, 586.

alternatives. With Paget believing that all students drank at least 2d of beer a day – more than the national average in 1845 – he estimated that they spent between 3s 5d and 4s per week on food.[105] This was certainly far more than Thomas Wakley, founder of the *Lancet*, lived on when he was a student, but was close to the amount Mrs Rundell, in her popular *A System of Practical Domestic Economy*, recommended be spent in a household of five with an income of 33s per week. From these rough estimates, the average expenditure on food by students at St Bartholomew's matched the weekly income of a skilled industrial worker.[106]

Not all students were so well placed. Horder remembered that when he was a student he 'had to find the cheapest lunch I could' and often dined on prunes: 'I used to eat about half a pound of them – nothing else – most days walking round St Paul's Churchyard, dodging the horses and carts and hoping no one would see me.'[107] Food in College Hall was reported to be little better. Well-connected students frequently took advantage of the growing number of London clubs or joined the Savile Club, formed in 1868 to give middle-class men an opportunity to meet and dine. Poorer students relied on local inns or from the 1880s on the Aerated Bread Company, which opened a shop in West Smithfield as part of its metropolitan expansion. Here students could buy a roll and butter and a slice of cake for 5d.[108]

In 1910, an attempt was made to improve the situation with the formation of the 'The St Bartholomew's Hospital Catering Company Ltd'. The company eschewed profit for reasonable meals, any gain being used to improve catering.[109] Problems were quickly encountered over the quality of the food and dividends were not always paid. As the company expanded profits decreased, especially following the opening of a dining-room in Charterhouse. Pressure was applied on students to use the College's catering facilities and stricter supervision was introduced.[110] Students, having 'associated with one another at lectures during the morning', tended to lunch 'at outside places' however. This was hardly surprising given the quality of food available through the catering company.[111] The situation became alarming in 1938 when students complained of 'galvanised iron nails' in the dessert, dirt in the milk and 'large round worms' in the cod. Protests were

---

[105] John Burnett, *Plenty and Want: A Social History of Diet in England from 1815 to the Present Day* (London, 1979), p. 61; College minutes, 9 March 1843, MS 3.

[106] Charles Newman, *Evolution of Medical Education in the Nineteenth Century* (London, 1957), p. 47; Burnett, *Plenty and Want*, pp. 51, 63–5.

[107] Cited in Horder, *Little Genius*, p. 8.

[108] Catherine Phillips, *Robert Bridges: A Biography* (Oxford, 1992), p. 62; *St Bartholomew's Hospital Journal*, September 1950, p. 195.

[109] Girling Ball, 'History of the Medical College', p. 222.

[110] Board of directors for catering company, 15 May 1936, 11 February 1936, 10 November 1936, DF 213.

[111] Ibid., 27 September 1938, DF 213.

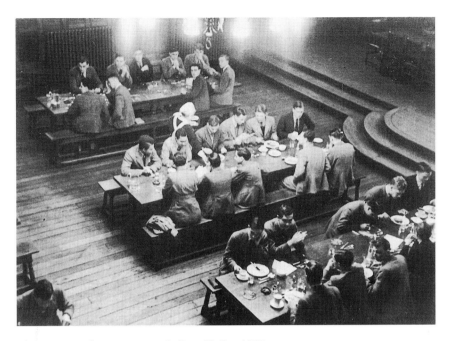

Plate 7.2 Students eating in College Hall, *c*.1937

made against the monotonous nature of the food, and complaints were voiced about price and quantity. Doubts were expressed about whether the company was non-profit making given that food was regularly felt to be expensive. Efforts were made to provide set meals and cheap lunches.[112]

Poor food was not the only difficulty facing students. Conditions in the College were often poor. Before the opening of the new lecture theatre in 1822, the existing accommodation was 'most inconvenient for comfort – or rather, comfortless – as the seats were without rails, and therefore each ascending row of students received the knees of those above into their backs, while they thrust theirs into those of the sitters below'.[113] Students remembered being frozen out of the deadhouse in winter, which was little more than 'a miserable kind of shed' in the 1830s. Conditions had hardly improved by the 1860s and with only two fires – mainly designed for ventilation to prevent the smell of preservatives and bodies from becoming overpowering – many students dissected in their overcoats.[114] The opening of new buildings between 1879 and 1881 improved conditions considerably.

---

[112] SU minutes, 1 October 1936, SU 11/2; Suggestions book, 4 November 1947, 8 January 1949, DF 207.

[113] Charles Lett Feltoe, *Memoirs of John Flint South* (London, 1884), p. 85.

[114] Paget, ed., *Memoirs*, p. 42; *Memoir of Howard Marsh*, p. 10.

The dissection room was enlarged (although it was still approached through an avenue of up-ended coffins) while the library and museum were extended. The addition of new subjects and the need to expand practical classes, mainly in the pre-clinical departments, saw all available space quickly used, leading to cramped conditions. The problem was not successfully solved until the opening of Charterhouse in 1935.

Where did these students live? One student in the 1850s believed that they were concentrated 'in the Borough of Pentonville, and in the obscure streets leading out of Gray's Inn Road' but the pattern of residence was more widespread, spreading as London grew outward.[115] College Hall proved popular and demand outstripped the number of rooms available. 'Gentlemen connected with the Hospital' also received 'Students to board in their houses'.[116] However, most found lodgings, or, if from London, lived at home. Students were caught up in the move to the suburbs, deserting rooms in the streets around the hospital that had dominated students' place of residence in the 1840s. They followed middle-class fashions as areas declined, moving from Cheapside, Clerkenwell and West Smithfield as poverty and overcrowding increased. Initially, students moved north to Islington before going to areas like Hampstead, Belsize Park and Finchley. The purchase of a sports ground at Winchmore Hill (see below) in 1893 provided a focus for students. A large contingent also went west with the growth of Kensington and Fulham in the 1860s and 1870s. A far smaller number found lodgings in Hackney, Stoke Newington and Dalston, then seen as 'handsome suburbs'; those with less money moved to the respectable working-class suburbs that grew up in northeast London after 1870.[117] However, areas like Clapham, Dulwich, Streatham and Norwood became possible as the railway carved up south London. Horse-buses, the growth of trams, railways, and the gradual opening of the Underground after 1873 made it possible to live further from the College. Geoffrey Bourne, for example, travelled each day 'by motorbus to Highgate . . . and thence by tram to Smithfield'.[118] The opening of a Metropolitan Electric Tramways line to Winchmore Hill meant quicker travel to the College from the housing around the sports ground, while the extension of the Underground network further shaped the residential patterns of students. However, for those who had to attend early morning ward rounds, a room near the hospital was still seen as essential.

[115] Ibid., p. 8.
[116] College Calendar (1884/5), p. 22.
[117] Student's signature book, 1842–1936, MS 1/1–4.
[118] Bourne, *We Met at Bart's*, p. 17.

'Not a place for trifling, but for the commencement of studies': the Abernethian Society and intellectual culture

The formation of the Hospital Medical and Philosophical Society in 1795 was intended to improve minds by providing an intellectual forum for the corporate mentality. It was established by Abernethy and Richard Powell, lecturer in chemistry, in response to the popularity of Abernethy's lectures. The Society gave an academic if not a social focus for the College. It was part of an expansion of intellectual and medical societies in the late eighteenth century stimulated by the London coffee-house culture and the 'fluid sociability of urban life'. Such medical societies placed a high premium on discussion and knowledge. For Susan Lawrence, they helped shape the metropolitan medical community by creating forums for 'the exchange of information, ideas, and cautious criticisms' that allowed practitioners and students to articulate, channel and define medical knowledge.[119] The Medical and Philosophical Society at St Bartholomew's reinforced the importance of hospital instruction and a masculine culture of learning. It provided a medium through which students and staff could discuss medical experiences and ideas.

Modelled on the society at Guy's (founded in 1771), of which Abernethy was a member, the Medical and Philosophical Society welcomed those 'who are, or have been, connected with St Bartholomew's'. After a patchy start during a period in which it was riddled with disputes, the Society was put 'into good order' by William Lawrence and Edward Stanley, both demonstrators of anatomy.[120] Meetings focused on clinical issues, giving members a chance to present cases, discuss problems and mix with the hospital elite. Medical politics were avoided as too contentious. Although staff dominated, students took part. They used the Society to learn or seek advice, especially as Abernethy was inclined to treat meetings as 'an extension of his lecture[s]'.[121] Supporters of medical societies argued that the presence of students and the encouragement given to their presentations was important to their future careers. It helped them 'acquire the art of thinking and speaking', and provided solutions or support in dealing with inconsistencies or difficult cases.[122] The Society gave students a platform: for the ambitious, it also offered an additional means of being noticed, improving the chances of a post. In collegiate terms, with speakers drawn from St Bartholomew's, it contributed to a sense of solidarity and strengthened ties.

[119] James E. McClellan, *Science Reorganised: Scientific Societies in the Eighteenth Century* (New York, 1985), pp. 41–54; Lawrence, *Charitable Knowledge*, pp. 260–3.
[120] Abernethian Society minutes, 30 October 1845, SA 1/7.
[121] Susan C. Lawrence, '"Desirous of improvement in medicine": Pupils and Practitioners in the Medical Societies at Guy's and St Bartholomew's Hospitals, 1795–1815', *BHM* lix (1985), pp. 93–4.
[122] Keetley, *Practitioner's Guide*, p. 37.

Following Abernethy's death in 1830 and a spate of illness, the Society declined. In response to trends towards professional association, it was re-founded by twenty-nine students in 1832 as 'a Society of Medical Pupils'. Renamed the Abernethian Society the model established before 1830 was retained.[123] Support for the Society was renewed, with papers addressing major medical issues and interesting cases in the wards. Membership fell again from the mid-1840s with the fortunes of the College, and 'owing to the fact that the Society is imperfectly known' and 'insufficiently appreciated'. To boost interest, its role in 'the diffusion of professional knowledge', and value as a 'pleasant relaxation from severer studies', was reasserted. Students were encouraged to join and a number of papers were published to raise the Society's profile. Improvements were made to the reading room, which was renamed the Abernethian Room and took on the atmosphere of a London club.[124] After a period of anxiety membership rose, soaring in the 1870s and 1880s as papers took on a scientific character and employed the new language of pathology and bacteriology that was beginning to enthuse staff in the College. Numbers at meetings tripled, averaging around fifty; over ninety members attended popular speakers where in the 1870s fifteen to twenty members had been common. Meetings were compared to an 'intellectual gymnasium', and speakers regularly declared that the Society aided the social and educational development of the College.[125]

From a high point in the 1890s, attendance declined until the mid-1920s. As the enthusiasm surrounding the bacteriological and pathological approach of the 1890s moderated, the Society lost ground as a hothouse of ideas. With students exposed to more pathology and bacteriology in classes, papers to the Society became less innovative and paid greater attention to cases in the wards, adopting a more empirical tone. The formation of a Students' Union (SU) in 1904 (see below) created a competing arena of sociability and reduced the Society's role in the social life of the College, altering its significance for students. With the intellectual and social impetus lost, student interest in the Society declined, only gaining momentum after the First World War.[126] Under the influence of the professorial units, it once more became an important focus for medical discussion. Debates on medical issues were introduced and distinguished speakers invited. The playwright Bernard Shaw, the Cambridge geneticist J. B. S. Haldane, the leading surgeon Berkeley Moynihan, and Almroth Wright were among those persuaded to speak and generated large audiences.[127] The Society became less of a

---

[123] Abernethian Society minutes, 23 November 1832, SA 1/3.

[124] William S. Savory, 'Introductory Address', pp. 1–2, SA 14/1.

[125] Abernethian Society attendance, SA 10/1–2; *Proceedings of the Abernethian Society* (1883/4), pp. 9–13, SA 13; Abernethian Society minutes, 8 October 1896, SA 1/13.

[126] Abernethian Society, SA 1/13–14.

[127] Abernethian Society attendance, SA 10/3–4.

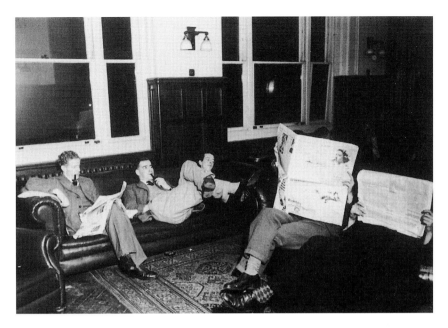

Plate 7.3 Students relaxing in the Abernethian room, *c.*1937

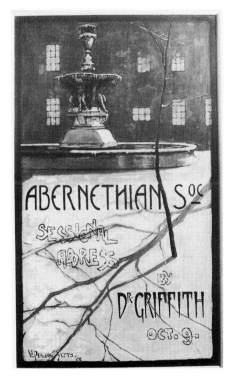

Plate 7.4 Poster for Abernethian Society sessional address, 1902

vehicle for the College and more a scientific forum, keeping students and staff in touch with clinical and political developments in medicine. If the Abernethian Society was no longer the centre of collegiate life, it had reacquired its role in the promotion of the College's intellectual identity.

'Play up! and play the game'

While College Hall and the Abernethian Society acted as mechanisms directed by the lecturers in promoting a corporate identity and discipline, leisure also played an important role. Before the 1890s, little attention was paid to sport as a way of inculcating discipline or identity, and student life at the College had no fixed social framework beyond the Abernethian Society. Formal social contact outside lectures and ward rounds was circumscribed. Social and sporting events were tangential to College life. In contrast to the paternalism of Oxford and Cambridge, or the political controls found in many European medical schools, lecturers at St Bartholomew's made little attempt to encourage student societies as a way of fostering character-building qualities. Students were left to their own devices, and though a collegiate identity developed from the 1850s it was largely two-dimensional, based on the common experiences of institutional study and the personalities of the lecturers. When societies were formed, the initiative was taken by students and owed more to local patterns of club formation and a continuation of experiences at public school or Oxbridge than it did to the College. With a student body increasingly spread across London; with teaching concentrated on an overcrowded site; and with limited funds for additional projects, it is no surprise that life at St Bartholomew's took time to develop the corporate student culture that evolved in English and Scottish universities in the late nineteenth century. Other London medical schools faced similar problems. Only with a rise in the age of students, a late Victorian boom in sport and moves by secondary schools to develop their own corporate life was a favourable environment provided for student societies. The creation of the Amalgamated Club and growing support for sport served to reinforce the collegiate identity, giving expression to solidarity, pride and identity.

When Frederick Farre entered St Bartholomew's as a student in the 1820s he remembered that there was no place where students could work quietly or socialise, although there was a room over a baker's shop near the hospital's gate, where 'we could sit during intervals of work and read the journals'. By the 1840s, the situation had improved with the opening of 'a convenient library and reading-room' which, it was anticipated, students would use 'advantageously' during the 'hours intervening between . . . Lectures'. Open daily until 7 p.m., students had to pay a subscription to use the room until 1880. Efforts were made to ensure that the library remained 'a place of study only' where 'conversation is not allowed', but students frequently ignored these rules.[128] With the College engaged in the business of education, the social provision for students was largely neglected. In the 1850s, the treasurer James Bently organised fortnightly dances in winter, while the apothecary held an informal dance in the Apothecary's Shop on New Year's Eve.[129] The opening of College Hall gave some focus for the associated life of the College, but what few clubs had been formed by the 1870s met 'in a very irregular manner'. When Walter Langdon Brown came to St Bartholomew's in 1894, 'amenities for the students were few' when compared to other London schools. The Abernethian Room offered some comfort and in 1891 the small theatre in the dingy library basement was converted into a smoking room.[130]

The lack of social facilities corresponded with the absence of institutional provision for sport. Notwithstanding growing interest and participation in sport in the urban middle class, the College remained preoccupied with providing training. Confident about the disciplinary structures already adopted, the lecturers as a collective body made little attempt until the 1890s to develop the flourishing sports culture found in elite schools and universities. Although an aura of masculinity was strong in London's medical schools, as institutions they were slow to adopt the games cult of the Victorian public school.[131] Hampered by a lack of facilities, the entrepreneurial nature of teaching, and their metropolitan locations where open spaces for recreation were restricted, London's medical schools made little provision for sport until the end of the nineteenth century. When sporting clubs were organised at St Bartholomew's the students took the initiative, occasionally in cooperation with individual lecturers. In the main, sport was fitted in between studies. It followed the same vogues embraced by the urban bourgeoisie and built on the experiences of former public school pupils, in a climate where opportunities and aspirations for leisure were expanding. Whether students founding clubs were inspired by pleasure, manly ideals of camaraderie or competition, a need to escape study, or health, it was through their efforts that sport came to play a growing part in the life of the College.[132]

While students had previously discharged their energies in walking, cricket, football and other sports on an individual basis, evidence suggests that rugby was the first sport to be organised at St Bartholomew's. Against the background of the Victorian sports craze and cult of athleticism, *ad hoc* rugby

---

[128] Frederick Farre, *On Self-Culture and the Principles to be Observed in the Study of Medicine* (London, 1849), pp. 8–9; College Calendar (1844/5), p. 17; ibid. (1880/1), p. 20.

[129] *St Bartholomew's Hospital Journal*, December 1898, p. 21.

[130] Ibid., June 1947, p. 59; Subcommittee, 9 November 1891, 24 March 1892, MS 34/1.

[131] See R. J. Holt, *Sport and the British: A Modern History* (Oxford, 1989); J. A. Mangan, *Athleticism in the Victorian and Edwardian Public School: The Emergence and Consolidation of an Educational Ideology* (Cambridge, 1981).

[132] For an overview of historians' views of why participation in sport grew, see N. Tranter, *Sport, Economy and Society in Britain, 1750–1914* (Cambridge, 1998), pp. 52–78; John Lowerson, *Sport and the English Middle Classes, 1870–1914* (Manchester, 1993), pp. 64–94.

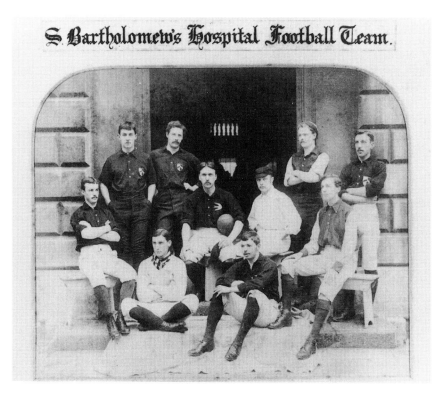

S. Bartholomew's Hospital Football Team.

Plate 7.5 Hospital rugby football team, c.1880

matches were held on a ground in Battersea in the 1860s. In 1875, a team was organised to compete in the inter-hospital rugby cup during a boom in club formation after the foundation of the Rugby Union four years earlier. After winning the cup in 1883, the team went into decline, raising concerns about the type of students entering the College. However, by this point the sporting culture that came to characterise London's medical schools had started to emerge at St Bartholomew's.[133] As national levels of participation widened, clubs were established. Caught up in the rhetoric that came to surround the benefits of sport to health and society, clubs at the College followed middle-class recreational patterns rather than a self-conscious adoption of public school or university sporting values. Underpinned by commercialisation and the development of standardised rules, they followed sporting fashions.[134] In response to the soaring popularity of cricket, a cricket club was established, though how much this also had to do with the success of the famous cricketer W. G. Grace, a former student, is uncertain. The displacement of prize fighting

---

[133] *St Bartholomew's Hospital Journal*, June 1951, p. 132.
[134] Lowerson, *Sport*, p. 96.

in the 1880s by amateur boxing under the Marquis of Queensberry rules encouraged the formation of a boxing club in 1888. Growing interest in soccer in churches, universities and public schools, as opposed to the more violent street football, saw clubs founded across Britain in the 1860s and 1870s, and an association football club was started at St Bartholomew's in 1879.

The initiative to found a club often came in response to the start of inter-hospital competitions. Drawing on intercollegiate matches at Oxford and Cambridge, competitions organised between hospitals attempted to re-create the same sense of cohesiveness among the London teaching hospitals. The Athletic Club, for example, was founded in 1867 at the same time as the Inter-Hospital Cup.[135] Encouraged by external competitions and sporting fashions, many of these societies had a patchy history, but they quickly came to play a growing role in the culture of the College, adding a sense of cohesion and pride. The Athletic Club's annual sports day, started in 1904, became one of the social events of the College year, while the successes of the Association Football Club in the London Cup attracted national attention and raised the profile of the College.

Although sporting societies dominated, other clubs were established. Students from Oxford and Cambridge formed separate societies so that 'those members of the university already at the Hospital might have an opportunity of making the acquaintance of the newcomers'.[136] The Music Society, created after a successful concert in 1878, and the Amateur Dramatic Club (ADC), formed in 1883, had a greater impact on the cultural life of the hospital. Since the mid-nineteenth century, ward entertainment and plays had become part of the annual ritual of individual hospitals. Societies and clubs evolved around these activities, influenced by the growth of bands and local orchestras. Some institutions even built stages to accommodate them. Facilities at St Bartholomew's were not so organised, but both the Musical Society and the ADC played an important role in providing entertainment for patients and staff. Although not at first part of the College, the Musical Society and ADC involved students from the outset in putting on regular concerts, ward entertainments and plays that had more in common with 'low' musical-halls than West End theatres.[137] With a repertoire that consisted mainly of farces and contemporary satires that matched general Victorian tastes, the ADC's plays and Christmas shows proved popular. Gradually it assumed a more definite student character, so that by 1921 it had become 'composed entirely of [clinical] students', and the type of plays and comic sketches (often lampooning senior staff) came to reflect this.[138] The ADC was less successful at involving pre-clinical students, who wanted more than

[135] 1904/5 *Yearbook*, SU 12; 1923/4 *Yearbook*, SU 12.
[136] Cambridge Graduates Club, SC 1/1–2.
[137] 1904/5 *Yearbook*, SU 12.
[138] ADC, 15 October 1928, SU 51/1.

Christmas shows. In 1935, a competing pre-clinical drama society was formed to stage a *A Doctor's Dilemma* in aid of the College's building appeal. After suggestions of a joint performance, amalgamation was suggested and the ADC finally became part of the SU as the Amateur Dramatic Society.[139]

The fitful development of sport at St Bartholomew's became a source of anxiety and a focus for organisation in the 1890s. Concern was stimulated by events at Oxford and Cambridge, not by the short-lived attempts to unite students in London or the growing interest in student participation spreading out from Scotland.[140] With efforts to organise the clubs in 1892, Oxbridge students came to play a central role in shaping the structure, if not the nature of sporting provision at St Bartholomew's. A series of defeats in inter-hospital competitions raised doubts about the sporting vigour of the College that offended the growing sense of institutional pride generated by the societies. Students from Cambridge were disgusted by the *ad hoc* arrangements and lack of cooperation in an environment where societies competed with each other for members. They found life at the College very different from Cambridge, where afternoon walks and exercise were features of academic life. Sport had been 'domesticated' at Oxford and Cambridge in the mid-Victorian period, tied up with efforts to reform the collegiate system and strengthen a sense of community. Amalgamated clubs had been formed in the 1880s to group together disparate societies.[141] Coming from this environment, students from Oxbridge found the situation at St Bartholomew's Byzantine. There was no sense of organisation, and membership of more than one club could prove expensive. Each club collected its own subscription, resulting in frantic labours before the start of each season to raise enough money to pay for the annual expenses. An overcrowded timetable and the fact that many students lived at home or in lodgings prevented coordination, but with pressure mounting for a common sports ground, which no individual club could afford, the need to organise became pressing. Although the Abernethian Society had discussed the need for a 'Students Club' in 1885, it was students from Cambridge who successfully campaigned in 1892 for the formation of an amalgamated club modelled on the Oxbridge system.[142]

Like its counterparts at Oxbridge, the Amalgamated Club was formed for 'financial purposes', not to articulate student opinion. Not every society was included and tensions existed with the Abernethian Society, which remained on the periphery.[143] To give a voice to the Club, the *St Bartholomew's Hospital*

[139] Ibid., 6 June 1935, 22 October 1935, 19 February 1936, 5 March 1936, SU 51/1.

[140] Eric Ashby and Mary Anderson, *The Rise of the Student Estate in Britain* (Basingstoke, 1970), p. 40.

[141] H. S. Jones, 'Student Life and Sociability 1860–1930', *History of Universities* xiv (1995/6), pp. 228–9; Peter Searby, *A History of the University of Cambridge, 1750–1870* (Cambridge, 1997), pp. 641–8.

[142] Abernethian Society, 9 February 1885, SA 2.

[143] *The Amalgamated Clubs of St Bartholomew's Hospital* (London, 1893), p. 5.

Journal was established. The lecturers gave their support. A rhetoric that stressed the beneficial nature of sport to young men and society had come to influence staff who were also concerned about competition. Lecturers feared that St Bartholomew's would lose students if efforts were not made to improve the sporting and social environment of the College.[144] A student union had been formed at the Westminster in 1886 and Guy's had established a similar Club's Union in 1891 and opened a sports ground at Honor Oak Park. These efforts had followed a wave of concern that students were being neglected to their detriment.[145] The lecturers therefore agreed to collect the membership fee.

Despite prophecies of disaster, membership grew, forcing the issue of a sports ground. With more students participating, it became progressively harder to find suitable pitches to rent, frustrating the activities of the clubs. The lecturers, after months of investigating possible sites, intervened in 1893 hoping that new facilities would improve the athletic prowess of the College. Land for a sports ground was bought at Winchmore Hill, near Edmonton on the outskirts of Northeast London. Its suburban location reflected middle-class leisure patterns and restrictions on recreational space nearer to the College. The site was fenced and drained, a pavilion built and the new ground was formally opened in 1895.[146] Trevor Lawrence, treasurer of the hospital, was optimistic that it would 'bring students together in that corporate life which was so advantageous to bodies of young men engaged in similar studies'.[147]

Lawrence's ambitions for the Club went unfulfilled. Although it successfully ran sporting fixtures, its outlook was limited to athletics, football and rugby. No corporate student body had been formed and those not interested in sport felt excluded. The position at St Bartholomew's contrasted with efforts in the provinces and in London where students were also beginning to organise in the 1890s. With the formation of corporate student bodies across the country, pressure mounted for better facilities and accommodation for students in the College.[148] The two issues – lack of accommodation and the absence of an *esprit de corps* – came to a head in 1903. Disputes over the planning of a new outpatient block became a vehicle through which calls for more student accommodation were made. Plans for the new block included suggestions that better accommodation should be included for the Abernethian Society, and the lack of unity in the existing Club motivated a group of students to campaign for a corporate body. The

[144] *St Bartholomew's Hospital Journal*, November 1932, p. 25.

[145] H. C. Cameron, *Mr Guy's Hospital, 1726–1948* (London, 1954), p. 277; *The Times*, 20 August 1886, p. 13.

[146] House committee, 8 March 1894, HA 1/27.

[147] *BMJ* i (1895), p. 1343.

[148] *St Bartholomew's Hospital Journal*, March 1933, p. 110; Ashby and Anderson, *Student Estate*, pp. 45–6.

need for a union was declared at a general meeting in 1904.[149] It was agreed that an executive committee be formed acting in cooperation with the lecturers to represent students on matters concerning their welfare and to forge closer links between students and lecturers. Weakly reflecting the demands made at other colleges for student representation, the SU sought to promote 'social intercourse and unity of interest among its members' and to incorporate 'those clubs and societies which constitute the Amalgamated Clubs and such other clubs'. Despite the rhetoric, the SU did not aim to be an inclusive body. Although the Abernethian Society was merged with the SU, those societies connected to the hospital, such as the ADC, or of a political or religious nature, remained outside.[150]

The SU made a number of immediate improvements. A cautious policy saw rooms allocated in the new junior staff quarters when it was opened in 1907 as part of rebuilding surrounding the outpatient block. A common-room (called the Abernethian Room), an adjoining committee room or sitting-room and dining-room was set aside for the SU. Two years later, a rifle range was opened in the basement. The SU stimulated a greater interest in sport and was able to organise a dance and two 'smoking concerts' (where students were permitted to smoke), the former becoming a regular fixture of the College calendar.[151] The outbreak of war in 1914 limited the SU's activities. War was at first eulogised as a heroic vision of masculinity, with football applauded as training for military success. Even sophisticated Freudians were swept along by the cult of manliness, but at a practical level sporting fixtures under wartime conditions proved hard to organise. National restrictions on wartime life and the large numbers of young men who joined the forces dampened sporting and social activity. While the rifle club grew in size, fixtures were 'scratched' and garden parties, dances and sports days had to be cancelled with the threat of Zeppelin raids.[152]

The immediate aftermath of war saw a period of reconstruction with returning ex-service men more used to the corporate life of the army. Nationally a more sombre mood encouraged a boom in 'more refined pleasures': theatre-going, reading and the cinema.[153] At St Bartholomew's, however, strenuous efforts were made to revive and extend the prewar College culture. Dances were resumed and increasingly pandered to new musical trends embodied in the Charlestone. The 'Past & Present' cricket match between staff and students and the garden party were revived, the latter turning into an annual ball. Hospital colours were reintroduced and an 'official Hospital blazer' of white and black striped flannel was designed which

---

[149] 1904/5 *Yearbook*, SU 12.
[150] Constitution and laws, SU 13/1.
[151] 1904/5 *Yearbook*, SU 12; SU minutes, 6 October 1911, SU 11/1.
[152] Ibid., 5 October 1914, 6 March 1916, SU 11/1.
[153] James Walvin, *Leisure and Society, 1839–1950* (London, 1978), p. 132.

could be worn by any member of the union, and provided a uniform and an identity that appealed to those who had left the armed forces.[154] At Winchmore Hill a new stand was opened, and a 'freshers' tea' was started in 1924 to welcome new students. By the late 1920s universities and medical schools were competing to offer a range of extra-curricular activities to attract students, a policy encouraged by the UGC to build up student numbers.[155] At St Bartholomew's individual clubs grew in size. New ones were formed, encouraged by an upsurge in outdoor recreational activity and the sporting success of the College.[156] Whereas the SU was willing to recognise sports clubs, it was less responsive to political or religious societies. As one Edwardian student at the Middlesex noted, 'politics had no interest for us simply because it made no difference to our lives'. At St Bartholomew's the SU cast itself as an apolitical body. It avoided taking a stance on religious or moral issues. Although the aim was to include all students, the SU remained predominantly interested in sport.[157] It was isolationist and resisted efforts to promote student cooperation at a metropolitan or national level, opposing the NUS and the University of London Union.[158]

The activities of the SU were scaled down during the 1930s with the onset of the Depression. Under the influence of Wilfred Shaw, president of the SU and demonstrator of practical midwifery, money was saved whenever possible. However, further facilities continued to be added, largely through the efforts of the College in a climate where most civic universities were under pressure to supply or extend student facilities. Building at Charterhouse saw the opening of a dining-hall, gymnasium, squash courts and common-room.[159] A year later, a new sports ground was bought on the Foxley Estate near Chislehurst in Kent to take account of the increased popularity of sport as part of a wider fitness craze and the growth of the sporting societies at St Bartholomew's.[160] Money was borrowed to build a pavilion and the SU was charged a higher rent. In June 1938 the pavilion was completed, and after the grounds had been levelled and returfed, three rugby pitches, and a football and hockey pitch were opened. Local residents were invited to the opening ceremony in an effort to 'foster association' and with the hope of securing donations. Other sports facilities followed.[161]

---

[154] SU minutes, 21 June 1921, SU 11/1.

[155] See UGC Report. Academic Year 1928–29 (London, 1930).

[156] SU minutes, 14 July 1932, 16 March 1922, 6 September 1924, 15 June 1926, SU 11/1.

[157] BMJ ii (1969), p. 629.

[158] SU minutes, 11 April 1922, 17 May 1929, 4 June 1929, SU 11/1; SU minutes, 25 June 1937, 4 February 1938, 24 June 1938, 29 May 1940, SU 11/2.

[159] SU finance committee, DF 316.

[160] Executive committee, 9 December 1936, MS 30/1.

[161] Ibid., 9 June 1937, MS 30/1; AGM of College governors, 27 January 1937, 26 January 1938, MS 27/1.

A corporate identity

By the outbreak of war in 1939, the College had acquired not only a physical structure divided between two sites, but also a strong sense of corporate and collegiate identity. The numerous hospital traditions and sense of history surrounding it fused with this identity. Much of this structure had evolved since the 1880s although the College's reputation, strength of leading lecturers like Abernethy and Paget, and the common experiences of the wards and lectures, had already laid the foundation. From the 1880s onwards, the trend towards increasing student numbers encouraged the lecturers to support student efforts to construct a framework for the sporting and social life of the College. While students had previously protested against inadequate teaching, by the 1890s they had begun to press the College for better facilities. The lecturers were now keen to support these claims. Attention had already been turned to the disciplinary structure to raise the educational standing of the College and to meet professional concerns about discipline, and the early foundation of the Abernethian Society had helped articulate the intellectual culture of the College beyond the lecture theatre and wards. Such a framework countered the trend towards residential dispersal as more and more students came to find lodgings in London's growing suburbs. Divisions did exist between pre-clinical and clinical students, a trend strengthened by the relocation of the pre-clinical departments to Charterhouse in 1933, but even these divisions existed within an overall collegiate identity. Students could now boast a large sports ground, an active (if isolationist) SU, a large number of clubs, and modern accommodation for meeting, eating and talking. The establishment of a student health service in 1938, and the creation of a hardship fund, pointed to the College's increasingly active role in student life beyond an interest in discipline and academic performance. Between 1788, when the first systematic courses were offered, and 1939, St Bartholomew's had become one of London's largest medical schools with an active student body and a set of values that were intimately associated with the idea of a 'Bart's man'.

Part III

War and reconstruction 1939–68

8

A college at war

In 1938, St Bartholomew's started planning for the future. Rebuilding of the pre-clinical departments at Charterhouse had left the College financially overstretched. The 1930s had seen the number of academic and research staff rise and a concerted effort to appoint and endow chairs. Facilities for students had been improved and, with a rise in the number of applicants, the College had become more selective. However, problems remained, especially in obstetrics where teaching was deficient. Debates about the College's 'future policy' aimed to resolve these problems and extend professorial teaching but they were cut short by war in September 1939.

Although plans had been made for teaching during wartime, the College was still unprepared for what was to happen between 1939 and 1945. War left a legacy of structural and teaching problems that were overcome only gradually. Questions about the College's future merged with debates on how medical education should be organised and healthcare delivered. While agreement was reached on the need for reform, the process of achievement was fraught with difficulties. In the mythology of the welfare state, the Second World War created a common bond of citizenship and new middle ground that laid the foundations for the welfare state. Reality was more complex. At St Bartholomew's war produced dislocation and disruption as teaching involved sending students to four different sites in and around London. The devastation of Charterhouse by bombing encouraged a gloomy view of the future, and the protracted planning of a national health service was greeted with apprehension and, in some quarters, resentment. The College's history between 1939 and 1948 was more than just a question of struggling on gallantly in the face of bombing, makeshift arrangements and uncertainty. It was also a history of intense planning; of adaptation to a set of circumstance which many came to see as unavoidable.

Planning for war

Preparations for war started at the Home Office in 1935, but it was not until 1937 that the Ministry of Health gave serious consideration to the issue of wartime medical care. Blitzkrieg bombing in Spain, and Germany's *Anschluss* with Austria, had increased international tension, and elements in the civil service began to think about the possibility of another war, despite a policy of appeasement. The organisation of healthcare in event of war was transferred from the Home Office to the Ministry of Health and discussions were begun over what was to become the Emergency Medical Service (EMS). Lessons had been learned from the First World War, but it was fear of air raids that focused attention, encouraging planning for the treatment of casualties rather than the establishment of a comprehensive health service.[1] A dismal picture was presented. Experts were consulted, including the recently knighted William Girling Ball, the forthright dean at St Bartholomew's, who was committed to developing closer links with the University of London and between medical schools.[2] Planning and the 1938 hospital survey revealed overlapping yet inadequate healthcare facilities. The organisational task was immense. The EMS challenged the 'mixed economy' of interwar medical services. It created a regional framework in which hospitals were managed by their existing administration but where the Ministry of Health dictated the role each hospital should play. Permanent posts were frozen and long overdue surveys were conducted into hospital provision, prompting hurried programmes of improvement as new services were created in a bid to provide uniform conditions. Standards were raised and beds were pooled for the 1.2 million casualties estimated in the first sixty days of an aerial attack, but regional inequalities remained.[3]

The traditional hostility of voluntary hospitals to any government scheme slowed down planning in London. By January 1939 medical schools had become alarmed about the lack of progress. A meeting of metropolitan deans pressed for the creation of a Deans' Committee to organise a sector system in London.[4] The Ministry agreed. Girling Ball played a central role in establishing the EMS in London, but not all were satisfied. Some of the governors and staff at St Bartholomew's joined in complaints about the lack of a central organisation or 'man of standing to take control of the whole organisation'.[5] Anxiety mounted with delays in preparations and disagreements over catchment areas. The Ministry of Health had to bully doctors into restricting private practice and was forced to reach a compromise. Despite complaints that the voluntary hospitals dominated the EMS, little attempt was made to encourage integration with the medical services provided by the London County Council (LCC). London was divided into ten sectors, each based around a teaching hospital. St Bartholomew's (with

---

[1] C. L. Dunn, *Emergency Medical Services*, 2 vols (London, 1952), Vol. i, pp. 7–8.

[2] Girling Ball had been involved in the territorial wing of the Royal Army Medical Corp and was responsible for the management of the military wards at St Bartholomew's between 1914 and 1918. As dean of the University of London's Faculty of Medicine, he represented the interests of the London medical schools, and as a consultant surgeon to the Royal Air Force he was familiar with military demands.

[3] Frank Honigsbaum, *Health, Happiness and Security: The Creation of the National Health Service* (London, 1989), pp. 17–18; Brian Abel-Smith, *The Hospitals, 1800–1948: A Study in Social Administration in England and Wales* (London, 1964), pp. 425–7.

[4] Medical Council, 20 November 1939, MC 1/11.

[5] *The Times*, 14 June 1939, p. 16; ibid., 29 June 1939, p. 15.

the Royal Free) was placed in Sector 3 and designated a casualty receiving hospital, with Friern, New Southgate and Wellhouse hospitals designated advanced base hospitals. The headquarters were located at Mill Hill: Girling Ball was appointed Sector group officer and St Bartholomew's became the hub of Sector 3.[6]

There were problems over what to do with medical students. The University Grants Committee (UGC) was anxious that teaching should not be disrupted, but in London this presented difficulties. With the University insistent that casualty hospitals were unsuitable for teaching, and with the number of beds in central London dramatically reduced, both the UGC and the University argued that medical schools should be evacuated. Those running London's teaching hospitals were not convinced: when no agreement was reached, they started to make their own plans.[7] At St Bartholomew's provisional arrangements for the teaching in wartime had been made in 1937. By March 1939, as the international situation deteriorated, serious attention turned to how pre-clinical teaching could be carried on during wartime. Staff expected a considerable reduction in teaching, predicting that most of the responsibility for continuing medical education would fall to the heads of department. Special courses were planned in first aid, air-raid precaution and the treatment of fractures.[8]

These arrangements were immediately superseded when war was declared. After consulting the University, it was resolved that all pre-clinical students at St Bartholomew's and The London be sent to Cambridge. How this was achieved was left to individual colleges to decide: St Bartholomew's approached Queens' College and The London St Catherine's College, and both agreed to work together. The University went into exile and the College joined various government departments and other colleges of the University in Cambridge.

With the pre-clinical departments transferred to Cambridge, Charterhouse was closed and Finsbury Borough Council took over the car-park to build an air-raid shelter. Much of the remaining ground was placed under cultivation by Charles Harris, the warden, in a patriotic bid to make the College self-sufficient.[9] Other colleges across the country were engaged in similar activities. After detailed negotiation with Cambridge, it was decided that the College would have access to the University's laboratories for anatomy, physiology and biochemistry.[10] Help was also secured from the Leys School in Cambridge, which offered facilities for the First MB classes. When the school was taken over by the EMS, all First MB teaching was transferred

---

[6] Dunn, *Emergency Medical Services*, Vol. i, pp. 45–7, 168.

[7] Girling Ball diary, f.6.

[8] College committee, 1 March 1939, MS 29/1.

[9] Ibid., 19 October 1939, MS 29/1.

[10] 1939/40 annual report.

to Cambridge and the Cavendish Laboratory.[11] Although students felt they could boast of having worked in the famous Cavendish Laboratory, it was apparent that 'beautiful laboratories and Bart's students are incompatible'.[12] Even after six months of war, the arrangements continued to be seen as temporary, and with no air raids staff began to protest against their enforced exile from London.

One hundred and sixty pre-clinical students were advised to attend Queens' College, Cambridge from 18 September 1939, fifteen days after Chamberlain had broadcast the news that Britain was at war with Germany. Queens' had grown from one of the smallest colleges in Cambridge to one of the largest after a series of reforms in the late nineteenth century.[13] By moving the pre-clinical students to Queens' it was believed that a collegiate life would be maintained in an environment where students from St Bartholomew's would be working alongside students from other London hospitals. Students were reassured that they would continue to be taught by 'Barts teachers' and would remain 'Barts men'. There was a price. The cost of education in Cambridge had remained high throughout the interwar period and students from St Bartholomew's were expected to pay extra for board and lodging in addition to their fees. Rooms could not be provided immediately, and those with camp beds were advised to bring them.[14] By October 1939, 176 students from St Bartholomew's had taken up residence at Cambridge. Frank Hopwood, professor of physics, went as subdean, taking with him Hamilton Hartridge, professor of physiology, William Hamilton, professor of anatomy and Arthur Wormall, professor of biochemistry, along with twelve junior staff and a secretary.[15]

Clinical students presented a greater problem. At the outbreak of war they were given three months' leave during which time the EMS was finalised and hospital beds cleared for the expected casualties. An official moratorium on teaching did not see a temporary end to instruction. Girling Ball was clear that 'as a matter of fact there is teaching going on in most Hospitals' and it was decided that this would be 'counted to the credit of the students'. He was anxious to get students of the same year together as quickly as possible. Tentative arrangements had been made to send students to Hill End Hospital, St Albans and to Friern Hospital. However, with war, students were initially divided between a small contingent working at West Smithfield with the rest scattered through the twenty-three hospitals in Sector 3.[16]

[11] Ball to Staff, 14 November 1940, DF 21.
[12] *St Bartholomew's Hospital Journal*, March 1941, p. 120.
[13] Christopher N. Brooke, *A History of the University of Cambridge* (Cambridge, 1993), pp. 193–4.
[14] Ball to College, 9 September 1939, DF 38.
[15] Executive committee, 8 September 1939, MS 30/1.
[16] Ibid., 11 October 1939, MS 30/1.

A workable scheme was finally established in December 1939 when students were concentrated in three hospitals. The absence of air raids gave an opportunity for reorganisation. The number of specialist departments was drastically reduced, so that instruction in them could be covered in three months. First-year clinical students were sent to Hill End (formerly the Hertfordshire County Asylum) and the smaller Cell Barnes Hospital, two-and-a-half miles from St Albans for the 'fundamentals of Medicine, Surgery and Pathology'. Second-year students remained at St Bartholomew's and third-year students were sent to Friern (formerly Colney Hatch), a mental hospital built in the 1840s and renowned for its central corridor that stretched for well over a quarter of a mile. Its proximity to St Bartholomew's and poor condition ensured that students spent a large portion of their time attending the outpatient departments at West Smithfield. The distance of Hill End and Cell Barnes from London made billeting essential. Despite difficulties, Harris 'hoped that as many as possible will avail themselves of these billeting arrangements so that the work of each Hospital may be effectively carried out'. Government funding, in return for assistance in the Sector hospitals, kept costs down. The situation was different at St Bartholomew's. Those working at West Smithfield were expected to find their own accommodation, though a limited number of rooms were made available in the west wing in a warren of plywood cubicles on condition that students 'undertake certain obligations'.[17] Moving students between sites required careful planning.

A divided college

The war presented both a threat and a challenge to voluntary hospitals and accelerated 'the process of co-operation with state officials'.[18] Although demand for services through the EMS created staffing problems, London's hospitals took full advantage of the service. With an estimated £100,000 a week allocated to keep beds empty, teaching hospitals welcomed the money to raise income when casualties failed to meet projections. The rising cost of medical education and growing demands from clinicians for salaries had produced a deficit in ten of London's twelve teaching hospitals.[19] EMS funds were used to reduce waiting lists, although for civilians admission remained problematic and cases were prioritised, creating anxieties at St Bartholomew's about the speed at which beds were emptied.[20] Gradually

---

[17] Harris to College, 5 March 1940, 22 December 1939, DF 29.
[18] Frank K. Prochaska, *Philanthropy and the Hospitals of London: The King's Fund, 1897–1990* (Oxford, 1992), p. 134.
[19] *Hospital*, October 1939, p. 345; Honigsbaum, *Health, Happiness and Security*, p. 16.
[20] Clerk to Aylwen, 19 February 1940, HA 16/11.

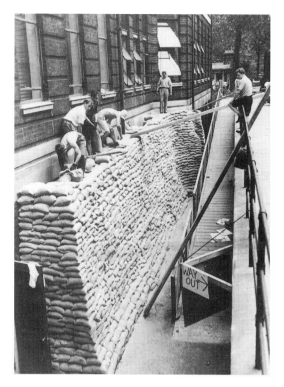

Plate 8.1 Sandbags being placed by students outside King George V block, 1939

services for the civilian sick were extended as they returned to London after the first wave of evacuation. The effect was to reduce the length of stay in teaching hospitals. For medical schools, it meant a limitation of clinical material for instruction.[21]

Patients were evacuated from London's hospitals once war was declared. At St Bartholomew's porters carried stretcher cases, while students were engaged in stacking sandbags and working on structural defences.[22] Wards were reorganised following a pattern common to many London hospitals. The student common-room was converted into a gas decontamination department and a 'casualty clearing station' was established in the basement of the outpatient department below 'six floors of steel and concrete'. One student remembered that the walls were whitewashed and that crickets lurked between the brickwork, requiring those on night duty to remove them with sinus forceps to prevent the noise from becoming intolerable. Staff were kept to a minimum, and most of the patients, staff and students were

[21] Abel-Smith, *Hospitals*, pp. 435, 431.
[22] General court, 23 November 1939, HA 1/31.

evacuated to the Sector hospitals. Work at West Smithfield continued at a reduced level, but the experience was seen as vital for students who were exposed to acute cases not seen in the Sector hospitals.[23]

Despite official optimism, teaching in all London's medical schools was frequently disrupted and housed in unfamiliar or ill-equipped buildings. Considerable time was wasted travelling between sites in and around London. At St Bartholomew's conditions were at first felt to be in 'turmoil'. Money had to be spent on equipping laboratories in the Sector hospitals and staff were asked to forgo fees if possible, creating tension over the salary that continued to be paid to Girling Ball as dean.[24] Even after some stability had been achieved, clinical instruction remained erratic. Makeshift teaching arrangements were felt to be 'not very good' and George Aylwen, treasurer of the hospital since 1937, had to be constantly reminded not to treat the clinical staff like children.[25] Teaching had to be matched to commitments in the EMS, while the position of Hill End in the service, with its large orthopaedic department and special departments for head, chest, maxillio-facial surgery and burns, created further difficulties. In the face of opposition from Aylwen, and reports that facilities were of 'a very low standard for students and nurses', outpatient clinics continued and were supplemented by *ad hoc* arrangements for outpatient teaching at Hill End.[26] Students were asked not to 'complain if you do not find everything that you expected', especially as neither Hill End nor Friern had been designed for teaching.[27] To end this, a building at Hill End was converted into a teaching laboratory and new common-rooms were added. Hill End quickly became known as 'Barts in the country', especially once the museum and pathological teaching were centralised there after the start of bombing on London. With only 40 per cent of admissions made up of casualties, it took patients similar to those admitted to St Bartholomew's before 1939.[28] This gave students 'very fine opportunities of being taught practically to deal with the problems of war surgery'. However, treatment at Hill End was not always along modern lines. Traditional methods continued to be used, and during severe air raids on London and after Dunkirk the hospital became overstretched, making it difficult for students to receive instruction.[29]

Rather than allowing students indefinite leave to join the services, a condensed curriculum was adopted on the advice of the General Medical

---

[23] William Girling Ball, *St Bartholomew's Hospital in the 'Blitz'* (London, 1943), pp. 1–3; Brendan Webb, 'Barts in Wartime', *St Bartholomew's Hospital Journal*, winter 1998, p. 20.

[24] College committee, 19 October 1939, 1 May 1940, MS 29/1.

[25] Girling Ball diary, 28 November 1939, f. 11.

[26] College committee, 9 October 1940, 13 November 1940, 8 January 1941, MS 29/1; Medical Council, 14 January 1942, MC 1/11.

[27] *St Bartholomew's Hospital Journal*, November 1941, p. 28.

[28] Dunn, *Emergency Medical Services*, Vol. ii, p. 229.

[29] 'Life at Hill End', *The Hillender*.

Council (GMC) to meet the demand for medical manpower. Students subsequently spent less time training and more time sitting examinations.[30] More innovative teaching techniques were adopted to take account of disruptions, wartime medical care and a reduction in staff. Lantern-slides, for example, were used to a greater extent to teach radiology, and teaching collections were improved. The pathology course was condensed into three months to get around the difficulties created by inadequate accommodation and a shortage of demonstrators.[31] Extra classes were added in resuscitation, treatment of traumatic shock, and techniques of giving and taking blood to prepare students for wartime medical demands. Lectures in therapeutics, and the first lecture course in rehabilitation, were added.[32] In some areas the College was forced to rely on other schools to fill gaps. Students were sent to Clare Hall, South Mimms for tuberculosis instruction. A close partnership was built up with The London, which agreed to provide joint pharmacology lectures. The College cooperated in other areas: from 1940 it agreed to teach first-year Cambridge medical students after the University's teaching staff was cut.[33]

Girling Ball felt that arrangements, after some teething troubles, 'worked well' and recognised that staff were making considerable sacrifices. Many were separated from their families and were working 'at some financial loss' with little prospect of promotion after the University decided to suspend all new professorial appointments.[34] By 1945, the number of clinical teachers had fallen to three-quarters of the College's prewar level. Junior staff were hardest hit, ensuring that demonstrations were not always possible, especially in pathology.[35] Lecture rooms were invariably too small and lectures were regularly cancelled. A lack of coordination between Hill End and West Smithfield ensured that while some subjects were omitted, others were repeated.[36] Complaints quickly emerged. Feuds erupted between staff over which site was better organised. Overcrowding, initially caused by an overlap of students after teaching had been suspended for three months and then by the lack of serviceable lecture theatres, was a source of considerable anxiety. Students compared ward rounds to a scrum and it was only in 1942 that overcrowding was reduced with a fall in attendance. Clinical work was hampered by the shortage of acute cases. Staff were therefore delighted when in 1943 the governors agreed to reopen the outpatient departments after air raids stopped. However, students were frustrated by the increased number of

[30] Executive committee, 10 July 1940, MS 30/1.
[31] College committee, 12 February 1941, MS 29/1.
[32] Ball to College, 6 July 1942, 1 May 1943, DF 18; Harris to Ball, 7 May 1943, DF 18.
[33] Tutors committee, 24 January 1941, DF 78; 1939/40 annual report.
[34] Executive committee, 12 June 1940, MS 30/1.
[35] College Calendar (1945/6).
[36] Letter to Harris, 13 October 1941, DF 18.

lectures and demonstrations, which were used to supplement the limited clinical material available for teaching.[37] At Friern, they were 'starved of good teaching material'. Although twelve wards were taken over by the EMS, the remainder of the hospital continued to be used for psychiatric patients. To compensate, students were required to split their time between the wards and attendance at St Bartholomew's. Nurses at Friern (as in many institutions taken over by the EMS) did not adjust readily to the hospital's change in status. They resented the students, who frequently complained that they were depressed by the mental hospital atmosphere.[38] Problems were also encountered at Hill End where the existing medical officer resented staff from St Bartholomew's. Accommodation was cramped and the wards were seen as 'Victorian mahogany monstrosities'. Lectures were given in the pathology department and nurses' home (which the nurses continued to use in the mornings) where there were insufficient chairs, not enough room and inadequate ventilation, especially in summer.[39] The College felt it could do little and tried to make the best possible use of the facilities available, not always with success.

Corduroy trousers, prunes and 'all pervading' gloom: Bart's students at war

In September 1939, Girling Ball reminded students of their national duty and the need for discipline. They were told not to move around more than was necessary and those found not to be working sufficiently hard were threatened with military service. This was a far more effective incentive to study than the threats of being sent down used before the war.[40] Despite exhortations to work, incidences of undefined misbehaviour and petty crime increased. Five students had to be suspended in 1942 after giving false evidence to a court and a greater number of students were called before the discipline committee for theft, especially of College property, than before 1939. Mass Observation recorded similar increases in theft and petty crime and a rise in juvenile delinquency. To help '[stamp] out this in the future', the names of those called before the discipline committee were published, but in general the College recognised that a more lenient attitude was required during wartime.[41]

---

[37] 1942/3 annual report.
[38] Ball to University of London, 14 November 1940, DF 21; Medical Council, 27 May 1942, MC 1/11; St Bartholomew's Hospital Journal, April 1941, p. 146.
[39] 'Life at Hill End'.
[40] SU minutes, 23 September 1939, SU 11/2.
[41] Discipline committee, 1 January 1942, MS 32/3; ibid., MS 32/4; SU minutes, 11 August 1942, SU 11/2.

For all the difficulties students created, they made an important contribution to wartime clinical care. Initially, 140 worked in the outpatient department at West Smithfield but a reduction in the number of patients saw this cut to seventy, forcing the College to send students earlier to Friern.[42] To answer the shortage of clinical staff, unqualified house officers were appointed in 1941 from those students in the last three months of their clerking. Although numbers were kept to a minimum, staff shortages saw unqualified students undertaking more work than most house officers had before the war. In 1942, a sudden service demand for qualified doctors saw students moving from fire-watcher to houseman overnight without the prewar formality of examination or registration.[43] Students organised themselves and helped the hospital in other ways. Some were required to dig potatoes; others acted as porters and five were constantly employed as fire-watchers. Accommodation was provided in the west wing in temporary rooms previously used by the nurses. The work was cold and wet, and a rota was devised so that every student at West Smithfield had a free twenty-four hours every ten days. Most students volunteered and spent between six and nine months at West Smithfield. It was quickly found that some were applying only because they wanted to live in the hospital, 'not because they specially want to do any work either for the Hospital or for the City of London'.[44] Although rooms in the west wing were sparse, it did provide a return to a style of collegiate life not seen since the closure of College Hall in 1923. However, conditions were not ideal and led to the rapid spread of glandular fever and German measles. When all the windows were blown out the risk from flying glass was reduced, but the rooms became cold. The wiring was unsuitable for anything more than a light, a bedside lamp and a radio and electric fires were therefore banned. Student ignored the prohibition and in winter ran fires from the light fittings.[45]

In the first months of war – the 'bore war' effectively captured by Evelyn Waugh in *Put Out More Flags* – with no air raids, little obvious danger and 'enforced non-combatancy', student life was seen as irksome.[46] Parts of the hospital took on an 'all-pervading gloom' with the windows blacked out for air raids. At the 'evening meal no sound is heard but the sound of mashed potato being dispensed'. Students complained that they felt ashamed of their inactivity when those of military age were being enlisted, but for many life at first went on as normal.[47] The start of air raids in September 1940

[42] College Council, 23 October 1940, MS 28/2.

[43] College committee, 9 July 1941, MS 29/1; *St Bartholomew's Hospital Journal*, summer 1988, p. 15.

[44] Harris to Ball, 9 September 1941, DF 29.

[45] Ibid., 7 November 1940, 2 December 1942, DF 29.

[46] Cited in Peter Clarke, *Hope and Glory: Britain, 1900–1990* (London, 1997), p. 192.

[47] *St Bartholomew's Hospital Journal*, April 1940, p. 116; 'Shreds', ibid., June 1940, p. 151.

dramatically changed the situation. Looking back, one member of staff remembered that

> from then on till the end of the War in Europe no inhabitant of the West Wing went to bed at night sure that he would not be called up after the briefest rest to carry out his work of stretcher bearing, in assisting in the resuscitation room or in the operating theatres or in the wards or a combination of all four.

It quickly became common for those in 'the West Wing to be working every night of the week' and the direct and indirect effects of the bombardment took their toll. Surprisingly none were killed or seriously injured even when, during the severest bombing raid of the Blitz in May 1941, three direct hits destroyed six student rooms. Sleepless nights led to chronic tiredness, however. Onerous restrictions were now placed on students' movements and a routine developed. With the renewed threat of aerial attack in 1944, students slept in corridor bunks or in the hospital's basement.[48]

At Cambridge, life for the pre-clinical students was less fraught or depressing. Students here were felt to form a heroic band 'who played hard, teasing the Proctors as they nightly strode ungowned between the "Waffle", the "Whim" or the Blue Bore'.[49] The Second World War had a less dramatic impact on Cambridge than the First. The mood was less optimistic about a short war, and if students remained patriotic they no longer adopted the same raucous jingoism. Life at Cambridge, where corduroy trousers were all the rage and academic dress was gradually relaxed, was relatively unaffected. Medical and science students were allowed to complete their studies and in the early years of the war, most other students continued to study for two years before being called up. For many, war meant more time spent dining in college, restrictions on travel, rationing and a period in the Home Guard.[50]

Initially, students from St Bartholomew's found it difficult to adjust to life in Cambridge. At Queens' a blackout was strictly enforced, women guests forbidden after 7 p.m., and students were encouraged 'not to wander about or congregate in the streets after dark'.[51] At first, conditions were cramped: with so many non-Cambridge students present accommodation was at a premium. Most of those from St Bartholomew's were 'inadequately housed' in Queens' where preference was given to its own undergraduates. Students were required to share rooms and many were forced to bring their own mattresses. At first this created tension. Queens' was accused of being undemocratic and

---

[48] Ibid.
[49] Ibid., summer 1993, p. 14.
[50] For Cambridge during the war see A. S. F. Gow, *Letters from Cambridge, 1939–1944* (London, 1945).
[51] Cited in John Twigg, *A History of Queens' College, Cambridge, 1448–1986* (Woodbridge, 1987), p. 356.

of subjecting its visitors to 'medieval discipline'.[52] With a large number leaving Queens' to find better lodgings, the atmosphere became less strained. Relations between the two colleges improved; when Queens' compared its wartime experiences to those of other Cambridge colleges, it felt that 'remarkably happy relations' had existed 'which must have been unique in the story of evacuation to Cambridge'.[53]

However, complaints continued to mount about the cost of living: one student protested that the expense of studying in Cambridge had forced him to give up medicine; others found part-time jobs. Complaints were not ignored. Aware that the financial position of many parents had been dramatically altered by war (especially those on military pay with their families on separation allowances), every effort was made to reduce the cost of study in Cambridge. When circumstances dictated, the College agreed either to pay half the cost of lodgings or to cover the entire cost. It was also agreed that aid be extended to clinical students 'in the same way that they are helping Cambridge students'.[54] Despite the College's efforts, living expenses continued to rise and the quality of the food declined. Students tended to eat at least one meal a day in Queens' and one student remembered spending the rest of the time living on 'bread, margarine and marmalade, with buns from Fitzbillies'.[55] Many complained that they did not get enough to eat as rationing signalled both privation and 'fair shares' in food allocation. Those using the catering facilities at St Bartholomew's quickly became bored with the endless mashed potatoes that seemed to be served with every dish and criticised rising prices and falling quality.[56]

In an attempt to bolster morale, every effort was made to maintain the associate life of the College. In West Smithfield, Christmas shows continued in the wards even when 'under fire'.[57] Fortnightly concerts were organised in a 'little makeshift theatre'. A private pub was opened in 1941 in the basement of the old casualty department with help from Whitbred's. One student claimed that the bar, called the 'Vicarage' because it was run by the padre, was the inspiration of Harris who felt it was too dangerous for students and staff to continue to visit the White Hart and Admiral Carter on Giltspur Street. Early enthusiasm ensured that the 'Vicarage' was an important source of entertainment for staff and students, and many resented its closure when the College started to admit women. Patients were also reassured: those working in the hospital were required to write their locations on a blackboard and the

[52] *Dial*, Michaelmas 1939, pp. 1–3.
[53] Executive committee, 11 October 1939, 12 June 1940, MS 30/1; Twigg, *Queens'*, p. 359.
[54] Harris to Ball, 29 December 1939, DF 29.
[55] *St Bartholomew's Hospital Journal*, summer 1993, p. 14.
[56] Suggestion book, DF 207.
[57] *St Bartholomew's Hospital Journal*, February 1941, p. 86.

constant reference to the 'Vicarage' suggested a different image.[58] Sports equipment was transferred between sites and new pre-clinical clubs were established at Cambridge. Others were amalgamated with Cambridge University societies and a fencing club was formed at Hill End, which also maintained an active music society and cricket team. Most of the sporting and social activity was concentrated at Cambridge and Hill End as they were relatively unaffected by bombing, and the distance of the Sector hospitals from the sports ground at Chislehurst made it difficult to reach. Fixtures were scaled down, though students at West Smithfield welcomed the afternoon matches organised by the football club as an opportunity to escape from the hospital.[59]

To compensate for the wartime dislocation, a Hill End-Bart's Club was formed to keep 'the party happy in the rather out of the way spot in which the Hospital is placed'. Regular 'Prunes' (or dances) were held on Fridays after the reception hall was opened in 1940. As the gramophone society held twice-weekly concerts, the year students spent at Hill End seemed filled with 'dances and concerts and plays and one thing and another'.[60] Scottish dancing proved particularly popular but debates were less successful. The Abernethian Society fell into decline since students preferred more distracting forms of entertainment. Life was more sombre at Friern. Students did not always adjust to working at a former mental hospital and felt isolated from the school-like activities that characterised Cambridge and Hill End. There were no arrangements for organised sports, although they were able to use the tennis courts and billiard room at certain times. In the villas, with their parsimonious board, a formal atmosphere prevailed. Intense revision courses and final examinations contributed to the sombre environment.

By 1942, St Bartholomew's, Friern and Hill End had all temporarily succumbed to a more resigned attitude and it was felt that the 'spark' had gone out of the students after military defeats in North Africa. A better record of sporting achievement and a series of military successes dispelled this feeling in the following year. Critics, however, continued to feel that 'Bart's is no longer interested in sport' and that apathy prevailed.[61]

'An awesome and awful sight'

German attacks in 1940 and 1941 destroyed and damaged vast numbers of houses and businesses in London. The heaviest raids came in the summer of

---

[58] *Evening News*, 7 October 1939; *Guide and Ideas*, 6 January 1940; *St Bartholomew's Hospital Journal*, summer 1981, pp. 33–4; ibid., summer 1988, pp. 16–17.
[59] Cricket Club minutes, 19 November 1941, SU 41; Association Football minutes, 10 July 1941, SU 61.
[60] *St Bartholomew's Hospital Journal*, November 1941, p. 25; ibid., September 1943, p. 217.
[61] Ibid., March 1942, p. 111; 'Planning for Sport', ibid., August 1944, pp. 119–20.

1940 and by June 1941 more than two million homes had been destroyed, 60 per cent of them in London.[62] 20,000 had died and a further 25,000 were injured.[63] Although London's hospitals were not overwhelmed by a massive influx of casualties, they seemed vulnerable to German attack. By the end of 1940, thirty-five hospitals reported severe bomb damage; the number had risen to forty-three by July 1941. Only St Mary's in Paddington did not have to reduce its number of beds.[64]

Neither the hospital nor the College was under any delusions about the dangers presented by their location. By May 1941, St Bartholomew's stood 'with St Paul's Cathedral, the Old Bailey and the General Post Office in an almost completely devastated area between Holborn and Moorgate'. Early raids created a mood of excitement among the students who had found inactivity tiresome. Bomb damage was at first dismissed with bravado as removing buildings that 'needed demolishing anyhow'. As the 'Battle of London' continued, the situation worsened.[65] On many nights, the hospital was surrounded by fires. On 29 December 1940, 'the commercial heart of the capital was wrecked by hundreds of incendiaries. Churches, banks, offices and houses caught fire, creating a massive conflagration.'[66] At St Bartholomew's half the patients were evacuated to Friern and damage was avoided only by a change in wind direction. Although the hospital was reduced to 345 beds and suffered financially through a loss of rental income, it escaped serious damage. The College was not so fortunate. In the first months of bombing, the lecture rooms were practically demolished. From October 1940, incendiary bombs started to fall in Charterhouse and low water pressure made fires difficult to extinguish. The physiology block was among the first to be gutted and was virtually demolished by successive raids.[67] Debris from bombs falling in Aldersgate and St John's Street smashed windows, covering Charterhouse in brickwork, glass and window frames.[68] Girling Ball felt that he would quickly have 'no College to be dean of'. By January 1942,

> the Inorganic Chemistry Laboratory, the main part of the Physics Laboratory, practically the whole of the Physiological Laboratory, the Pharmacology Laboratory, the Library, the Students' Common Rooms, the Cloakrooms and the College Dining Hall . . . [had] gone.[69]

[62] Angus Calder, *The People's War: Britain, 1939–45* (London, 1992), p. 223.
[63] Roy Porter, *London: A Social History* (London, 1994), p. 340.
[64] Dunn, *Emergency Medical Services*, Vol. i, pp. 115–18.
[65] *St Bartholomew's Hospital Journal*, October 1940, p. 1.
[66] Porter, *London*, p. 229.
[67] Girling Ball diary, 25 September 1940, f.54; Ball, *St Bartholomew's Hospital in the 'Blitz'*, pp. 4–5, 9.
[68] Damage summary, DF 31.
[69] Ball to Jameson, 15 January 1942, DF 26.

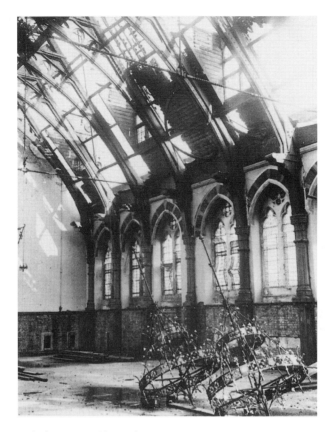

Plate 8.2 Bomb damage to Charterhouse

Repairs were made to prevent further deterioration and parts of the College were put to other uses: the Charterhouse Cold Storage Company, for example, stored sugar in the dissecting room.[70] In the hospital, the clinical lecture theatres were 'completely destroyed', with 'glass strewn everywhere; great chunks of masonry all over the place'. At Friern, where windows were smashed, teaching was disrupted.[71] Having worked so hard to develop Charterhouse, Girling Ball took the destruction personally. He was infuriated that he had spent 'all these years raising the College to one of high eminence and now that damned swine has destroyed it beyond repair'.[72]

[70] Harris to Ball, 19 April 1945, DF 37.
[71] Ball to Jameson, 15 January 1942, DF 26; General court, 28 November 1940, HA 1/32.
[72] Girling Ball to University, 30 December 1940, DF 32.

A question of reconstructing

The extent of the damage raised questions about the future of the College. Girling Ball was optimistic about the clinical school, believing it could 're-start at Bart's if the War came to an end', but feared for the pre-clinical school. The surviving buildings were 'not of sufficient size' to continue teaching and there was no laboratory accommodation left standing. Despite reluctance to think about the postwar situation, planning began in 1942 when a decline in air raids gave the College a breathing space. Elsewhere, reconstruction was discussed more seriously following the victory at El Alamein and Churchill's pronouncement in November 1942 that 'it is not the beginning of the end but it may be the end of the beginning'. The need for educational reform had been gathering momentum since 1940 and a growing body of literature highlighted a change in thinking on higher education. Pressure to expand the university sector was part of an overall drive to improve the educational performance of the country.[73] In medicine, the appointment of the interdepartmental committee on medical schools in 1942 focused debate. At the University of London, postwar planning started in earnest in the following year. The dispersal of medical students and the loss of teachers (especially in the clinical subjects) made universities anxious about medical education. Deterioration was feared, especially as interwar efforts at reform had proved stillborn. Although the number of professorial appointments had risen, the changes called for by the Haldane Commission in 1913 had not materialised. Students complained that training was geared towards interesting rather than typical cases. Calls were made for medical education to be made more practical, more relevant to general practice, or more academic, and a growing consensus emerged that the gap between pre-clinical and clinical years had to be bridged. How to alter medical education 'to provide a better scientific and general training' without adding to an already overcrowded curriculum, and how to foster 'a more organised and integrated approach', became recurrent themes.[74]

Initially the College stood apart from these debates, wrestling with the practical difficulties caused by bombing. As other schools started to return to London, staff at St Bartholomew's discussed the possibility of using temporary huts and renting space in nearby buildings. Consideration was also given to 'a temporary fusion . . . with some other Medical College'.[75] However, in the long term, rebuilding was seen as the only answer. With the postwar intentions of the Ministry of Health unclear and lecturers anxious that

---

[73] Robert G. Burgess, 'Aspects of Education in Postwar Britain', in *Understanding Postwar Britain*, ed. James Obelkevich and Peter Catteral (London, 1994), pp. 131, 136.
[74] John Ryle, 'Future of Medical Education', *BMJ* ii (1941), p. 323; Donald McDonald, 'Future of Medical Education', ibid., pp. 327–9.
[75] Ball to Jameson, 15 January 1942, DF 26.

students would be quickly 'turned out' of Cambridge at the end of the war, Girling Ball looked for reassurances. A survey into London's hospitals for the Ministry of Health in 1942 had created alarm. The press claimed that those conducting the survey were eager to destroy the London voluntary system and predictions were made that some hospitals would disappear or be relocated.[76] Although interest in restructuring the geography of institutional healthcare had been voiced before 1939 and a number of schemes had been put forward, in 1942 it was uncertain which institution would be affected. Girling Ball approached the Ministry of Health for reassurance that St Bartholomew's would remain where it was at 'the centre of the hub of the British universe of medicine'. Wilson Jameson, chief medical officer of the Ministry of Health and Board of Education, could not offer any firm guarantees. Much was felt to depend 'on the organisation of pre-clinical teaching and the desirability of residential hospitals for medical students only'.[77] The University of London proved more helpful. It pressed the UGC to ensure that evacuated medical schools would regain possession of their buildings and that those which had suffered severe damage would be given priority in obtaining materials and labour for reconstruction.[78] Cambridge was also sympathetic to the College's position. However, a rise in student numbers strained the availability of lodgings, and Cambridge felt unable to promise to accommodate students from St Bartholomew's after the war. With an estimate that rebuilding would take at least three years, anxiety mounted about the College's future.[79]

Negotiations with the War Damage Commission were protracted, in part because the College intended to make alterations rather than just rebuild. It was admitted that 'the requirements of the future open up such an enormous prospect that it is difficult to limit one's desires'. Staff recognised that work on Charterhouse in the 1930s had produced an awkward arrangement and that many of the original buildings were 'not designed for their present purpose'. Reconstruction was seen as an ideal opportunity to redevelop Charterhouse.[80] There was a sense of urgency to these discussions as it was widely realised that a lack of accommodation made early rebuilding essential. Sir Walter Moberly, chair of the UGC, agreed, but was unprepared to commit the UGC while the nature of medical education in London remained in flux. He therefore envisaged an interim period of two to three years during which time the College could be rebuilt. The University of London gave its support and

---

[76] Cited in Geoffrey Rivett, *The Development of the London Hospital System, 1823–1982* (London, 1986), pp. 249–50.
[77] AGM, 28 January 1942, MS 27/2; Ball to Jameson, 15 January 1942, 3 December 1942, DF 26; 1941/2 annual report.
[78] University to Ball, 3 February 1942, DF 32.
[79] Ball to Bonavia, 10 November 1941, DF 21.
[80] 'Proposed New Medical College Buildings' (London, 1942).

University College unofficially offered to take 'a number of students for anatomy and physiology' during rebuilding.[81] The War Damage Commission was not so easily convinced. It was only prepared to cover the expense of returning St Bartholomew's to its 1939 'pre-damaged form'.[82] The College agreed in principle.

With clear plans formulated for rebuilding, attention turned to emergency repairs so that teaching could resume in some form in London after the war. An effort was made to 'squeeze' returning students into existing buildings amidst fears that this would 'lead to bad teaching and inefficient education'.[83] With money for emergency repairs slow to materialise, damaged buildings continued to deteriorate. At the same time, the cost of repairs trebled as the shortage of building materials intensified. By 1944, with concern mounting about Cambridge's willingness to house pre-clinical students, and with the gradual demobilisation of doctors, the need to make repairs and provide temporary arrangements became matters of urgency.[84] When it became known that a decision had been made to finish rebuilding Birkbeck College in Bloomsbury after construction had been abandoned in 1939 staff at St Bartholomew's were 'rather up in arms'. They felt that preference was being given to other schools to the detriment of the College and were mollified only once it became clear that Birkbeck was to be completed and then handed over to the government for three years. This was a price they were not prepared to pay.[85] Delays continued and the destruction caused by German V1 flying bombs and V2 rockets ensured that a licence for essential repairs could not be granted immediately. Although flying bombs caused only superficial damage at St Bartholomew's, elsewhere they had a devastating effect. V1s damaged over 1.25 million London houses, with the Blitz responsible for the destruction or damage of 3.5 million homes. In the City, 225 acres were virtually reduced to rubble.[86] Given the London-wide destruction, the War Damage Commission and the Ministry of Works and Planning did not see the College as a priority.

Girling Ball was infuriated by constant requests for a decision about when pre-clinical teaching would restart in London and wished that the staff would 'stop this grousing' and realise 'the trouble I have taken to get the return to Bart's'.[87] John Venn, dean of Queens' College, had informed him that 'until our men start to return, we are very ready to keep Barts here', but was clear that 'as soon as the balloon comes down we shall want every bit of

---

[81] Executive committee, 15 July 1942, MS 30/2.
[82] Robinson to Ball, 12 October 1942, DF 30.
[83] Ball to University, 27 May 1942, DF 32; College committee, 14 April 1943, MS 29/2.
[84] Ball to War Damage Commission, 14 October 1944, DF 30.
[85] Claughton to College, 12 May 1944, DF 32; Ball to Venn, 13 May 1944, DF 34.
[86] Porter, London, p. 341.
[87] Ball to Venn, 26 May 1944, DF 34.

accommodation'.[88] From January 1945 onwards, the College was under increasing pressure to find a home for its pre-clinical students. It was only in July that this was finally made a priority by the War Damage Commission. The situation had already become desperate. Friern was due to close in October and, with Cambridge unable to offer accommodation beyond January 1946, 200 pre-clinical students and 400 clinical students were expected to return to West Smithfield for teaching in 1946.[89] The sudden need for Girling Ball to take sick leave and quarrels between the pre-clinical and clinical staff added further complications as departments were gradually transferred back from the Sector hospitals.

The reform of medical education

In the debates over the postwar reconstruction of healthcare, teaching hospitals were placed in a unique position. In earlier plans they had either been excluded as too problematic or made the centre of proposed regional structures. Ernest Brown's statement to the House of Commons as Minister of Health in 1941 on the government's aim to create 'a comprehensive hospital service' after the war stimulated debate, not least at Hill End where the Debating Society discussed the idea of a state medical service.[90] The position of teaching hospitals in any service was recognised as an important issue, and at the last minute it was announced that special arrangements were being considered for them. Special consideration was quickly translated into an interdepartmental committee under Sir William Goodenough, deputy chairman of Barclay's Bank and highly active in the Nuffield Provincial Hospitals Trust, which had investigated the structure of healthcare before the war.

Interest in education was growing with pressure for greater equality of opportunity. Funding had risen as universities adopted an expansionist policy. Emphasis was once more placed on the need for closer links with industry. However, the system remained confused. The need for an inquiry into London's teaching hospitals had been suggested before the war by Sir Frederick Menzies, chief medical officer of the LCC, and by the University of London in 1936 after the ambitions of the Haldane Commission had been frustrated by institutional and government inertia.[91] With the British Medical Association (BMA) already investigating medical education, and with a growing demand for a reformed curriculum, the Goodenough committee built on existing concerns and returned to ideas addressed by the

---

[88] Venn to Ball, 3 March 1944, DF 34.
[89] Ball to University, 17 January 1945, 22 March 1945, DF 30.
[90] Rivett, *Development of the London Hospital System*, pp. 242–7; *St Bartholomew's Hospital Journal*, February 1941, p. 97.
[91] Honigsbaum, *Health, Happiness and Security*, p. 16.

Haldane Commission. Membership of the committee was dominated by academic clinicians and their supporters, who had been selected because they were sympathetic to the government's objectives on healthcare and medical education. Goodenough favoured regionalisation, and witnesses were advised that the committee intended to look at 'the organisation of medical education and its relation to the Universities on the one hand and to the hospitals on the other' and not at the curriculum. In adopting an academic model, the committee was asked to address:

> the proper organisation and distribution of medical schools; the appointment and remuneration of teaching staff; the provision of an adequate range and variety of 'cases' for study and of suitable laboratory accommodation and equipment for teaching and research, including the possibility of linking hospitals for educational purposes.[92]

Against this national remit, the committee was expected to pay special attention to two London problems: the organisation of pre-clinical teaching, and the possible amalgamation of teaching hospitals. Although it quickly became clear that 'some of the failings from which the London medical schools are alleged to suffer exist in most other medical schools in the country', throughout the deliberations the problems attributed to London were believed to be the most complicated issues the committee would have to address.[93]

At St Bartholomew's attention had also turned to reconstruction in 1942 and discussion was in part inspired by national debates about healthcare and medical education. Wartime conditions had accustomed staff working in the EMS to a salaried service and lecturers gave their tentative support to the idea of full-time clinical teachers. They realised that to promote high standards adequate wages were necessary to ensure that staff did 'not have to seek work elsewhere to supplement their incomes'. Whether medical schools should appoint full-time clinical lecturers freed from private practice had been a source of friction in the interwar period as full-time academics and part-time consultants fought over who controlled medical education. Staff at St Bartholomew's had already accepted the principle in 1919 with the professorial units. They had also made financial sacrifices during the war, and with uncertainty about the future structure of healthcare full-time appointments promised some security. The Goodenough committee and debates in the University of London gave a further context for discussion. Even before the war, the College had started to address these concerns and a report on the College's 'future policy' had been prepared in 1938. Many of its suggestions were taken up again in 1942. To revise the existing report, a

---

[92] Wellcome: Farrer-Brown to Lewis, 28 October 1942, PP/LEW/D.6/3.
[93] PRO: Farrer Brown to Hill, 19 May 1943, MH 71/65.

policy committee was appointed to plan for the 'next ten to twenty years'. All departments were consulted. The resulting interim report reflected enthusiasm in the Hospital and the College for greater cooperation and suggested how clinical departments could be reorganised to promote better teaching. From the start, it was considered imperative that the hospital and College remain on their existing sites, with the College providing 'facilities for teaching the subjects for the whole medical curriculum'.[94]

Using material collected by the policy committee, the College made its suggestions to the Goodenough committee. Although St Bartholomew's wanted to stress its unique position, other witnesses felt it was 'in much the same position as the other schools'.[95] The College's recommendations closely matched the policies of the University of London and built on the lecturers' hopes for the future. The position of Charterhouse was defended and staff asserted that 'all branches of its teaching should be of University standard'. St Bartholomew's had already tentatively embraced a university model and wanted to see this extended, arguing that 'a College without such Units must lose a great deal'. However, deficiencies were admitted. The hope was that reform would ensure that the professorial units would be less isolated and play a greater role in teaching. The need for more laboratory accommodation and research in medical schools was reasserted and the realities of the postwar situation were anticipated.[96] The lecturers recognised that the major problems facing the development of medical education would be funding and accommodation. This was clear at St Bartholomew's and the extensive war damage was highlighted. Support from the UGC was acknowledged as a prerequisite for development, along with the need for regionalisation and links with LCC hospitals to extend teaching. Under the EMS, the lecturers had adjusted to working in a region and found the teaching links established with St Andrew's, St Giles, Hackney and Bethnal Green hospitals in the 1930s advantageous.[97] However, staff wanted to maintain control and supported regionalisation as a way of assuring an appropriate level of clinical material.

Throughout the College's evidence, emphasis was placed on the institutional structure of medical education. Interest had been expressed in establishing closer links between pre-clinical and clinical teaching and in developing specialisation, but unlike other institutions giving evidence, the College was less concerned with the structure of the curriculum.[98] Lord Moran at the Royal College of Physicians interpreted the Goodenough committee as 'an appeal for a reformation of the current system' and the

---

[94] Policy committee interim report, MS 9/11.
[95] Wellcome: Draft memorandum, PP/LEW/D.6/3.
[96] Evidence to the interdepartmental committee on medical education, 1943, DF 24.
[97] College committee, 2 October 1946, MS 29/2.
[98] Memorandum, DF 193.

Royal College appointed a committee to investigate as part of a wholesale programme of studies on medical reform. Moran felt that the inter-departmental committee aimed merely to 'tidy the curriculum' when what was needed was radical reconstruction.[99] At University College, a more theoretical system, linked to vocational teaching within a simplified curriculum, was called for as a solution to the haphazard system that characterised teaching.[100] Elsewhere greater emphasis was placed on the need to coordinate facilities for research. Differences also existed over the extent and nature of regionalisation. University College in particular was not convinced that teaching hospitals should be integral to any regional structure, a view shared by the British Hospitals Association.[101]

In 1944, the Goodenough committee presented its final report. Efforts had been made to arrange the evidence to help the committee come to its conclusions and most of its members had clear ideas on how medical education should be structured.[102] The report concluded that 'although the nation is justified in taking pride in the reputation of British medical practice and of traditional British methods of education, there is an urgent need for radical improvements'. In a visionary plan for the better health of the nation, the report argued that 'carefully conducted medical education is the essential foundation' of the comprehensive health service envisaged after the war. The committee felt that 'medical education cannot be regarded as merely incidental to hospital service'. The ideas outlined in the government's 1944 White Paper on healthcare for a merger of teaching and non-teaching staff was rejected in favour of a 'series of educational associations with all the major hospitals in a wide area around'.[103] The Goodenough committee was clear that teaching hospitals had a major role to play.

The Goodenough report returned to the issues stressed by the Haldane Commission. Once more, the need to shift teaching from a vocational system dominated by the need to amass factual knowledge to a more science-based course was asserted. Like the Haldane Commission, Goodenough's committee felt that this could be achieved through professorial units, arguing that 'whole-time professors in the clinical subjects should be the academic heads of their departments, with a measure of control over the planning of the teaching work of their non-professorial colleagues'. Medical education was to be organised on a university model, with salaried clinical teachers appointed and pre-clinical departments dovetailed with university science departments.

[99] *Committee Reports of the Royal College of Physicians* (December 1942 to April 1947).
[100] Wellcome: 'A Preamble on the Present Needs of Medical Education', 1943, PP/LEW/D.6.2.
[101] Wellcome: Lewis to Goodenough, 29 January 1943, PP/LEW/D.6/3.
[102] PRO: Goodenough committee, MH 71/65–6.
[103] *Report of the Inter-Departmental Committee on Medical Schools* (London, 1944), pp. 11, 8–9.

However, university-managed teaching hospitals were rejected. Instead, support was given to 'university teaching centres' with one hospital at the centre directing services. If this was a repetition of the Haldane Commission's findings, the concept of university education had changed since 1913.[104] The ideal of the liberal university had been replaced by a view that was both technological and democratic. Universities were beginning to be seen in a more practical and utilitarian light: medicine fitted perfectly with this model.[105] The Goodenough committee therefore favoured a revised curriculum that had a more educational content. To promote a 'healthy nation', the committee argued that training had to be geared to the needs of general practice. For the Goodenough committee, this could be achieved by placing greater stress on child health, psychiatry and social medicine.[106] In support of its aims, it called for a 'coherent unification of medical knowledge' within 'an atmosphere of specialisation'.[107] Social medicine had taken root in the 1930s and called for a broader view of healthcare and medical training, a theme intimately related to wartime discussions on health planning and reconstruction. In many ways, it marked a revival of the notion of the whole patient linked to preventive medicine, and an awareness that doctors should be familiar with both health and sickness.[108] Members of the committee were strongly influenced by these ideas and incorporated them into the final report. To ensure that social medicine permeated medical education, the report recommended closer integration of pre-clinical and clinical subjects, returning to suggestions made before 1939.[109]

The recommendations of the interdepartmental committee for university-centred education as part of a reformed health service were linked to a reform of the examination system, compulsory hospital appointments after qualification, and a comprehensive programme for training specialists. Postgraduate study was constructed as one way whereby factual material could be reduced and new subjects added without increasing the burden on students. To provide doctors for the predicted expansion of postwar healthcare there was a need to expand student numbers, and the Goodenough committee recommended that the system of local authority grants should be extended to encourage this. The

---

[104] Ibid., pp. 12–13, 16–19.
[105] A. H. Halsey, *Decline of Donnish Dominion: The British Academic Professions in the Twentieth Century* (Oxford, 1992), pp. 48–9.
[106] *Inter-Departmental Committee on Medical Schools*, pp. 14–15, 28–9.
[107] Cited in Roger Cooter, *Surgery and Society in Peace and War: Orthopaedics and the Organisation of Modern Medicine, 1880–1940* (Basingstoke, 1993), p. 246.
[108] For social medicine, see Dorothy Porter, 'Changing Disciplines: John Ryle and the Making of Social Medicine in Britain in the 1940s', *History of Science* xxx (1992), pp. 137–64; Jane Lewis, 'The Public's Health: Philosophy and Practice in Britain in the Twentieth Century', in *A History of Education in Public Health*, ed. Elizabeth Fee and R. Acheson (Oxford, 1991), pp. 195–229.
[109] *Inter-Departmental Committee on Medical Schools*, pp. 14–15, 28–9.

committee anticipated that part of this rise could be met not by establishing additional medical schools but by making existing schools coeducational. The committee also called for links to be fostered with local authority hospitals. In arguing for fewer schools and for the removal of certain teaching hospitals to outside London, it was certain that clinical training would have to 'depend on groups of hospitals for clinical teaching facilities'. In outlining a comprehensive vision for medical education, the interdepartmental committee warned that 'the benefits of university life may have to be sacrificed' to the 'future hospital needs of London'.[110]

According to Rivett, the report was 'the most important statement on medical education since Sir George Newman's *Some Notes on Medical Education*' (1918), but at the time many felt it was nothing 'revolutionary'. The University of London had accepted the need for more professorial units in 1934 and had called for coeducation in 1942 (see Chapter 9). Most medical schools were keen to provide postgraduate training. Under wartime measures, junior doctors were required to spend six months in a general hospital after qualification and most medical schools were discussing how this might be extended.[111] In calling for an overhaul of the medical curriculum, the report was voicing a widely held opinion. Worries were aired about the idea of a free medical education and critics doubted that 'these and similar recommendations will . . . overcome the tremendous strength of tradition'. However, in returning to the hopes and aspirations of the Haldane Commission, the report elaborated a growing consensus.[112] For all the radical posturing of Moran, the Royal College of Physicians' investigation, published several months earlier, had come to similar conclusions. It admitted that the 'educational has been sacrificed for the vocational objective' and upheld the value of science, calling for closer integration of subjects in a university setting.[113] Both saw a need for a period of compulsory postgraduate study to provide the vocational element removed from undergraduate study.

The report had a mixed reception. Critics complained that University College had been unfairly represented and the other London schools excluded. The royal colleges welcomed the general conclusions, but disagreed with many of the recommendations and took issue with suggestions that the licensing system had to be changed. The BMA took a more positive stance. Although it argued that existing medical schools should not be incorporated, it generally agreed with the report.[114] At the Ministry of Health, the need to

---

[110] Ibid., pp. 20–3.

[111] PRO: Neville to Farrer Brown, 7 April 1944, MH 71/70.

[112] *BMJ* i (1944), p. 728.

[113] Royal College of Physicians, *Report on Medical Education* (London, 1944).

[114] PRO: Memorandum on the report of the interdepartmental committee, MH 71/59; Royal College of Physicians to Ministry of Health, 24 November 1945, MH 71/59; BMA observations on the report of the interdepartmental committee, MH 71/59.

implement the Goodenough report was accepted and pressure applied on the UGC and GMC.[115] It anticipated immediate postwar problems, seeing the report's findings as a series of long-term objectives that could be achieved by using UGC grants as a 'weapon' to promote reform. The UGC tried to side-step the issue, aware of the damaging effect withholding grants would have. However, it had already decided to increase funding to medical schools and withhold grants to those schools that did not admit women. The GMC was equally reluctant to enter the debate and felt that the issue should be left to individual schools to decide. Under pressure, however, it agreed to encourage reform and in 1947 presented plans for a revised curriculum. Effective action was hampered by the Treasury, which was 'not committed *on this report*' and was unprepared to meet the massive increase in spending the Ministry of Health believed was necessary.[116] Undaunted, Henry Willink, the Minister of Health, reinforced the findings of the report when he informed the House of Commons that the government attached 'equal importance to the revision of the medical curriculum, and acceptance of the principle of increased grants for medical education and research is dependent on the early completion of this process'.[117] The Goodenough report was virtually presented as a Cabinet edict. Alarmed, medical schools and the University of London reacted to the 'power of the purse' and grumbled about government interference. The University revised its existing postgraduate arrangements, establishing the British Postgraduate Medical Federation to provide the level of postgraduate training stipulated in the Goodenough report in anticipation of the training needs of the new NHS. At a school level, discussions were started on how the gap between pre-clinical and clinical subjects could be bridged and how the curriculum could be changed.

At St Bartholomew's, the suggestions contained in the Goodenough report that outpatient teaching should be undertaken, an introductory clinical course offered, incorporation with the University promoted, and schools reorganised around clinical units had been achieved before the war. The College had also partially adopted the style of teaching that the report endorsed and used its recommendations to help plan reconstruction, aware that future funding might depend on reform. Girling Ball recognised that further professorial units in medicine, surgery and midwifery had to be central to development, but other staff were reluctant to concentrate teaching in the hands of professors. They argued that the existing Boards of Studies already organised teaching and were worried that the 'influence of the whole-time professors on these Boards was increasing'.[118]

---

[115] PRO: Meeting of Goodenough committee with UGC, 25 July 1944, MH 71/59.

[116] PRO: Meeting of Ministry of Health with UGC, 11 August 1944, MH 71/59; Hale to George, 30 November 1944, MH 71/59.

[117] *BMJ* i (1945), p. 136.

[118] Notes on development policy 1945, DF 22; UGC Advisory committee on medical education, 26 June 1945, DF 22.

With the College divided, the University of London advised a cautious policy. It recommended that departments be strengthened before an effort was made to embark on 'new ventures'. However, it was acknowledged that universities would be called on to deal with a greater number of students and play a role in social and industrial reconstruction.[119] This created pressure for development that was not always compatible with the University's cautious stance. In November 1944, the University, bolstered by a rise in funding as part of the UGC's attempts to return universities to their prewar footing, recognised 'the financial difficulties' facing St Bartholomew's and agreed that these would be considered 'when it comes to making earmarked grants'. The promise of increased funding encouraged the College to submit a more coherent development policy in line with the recommendations outlined in the Goodenough committee.[120]

The need to recover 'from the damage and disorganisation' of war was central to the revised development policy. With facilities for clinical teaching split between Hill End and West Smithfield, new methods were seen as vital to take account of 'physical facts rather than logic'. The immediate task was to plan for the next five years, during which time it was anticipated that the hospital and pre-clinical department could be rebuilt. In line with the Goodenough report, the lecturers hoped to forge links between pre-clinical and clinical teaching to improve clinical training and develop opportunities for research. Efforts had already been made in this direction: courses in psychology were offered to pre-clinical students and a physiological approach to medicine was included in the introductory course. To improve cooperation, it was decided to re-establish the department of pharmacology and create academic units in therapeutics and applied pharmacology, which were also to be responsible for some pre-clinical teaching. It was anticipated that by encouraging clinical staff to teach pre-clinical students, the easier transition to clinical study that the interdepartmental committee argued was essential would be achieved.[121] The UGC recognised 'a hiatus between the pre-clinical and clinical stages in many medical schools' and welcomed the College's suggestions.[122] In other areas, the lecturers returned to earlier suggestions and proposed new departments for radiotherapeutics and paediatrics, matching the hospital's concerns that it was 'losing a great deal of prestige by the lack of certain Special Departments'.[123]

---

[119] Special committee, 26 October, 1 November 1945, DF 22; University to UGC, June 1943, DF 24.

[120] Logan to Ball, 2 November 1944, DF 24.

[121] Development policy, DF 20.

[122] Meeting with the UGC, 30 April 1947, DF 20.

[123] Development policy, DF 20; Medical Council, 26 June 1946, 23 October 1946, MC 1/12.

Although the development policy expressed the aspirations of the College in the immediate postwar period and the urgent need for rebuilding, the vision of the postwar structure of teaching was uncertain. As teaching hospitals faced an uncertain future, few were prepared to point out that the structure of training was in need of radical reorganisation.

'Health for all'

The physical devastation of London's hospitals created a considerable financial burden on the voluntary sector. The amount of money needed for essential repairs raised questions about their independence and softened opposition to a state system that promised to take over debts. The widespread destruction of hospital property and the extension of government control through the EMS created doubts that hospitals could return to their prewar position. Historians have traditionally seen the common experiences of war as producing mounting pressure for state intervention and the 1942 Beveridge report as embodying wartime aspirations.[124] The NHS did become a symbol for a more equitable social policy for which, many believed, the war had been fought. However, important groups in medicine and politics had already agreed the need, if not the nature of reform in the 1920s, bolstered by optimism about the effectiveness of medical care.[125] In the interwar period, enormous effort had gone into trying to redefine and change the contours of health provision. War reinforced this trend. The success of antibiotics in treating military casualties fuelled expectations of wider public benefits, while the EMS provided a blueprint for reform. 'It introduced hospital staff to public work on a salaried basis and help break down the traditional barriers between voluntary and public medical staff. . . . It established regional networks of diagnostic and treatment centres and set performance standards', but at the same time focused care on a 'more central curative based system based around a hospital structure' at the expensive of public health provision.[126] By 1941 it was clear that 'a reversion to the pre-war hospital world would probably be impossible at the end of the war' and that hospitals

---

[124] Derek Fraser, *The Evolution of the British Welfare State: A History of Social Policy since the Industrial Revolution* (London, 1984), pp. 207–39.

[125] For a discussion of hospitals and the NHS see Abel-Smith, *Hospitals*, pp. 440–88; Harry Eckstein, *The English Health Service: Its Origins, Structure and Achievements* (Cambridge, Mass., 1958); Daniel M. Fox, *Health Policies, Health Politics: The Experience of Britain and America, 1911–1965* (Princeton, 1986); Honigsbaum, *Health, Happiness and Security*; John E. Pater, *The Making of the National Health Service* (London, 1981); Charles Webster, *The Health Service since the War*, Vol. 1: *Problems of Health Care. The National Health Service before 1957* (London, 1988).

[126] Andrew Land, Rodney Lowe and Noel Whiteside, *The Development of the Welfare State, 1939–1951* (London, 1992), pp. 94–5.

had come to rely on government payments.[127] For Rosemary Stevens, it was never the end that was in doubt, only the means by which a service would be established.[128] It was here that the battles were fought.

Brown's statement to the House of Commons in 1941 stimulated debates on regionalisation and the repercussions this would have for London's hospitals. However, it was the publication of *Social Insurance and Allied Services* by William Beveridge, with its declaration of war on want, squalor, ignorance and idleness and its recommendations for a 'comprehensive national health service', which intensified public debate. Although the working class remained suspicious of social welfare and the middle class anxious about the use of taxation, the Ministry of Health was worried by the unexpected success of the report. In response, the Ministry began to develop proposals for a national health service. Hospital administrators, including Aylwen at St Bartholomew's, jumped to the defence of the voluntary system, believing it to be 'sound at heart'. Aylwen did reluctantly feel, however, that the EMS had 'provided ample evidence of the value to patients and hospitals alike of the greater co-ordination of their services'. He hinted at his willingness to cooperate with the LCC while maintaining the individuality of St Bartholomew's under the voluntary hospital system.[129] Doctors and lecturers at St Bartholomew's were less certain; they feared that Aylwen was 'putting his foot right into it'. Although welcoming further links with the LCC as a way to gain more beds for teaching, they worried about academic and medical freedom.[130] Feelings ran high and the pace of planning was stepped up in 1943.

In 1944, the government produced its long-awaited White Paper. Vague on all contentious issues, *A National Health Service* cautiously recommended a free medical service available to all, based on local authorities within which voluntary hospitals were guaranteed independence. The underlying principles of the White Paper had cross-party support and the document was greeted with enthusiasm by the press, public and local government. However, for voluntary hospitals it represented 'the stranglehold of local authorities' and they looked for ways to limit local government control.[131] The BMA agreed, having conveniently buried radical proposals made by its own commission into postwar healthcare. It remained committed to reform, but opposed the details of the White Paper, which appeared to threaten a

---

[127] Cited in Daniel M. Fox, 'The National Health Service and the Second World War: The Elaboration of Consensus', in *War and Social Change: British Society in the Second World War*, ed. Harold L. Smith (Manchester, 1986), p. 42.

[128] Rosemary Stevens, *Medical Practice in Modern England: The Impact of Medical Specialisation and State Medicine* (New Haven, 1966), p. 70.

[129] *City Press*, 7 May 1943; *Daily Sketch*, 17 May 1943.

[130] Girling Ball diary, 20 October 1942, f.134; General court, 27 November 1941, HA 1/32; *BMJ* i (1943), p. 493.

[131] Cited in Prochaska, *Philanthropy and the Hospitals of London*, p. 150.

salaried service, bureaucratic control and loss of clinical freedom. Staff at St Bartholomew's were equally hostile to the White Paper, if not the need for reform. Fearing centralisation and the danger of local government control, they pressed for 'freedom of expression in medical matters, freedom of speech and freedom of medical practice' to be preserved in any postwar settlement.[132] Outside the College, different ideas on how a national health service should be organised came into conflict and negotiations continued as politicians, civil servants, officials, doctors and hospital leaders worked to rebuild the consensus that made compromise possible. New proposals in 1945 gave voluntary hospitals a greater role in planning and made them into 'clearing house[s]' for each region, avoiding any direct financial relationship with local authorities. Disagreements had been compromised rather than resolved.[133]

The fragile balance was broken in July 1945 with Labour's landslide election victory. Electoral support for the party had grown in the last stages of the war as the Conservative Party was discredited and opinions shifted to the left. Clement Attlee formed a Labour Cabinet and Aneurin Bevan, Labour's new Minister of Health, set to work on healthcare reform. According to Charles Webster, the variety of ideas on state-directed healthcare made it impossible to suggest entirely new proposals and Bevan was able to put forward only 'fresh permutations of already known options'. His commitment to the idea of a national health service did not mean that he was unwilling to incorporate some of the earlier compromises. He rejected arguments that a health service should be local authority-based aware that doctors and medical schools found this the most objectionable aspect of the government's plans.[134] Although willing to compromise over local authority control, Bevan remained antagonistic to voluntarism and was determined to be ruthless in negotiations. He adopted a different course from that outlined by the White Paper and built on advice from civil servants in the Ministry of Health, already used to the EMS. Bevan believed that all hospitals should be nationalised and brought under the Ministry to ensure a single service with uniform standards. He argued that if voluntary hospitals were to be publicly financed they must also be publicly owned.[135]

Elements in the Cabinet were hostile to Bevan's proposals and the Conservative Party opposed those clauses that departed from the 1944 White Paper. Hospitals were divided. Nationalisation was seen as at least better than local authority control and opposition in the voluntary hospital community was not uniform. Although the British Hospitals Association saw in Bevan's scheme 'the mass murder of the hospitals', teaching hospitals were less hostile

---

[132] Medical Council, 31 March 1943, MC 1/11.
[133] Webster, *Health Service*, p. 80; Fox, 'National Health Service', pp. 48–9.
[134] Webster, *Health Service*, p. 80.
[135] Pater, *National Health Service*, p. 178.

to the Bill.[136] Henry Cohen, professor of medicine at Liverpool, in a consultation document for the Royal College of Physicians, noted that as long as the teaching hospitals were protected, it would be safe for the medical profession to leave the non-teaching hospitals to the 'mercies of the Regional Councils'.[137] Although William Goodenough noted that a convincing case has 'not been made for the transfer . . . of the ownership of all hospitals from local hands to central government', he reluctantly acknowledged the need for change along the lines proposed.[138] At St Bartholomew's Aylwen, believing that change was now 'inevitable', shifted his stance and began tentatively to support Bevan's proposals, rejecting opposition in favour of negotiation.[139] In offering support he hoped to negotiate a favourable position for St Bartholomew's, but was adamant that voluntary hospitals should not be subservient to local authority control.[140] Teaching hospitals saw some merit and more money in Bevan's scheme. They wanted to raise standards and agreed that the best way this could be achieved was through regional boards based on medical schools. Many deans had become convinced that a decentralised system was no longer desirable, and welcomed the Goodenough Committee's support for university teaching centres and cooperation with municipal hospitals. For those teaching hospitals earmarked for closure, it also provided a possibility to remain open.[141] Although the merits of a voluntary system continued to be defended, many connected to London's hospitals came to admit that the real debate was over how to 'arrange matters that all hospitals possess the maximum degree of . . . freedom compatible with a properly organised and efficient service', rather than over the need for a state-directed service.[142]

Teaching hospitals felt that there was still room for manoeuvre, and fresh negotiations followed. The King Edward's Hospital Fund for London, the self-appointed voice of the London voluntary hospitals, expressed reserved support for the National Health Service Bill as long as teaching hospitals were protected. It pressed its concern over the dangers of 'remote control' by anonymous boards and called for the need to protect endowments.[143] Aylwen shared these views and as chair of the Voluntary Hospitals Committee for London added further pressure. Already seen as sympathetic to reform, Aylwen asked whether existing boards and board members could be retained.[144] His stance was hardly surprising. St Bartholomew's was a wealthy

[136] Cited in Prochaska, *Philanthropy and the Hospitals of London*, p. 159.
[137] Wellcome: 'Notes on voluntary and municipal hospitals', GC/186/3.
[138] *The Times*, 6 April 1946, p. 5.
[139] General court, 25 April 1946, HA 1/32.
[140] LMA: Voluntary hospitals committee, 1 March 1944, A/KE/63/3.
[141] Honigsbaum, *Health, Happiness and Security*, p. 169.
[142] *The Times*, 9 April 1946, p. 5.
[143] Prochaska, *Philanthropy and the Hospitals of London*, p. 160.
[144] PRO: NHS Bill, preliminary papers, January to April 1942, MH 80/29; Representations for and against certain aspects of the NHS, April to May 1946, MH 77/78.

endowed hospital, proud of its history, and with an independent medical school.

The summary of the 1946 National Health Service Act revealed that Bevan had taken notice of these arguments. In the final drafting, concessions had been made to teaching hospitals. Bevan was guided in part by the recommendations of the Goodenough report and agreed that 'full and direct State control and regulation into the educational field' was undesirable. Teaching hospitals were given a privileged status under newly appointed governing bodies answerable not to the regional boards but directly to the Ministry of Health. They combined the functions of a regional hospital board with that of a hospital management committee, fitting with notions of a hierarchical system established before the war. Traditions and continuities were maintained: certain members of the old governing elite were re-elected and the new boards were comparable in size to the old governing bodies. Teaching hospitals acquired a degree of independence not achieved elsewhere in the health service.[145] Bevan's ideas were not new. A similar scheme had been outlined in 1942, but Bevan also allowed these new governing bodies control over the teaching hospitals' endowments while in other hospitals endowments were merged into a central fund.[146] Bevan freely admitted to the Institute of Hospital Administrators in May 1946 that 'teaching hospitals are going to be better off than ever they were before'. He warned, however, that any further opposition might result in modifications that were less to their liking.[147] Most teaching hospitals recognised that they had won considerable concessions. The compromise undermined regional planning and perpetuated divisions in the health service, but by winning over the teaching hospitals to his scheme, Bevan divided the voluntary hospitals. In the same way, he stuffed consultants' 'mouths with gold', so that they found it harder to oppose the Act in its final form.[148]

Regional divides

Difficulties emerged between the passing of the 1946 Act and its enactment on 5 July 1948. Bevan continued to fight with the BMA and general practitioners unconvinced about the merits of the new service. Surveys by the Nuffield Provincial Hospitals Trust revealed deficiencies in bed provision, which raised questions about whether the government could meet the 'newly

---

[145] Charles Webster, ed., *Aneurin Bevan on the National Health Service* (Oxford, 1991), pp. 36, 46–7; Webster, 'Conflict and Consensus: Explaining the British Health Service', *Twentieth Century British History* i (1990), p. 147.

[146] Wellcome: 'Skeleton scheme for discussion on hospital policy', GC/186/3.

[147] *Hospital*, May 1946, pp. 179–83.

[148] Abel-Smith, *Hospitals*, p. 480; Webster, *Health Service*, pp. 94–103, 107–20; Nicholas Timmins, *The Five Giants: A Biography of the Welfare State* (London, 1995), pp. 118–26.

assured right of all the population to hospital treatment'.[149] Teaching hospitals proved difficult, for many were not satisfied with the practical arrangements for the new service. Staff at St Bartholomew's half-heartedly claimed that they were 'opposed to the National Health Service Act' and would not 'contract with the Regional or Teaching Hospital Boards under this or an amended Act'. They also worried about the size of the new governing body and the extent of medical control.[150] The wider implications of the Act created further obstacles. However, with an immediate increase in student numbers at the end of the war and the need to define regions, decisions had to be made quickly.

University teaching hospitals, along the model outlined by Goodenough, were to be central to the new regions. This approach had been favoured by teaching hospitals, who saw a way of increasing access to teaching beds, and by the Royal College of Physicians and the King's Fund. This was no coincidence. Several members of the Goodenough committee were influential in both and played a prominent role in devising schemes for regionalisation.[151] Outside London, this created few problems: boundaries were easy to define and coincided with other nationalised undertakings.[152] However, how London was to be divided had troubled planners in the interwar period. London did not fit neatly into regionalisation and two possible approaches were suggested: either one massive region, or a sector system. The EMS was consulted and a 'London syndicate' formed to balance the capital's educational needs against a viable service and pressure from the LCC. Bevan refused to compromise. Having made concessions, he wanted medical schools at act as regional centres, believing that this would create the necessary concentration of specialist services and ensure that 'general practitioners are kept in more intimate association with new medical thought and training'.[153] Medical schools accepted the need to divide London into sectors, but had their own ideas over boundaries. St Bartholomew's wanted to extend its region west, The London argued for its own region, and King's felt that it should also be responsible for Croydon. With so many conflicting opinions, Bevan allowed a short consultation period. When no decision was reached, he unilaterally divided London into the four regions. St Bartholomew's and The London were allocated to the North East Metropolitan Region, a move which the College welcomed.[154] Sir Allen Daley as medical officer of health for the LCC was

---

[149] BMJ ii (1946), p. 270.
[150] College to Bevan, 7 April 1948, HA 35/26; Medical Council, 28 January 1948, MC 1/12.
[151] Wellcome: Royal College of Physicians Younger Fellows Club, 12 February 1941, GC/186/3.
[152] Webster, Health Service, p. 121.
[153] Webster, ed., Bevan, p. 67.
[154] Rivett, Development of the London Hospital System, pp. 271–7; 1947/8 annual report.

outraged and complained that London had been 'split into four in an extremely arbitrary fashion dictated solely by the need to apportion twelve teaching hospitals among the four regions'.[155]

Further discussions followed over the nature of teaching groups. Meetings were held between the London syndicate, the University and the LCC, which was keen to assert the importance of its hospitals for medical training. If the majority of schools in the syndicate did not want to become reliant on the LCC, they realised that LCC hospitals would have to be used.[156] The University supported the principles outlined by Goodenough, but had no clear policy of its own. St Bartholomew's and The London remained cautious, wanting to scale down plans for amalgamation. Although the College had worked with the LCC to overcome severe shortages of obstetric beds, it feared that closer association would slow rebuilding.[157] Staff worried that in using LCC beds they would be forced to 'improve the building up to St Bartholomew's standard', money that could be spent on the College. Experience quickly proved their concerns justified. At the Eastern Fever Hospital, Homerton, for example, repairs were estimated at £100,000. However, the need for more clinical beds tempered opposition. Once it became clear that services at Hill End would have to move to West Smithfield, negotiations were started with Daley at the LCC. Daley was respected in voluntary hospital circles and had kept himself informed of the Goodenough committee's work. Aware of the need to encourage practical links, he recommended that links should be established between St Bartholomew's and Bethnal Green Hospital. Despite being attacked for his tendency to side with voluntary hospitals, Daley was not prepared to cede complete control and pressed for joint clinical appointments.[158]

It was the Goodenough report that proved influential with its model of an undergraduate teaching hospital with 1000 beds.[159] It was felt that an opportunity could be taken to amalgamate smaller special institutions with teaching hospitals. Schemes from simple association to full absorption were canvassed. Bevan continued to favour amalgamation and was clear that teaching hospitals should not become district hospitals. He felt that exact functions should be determined by their educational needs.[160] After lengthy discussions, twelve undergraduate (representing 10,000 beds) and fourteen postgraduate groups were designated in May 1948 and 'consequently the Appointed Day arrived before the new management bodies had taken

---

[155] Cited in Rivett, *Development of the London Hospital System*, p. 275.
[156] College committee, 14 March 1945, MS 29/2.
[157] Board of Studies in Medicine, 15 July 1946, 19 May 1947, MS 103.
[158] Rivett, *Development of the London Hospital System*, pp. 261, 271–7; College committee, 2 October 1946, 7 May 1947, MS 29/2; Medical Council, 19 March 1947, MC 1/12.
[159] Webster, *Health Service*, p. 271.
[160] Rivett, *Development of the London Hospital System*, pp. 282–6.

effective control'.[161] Regions were forced to make concessions and teaching hospitals became groups of specialist units separate from the NHS. Designation remained controversial and left a legacy of ill-feeling. Teaching hospitals sought to absorb important non-teaching hospitals, exchanging them for unattractive alternatives. Initially St Bartholomew's was allocated the Alexandra Hospital for Children with Hip Diseases, Zachray Merton Convalescent Home, Northwood and the Metropolitan Hospital. Bethnal Green was not included, despite Daley's offer. Staff resisted the allocation of the Metropolitan Hospital, believing that it did not have suitable teaching accommodation, and argued instead that they should have control of the Eastern Fever Hospital. They were clear that whatever happened, they would not be able to 'supply all the additional teaching facilities required'.[162]

Conclusions

The NHS reversed interwar trends, deprived local authorities of control, and created a fragile system of healthcare that was from the start beset with economic problems. The 1946 Act was a compromise that did not guarantee administrative unity or a coordinated service. Hospitals dominated and general practitioners maintained their independence, leaving public health marginalised. In the new system, teaching hospitals acted like 'a select club of mandarins' and undue power was conceded to hospital consultants working in teaching hospitals. Regional board hospitals in turn resented what they saw as unjustified extravagance in teaching hospitals.[163] Although the organisation of healthcare had changed, the NHS saw significant continuities. The same was true of medical education. The Goodenough report endorsed suggestions that were already gaining acceptance. However, even with financial support from the UGC and a full endorsement from the Ministry of Health, the report represented a restatement of the parameters of reform rather than a blueprint for change. Pressure was applied to the GMC to devise a new curriculum and encouragement was given to postgraduate training, but the implementation of the report was left to individual schools and universities to decide.

At St Bartholomew's, teaching was adapted as temporary repairs and rebuilding were started. For the College, the NHS and the regional structure established in London was not ideal, but it did allow greater participation for the College in the hospital's management and created links with other non-teaching hospitals to compensate for the lack of adequate teaching accommodation on the island site at West Smithfield. It was the effects of

[161] Webster, *Health Service*, p. 123.
[162] College committee, 30 July 1947, MS 29/2.
[163] Webster, *Health Service*, p. 272.

war, rather than the situation created by the NHS and the Goodenough committee, that had a greater impact on the College. On the appointed day, the matter of greatest urgency was not the new NHS, but how to re-establish teaching and make the best use of the surviving facilities.

9

'No grounds for disqualification'

Women and medical education at St Bartholomew's

Women's struggle since the 1860s to gain access to medical education and equal opportunities in the medical profession has, in some respects, taken on a mythological quality. Invariably the story is one of a few dedicated women and their struggle against a male-dominated profession, which willingly constructed theories that played on social prejudices to support claims that women were either physically and mentally ill-suited to medicine, or ill-adapted to the 'strain' of education.[1] Professionalisation and occupational specialisation at the start of the nineteenth century had excluded existing female practitioners working in the domestic and community arenas, ensuring that the Victorian medical profession was a paradigm of male dominance. Women's challenge to it has been constructed as a 'gendered strategy of inclusion'; a 'usurpationary response on the part of an excluded group', but for much of the nineteenth century female students were excluded from London's teaching hospitals.[2] The First World War marked a turning point: seven of the twelve London schools agreed to take female students, although equal access proved temporary. New barriers were constructed that had less to do with pseudo-sexual physiology than with athleticism and arguments about accommodation. However, hostility within the profession was never uniform. Some doctors favoured opening medical schools and universities to women, and lecturers at St Bartholomew's were divided over the issue. Initially, the College inadvertently encouraged the movement by deciding in 1850 to accept Elizabeth Blackwell as a graduate student.

A female student 'in the wards'

Having graduated in America and spent time in Paris at the hospital La Maternité, Blackwell wished to follow her contemporaries and complete her

---

[1] See E. Moberly Bell, *Storming the Citadel: The Rise of the Woman Doctor* (London, 1953); Catriona Blake, *The Charge of the Parasols: Women's Entry to the Medical Profession* (London, 1990); Thomas N. Bonner, *To the Ends of the Earth: Women's Search for Education in Medicine* (Cambridge, Mass., 1992).
[2] Anne Witz, *Professions and Patriarchy* (London, 1992), p. 74.

training by walking the wards at a London hospital before entering general practice. Her cousin Kenyon Blackwell, a South Staffordshire ironmaster, interceded for her. He approached University College, Guy's and St Thomas's, which all suggested an application be made, but the warmest response was from James Paget, the warden at St Bartholomew's. Kenyon was convinced that Blackwell would find 'a powerful friend' in Paget, who hinted that other lecturers at St Bartholomew's shared his interest in her success.[3] It was Blackwell, however, who in 1850 asked permission to 'attend as a student in the wards and other departments'. The medical committee supported her request and gave her unlimited access to the wards for eighteen months.[4] The reason why is uncertain. Perhaps it was because Blackwell did not see herself as part of any movement and supported ideas that a woman's highest calling was to be a mother. Blackwell adopted a strategy used by early female doctors in claiming that she was merely channelling her maternal instincts into areas of medicine suitable for women. That Blackwell was already a talked-about medical graduate who had, to a limited degree, been accepted by the London medical community and had received encouragement from University College, Guy's and St Thomas's must also have swayed the staff at St Bartholomew's. There was some degree of sympathy in the College for her case.[5]

Blackwell was not welcomed unreservedly however. Conditions were imposed on her attendance: it was insisted that she could visit only those wards 'appropriate to females during the attendance of the Physicians and Surgeons'. In practice, this meant that Blackwell was excluded from the syphilitic wards. It was also decided that while she would be allowed to dissect, she could only do so in a room separate from the rest of the students, and would only be allowed to attend post-mortems performed on women. This, it was felt, would uphold notions of propriety and deal with the difficult problem of dissection with its 'very peculiar and precarious set of sexual-cultural meanings'.[6] In addition, Blackwell was granted permission to attend only those classes where the lecturer was willing to admit her.[7] By imposing these conditions, the lecturers created a sphere for Blackwell to work in that minimised her contact with male students, upheld their notions of decency and respected the attitudes of individual lecturers.

Blackwell was prevented from taking up her place immediately by an eye disease that had resulted in a partial loss of sight, and it was not until October

---

[3] Elizabeth Blackwell, 'A Reminiscence of Forty Years Ago', *St Bartholomew's Hospital Journal*, September 1894, p. 191.

[4] Medical committee, 11 April 1850, MC 1/1.

[5] Moberly Bell, *Storming the Citadel*, p. 35–6.

[6] Alison Bashford, *Purity and Pollution: Gender, Embodiment and Victorian Medicine* (Basingstoke, 1998), pp. 107, 117.

[7] Medical committee, 11 April 1850, MC 1/1.

1850 that she finally entered St Bartholomew's as a student. Paget assured her that she would be welcomed as a graduate student.[8] Despite the medical committee's ruling, she encountered opposition from Charles West as physician-accoucheur and lecturer in midwifery. West excluded her from the midwifery wards as he 'entirely disapproved of a lady studying medicine' and perhaps considered her a threat. The surgeons William Lawrence and Edward Stanley, and the difficult Clement Hue were more courteous but declined to admit her to lectures. It was George Burrows rather than Paget however who allowed Blackwell to make his wards 'my headquarters'. Burrow's support inclined Blackwell to limit her work to the medical wards, ensuring that she did not enter the surgical wards where a more masculine culture prevailed.[9] Paget's were the only lectures she attended. Writing in November 1850, Blackwell noted that the students 'politely step aside' to let her pass and appeared awkward around her. She hinted that her existence at the College was a solitary one, with an attendant showing her to a reserved seat in the lecture theatre.[10] Although not openly opposed,

> At first no one knew how to regard me. Some thought that I must be an extraordinary intellect overflowing with knowledge; others a queer eccentric woman; and none seemed to understand that I was a quiet sensible person who had acquired a small amount of medical knowledge, and who wished by patient observation and study to acquire considerably more . . . Mr Paget, who is very cordial, tells me that I shall have to encounter much more prejudice from ladies and gentlemen in my course. I am prepared for this.[11]

For Paget's wife, it was almost remarkable that Blackwell was 'quite unmolested' by the students.[12]

A bastion of opposition

Blackwell found St Bartholomew's less stimulating and exciting than her time in Paris and was sceptical of the methods taught. Knowing that her studies in London were not furthering her career, and worried about the cost of training at St Bartholomew's, she decided to return to America. After Blackwell's time in the hospital, the College quickly became a bastion of opposition to women doctors. Opposition stemmed largely from the

---

[8] Peggy Chambers, A Doctor Alone: A Biography of Elizabeth Blackwell, the First Woman Doctor, 1821–1910 (London, 1956), p. 81.
[9] Elizabeth Blackwell, Pioneer Work in Opening the Medical Profession to Women: Autobiographic Sketches (London, 1895), pp. 164–5, 172.
[10] Chambers, A Doctor Alone, pp. 83–4.
[11] Blackwell, Pioneer Work, p. 170.
[12] Stephen Paget, ed., Memoirs and Letters of Sir James Paget (London, 1901), p. 169.

students; staff generally adopted a more liberal attitude. While Paget remained sympathetic to women doctors (he viewed Blackwell's time at St Bartholomew's as a 'perfectly satisfactory ... experiment' that might be repeated), he was clear that it would only be appropriate for a 'lady' who had already undertaken most of her training.[13] Paget was not alone: George William Callender, Holmes Coote and Wilmot Parker Herringham was also sympathetic to female students. For much of the nineteenth century however, a majority of staff and students opposed the admission of female students, a view shared by large sections of the profession.

Although the 1858 Medical (Registration) Act did not aim to exclude women, London's medical schools and their students actively tried to prevent women from gaining those credentials that would allow them to become practitioners. In an overcrowded profession anxious about competition and incomes, female practitioners were seen as another threat. The aim was, as Frances Power Cobb noted, 'to keep ladies out of the lucrative profession of physician and crowd them into the ill paid one of nurses'.[14] The admission of female students also appeared to threaten the status of an already insecure profession. Medical schools, influenced by the fee-paying student body, resisted admitted female students and the same approach was adopted at St Bartholomew's.

When it was announced in 1865 that Miss Ellen Colborne had been admitted to 'the wards and to the Lectures of such members of the staff as may be disposed to allow of her attendance', a hasty meeting was convened by the students to see 'what measures should be taken to prevent if possible, the *lady* from becoming a Student'.[15] A petition 'signed by almost every man in the College' begged the lecturers to reconsider. William Savory, lecturer in general anatomy and physiology, subsequently informed the students that Colborne would probably not be admitted; the news was greeted with 'Loud cheers & clapping'. Savory's assessment proved incorrect. Two weeks later, Colborne started to attend lectures.[16] A determined feminist, Colborne was seen by contemporaries as part of a 'generation of "Women's Righters"'. Her actions were a strident challenge to the male atmosphere at St Bartholomew's and belonged with attempts to storm the citadels of all-male schools to secure an education that would allow women to qualify as practitioners under the 1858 Act. Colborne took her stance at a time when the issue of female enfranchisement and demands for women's secondary and higher education were creating considerable debate.[17] At St Bartholomew's the medical

[13] Ibid., pp. 174, 186–7.

[14] Frances Power Cobb, 'Medicine and Morality', *Modern Review* xi (1881), p. 323.

[15] Minutes of the medical officers and lecturers, 14 October 1865, MS 12/1.

[16] 'A Bart's Women', *St Bartholomew's Hospital Journal*, November 1931, p.32.

[17] Cited in Philippa Levine, *Feminist Lives in Victorian England: Private Roles and Public Commitment* (Oxford, 1990), p. 147; José Harris, *Private Lives, Public Spirit: Britain, 1870–1914* (London, 1994), p. 23.

theatre quickly became crowded with students 'who hooted, screamed, etc.'. Order was restored only after Colborne left to be interviewed by Callender who tried to persuade her to leave the College. However, Colborne was adamant. She persisted in her attempts to attend lectures. When she walked into one of Savory's crowded lectures her presence was so unsettling that Savory asked the students to vote whether they wanted him to continue: only two students voted in favour of carrying on 'under such circumstances'. Under such pressure, Colborne finally withdrew in January 1866.[18] The students' actions and the staff's reactions to them were not unusual. When Elizabeth Garret Anderson had attempted to study at the Middlesex Hospital five years before, she was met with a petition from male students who felt coeducation 'a dangerous innovation'. In Edinburgh, the efforts of a group of women led by Sophia Jex-Blake were greeted at first with 'petty annoyances' and then a student riot at Surgeon's Hall.[19]

For much of the nineteenth century, a large number of the lecturers and the majority of students at St Bartholomew's shared Thomas Laycock's view that he 'could not imagine *any decent women* wishing to study medicine'.[20] Burrows, Savory, Henry Power, Henry Butlin, Samuel Gee and Dyce Duckworth all openly opposed any extension of women's rights. Gee even persuaded John Wickham Legg to return from New Orleans in 1878 to vote against the proposal to award women licences from the Royal College of Physicians.[21] Others in the College equally subscribed to and helped construct social and biological views of women that showed them to be at the mercy of their reproductive organs or, if forceful, prone to hysteria.[22] From the late eighteenth century, doctors sought to confirm middle-class 'hegemonic definitions of femininity'. When the revised outpatient arrangements were introduced at St Bartholomew's in 1888, it was felt that they allowed female patients to 'have prepared and finished the mid-day meal and set their homes in order' before coming to the hospital.[23] Doctors argued that a woman's duty was to be both reproductive and domestic. Using menstruation and maternity as an argument, doctors asserted that women were intellectually and physiologically less robust than men, prone to illness and invalidism. A

[18] 'A Bart's Women', p. 32; Minutes of the medical officers and lecturers, 13 January 1866, MS 12/1.
[19] Cited in J. Manton, *Elizabeth Garrett Anderson* (New York, 1965), p. 351; See Sophia Jex-Blake, *Medical Women: A Thesis and a History* (Edinburgh, 1886).
[20] Ibid., p. 72.
[21] *St Bartholomew's Hospital Journal*, spring 1993, p. 21.
[22] See Frederick Carpenter Skey, *Hysteria: Remote Causes of Disease in General Treatment of Disease by Tonic Agency Local or Surgical Forms of Hysteria*, 2nd edn (London, 1867), pp. 77–84; Edward Rigby, *On the Constitutional Treatment of Female Diseases* (London, 1857).
[23] L. Nead, *Myths of Sexuality: Representations of Women in Victorian Britain* (Oxford, 1988), pp. 142–3; Medical Council, 9 June 1888, MC 1/2.

limited understanding of the role of menstruation made it easier for doctors to regard women as subject to their physiological functions. Medical science came to mediate and justify existing middle-class gender relations and masculine insecurities 'by confirming the threat of feminine disorder to the social and moral order'.[24]

New arguments were added in the 1870s after reformers had succeeded in opening the Cambridge lower examination to schoolgirls and examination results showed that women were as capable of passing as men. An expansion of women's role in public life and campaigns led by women against compulsory vaccination, vivisection and the Contagious Diseases Acts heightened concern. Encouraged by Henry Maudsley, and by Darwinian ideas, doctors asserted that menstruation rendered women vulnerable, while excessive study was dangerous to women's health. Education beyond a rudimentary level, it was felt, undermined girls' attachment to the home and held the risk of pathological menstruation or sterility.[25] Falling birth rates among educated middle-class women were used as justification. It was also feared that intellectual study would masculinise women, a concern adopted by the press in the 1890s in caricatures of female intellectuals as ugly, mannish and potentially sexually deviant.[26] In defence of their own position, doctors argued that the study of medicine presented a real danger that threatened to unsex women: a knowledge of the human body and its functions could debase and degrade women. Anatomy and physiology were believed to be particularly dangerous to female innocence, while the *Lancet* forcefully claimed that menstruation and pregnancy made women 'unfit to be entrusted with the life of a fellow creature'.[27] The medical and scientific codification of women as the weaker sex was in part a product of Victorian doctors' insecurity. Competition for patients and concerns about the profession's gentlemanly status bolstered fears about 'intruders from outside' and encouraged intense opposition to female doctors.[28]

---

[24] Barbara Harrison, 'Women and Health', in *Women's History: Britain 1850–1945: An Introduction*, ed. June Purvis (London, 1995), p. 157.

[25] Joan Burstyn, *Victorian Education and the Ideal of Womanhood* (London, 1980), ch. 5.

[26] Carol Dyhouse, *Girls Growing up in late-Victorian and Edwardian England* (London, 1981), p. 103; Dyhouse, 'Storming the Citadel or Storm in a Tea Cup? The Entry of Women into Higher Education, 1860–1920', in *Is Higher Education Fair to Women?*, ed. Sandra Acker and David Warren Piper (Guildford, 1984), p. 57; Joan Burstyn, 'Educators' Response to Scientific and Medical Studies of Women in England, 1860–1900', ibid., pp. 65–80.

[27] Jean L'Esperance, 'Doctors and Women in Nineteenth-Century Society: Sexuality and Role', in *Health Care and Popular Medicine in Nineteenth Century England: Essays in the Social History of Medicine*, ed. John Woodward and David Richards (New York, 1977), pp. 105–27; *Lancet* i (1858), p. 44.

[28] Cited in Harrison, 'Women and Health', p. 176.

Lecturers at St Bartholomew's were clearly sensitive to their male students' wishes, which were firmly opposed to female medical students. When the Cambridge Graduates Club decided to allow guests to attend its dinners in 1894, an all-male atmosphere was maintained and women were excluded.[29] St Bartholomew's saw itself as a collegiate male enclave like Oxford and Cambridge. The College was not alone. Although the 1858 Act permitted the registration of female doctors, they were practically excluded by the 'conditions imposed by the medical corporations and by the Universities'. In Parliament, attempts to break the male monopoly over medical education between 1874 and 1876 were firmly resisted and loopholes in licensing regulations closed.[30] Women's access to higher education was a slow process, but when progress was made in other areas of education (both secondary and higher), medical education was increasingly out of step. At the University of London, the medical faculty forced the issue when Convocation agreed to admit Edith Shove to its medical examinations. Alarmed by the prospect, a petition signed by 250 medical graduates protested against the decision. Savory at St Bartholomew's felt that with so many medical graduates opposed, 'was it right of the graduates of other faculties to force this strange innovation upon them?'[31] He was adamant that he would not examine female students and secured the adoption of a resolution that it was 'inadvisable' for Senate 'to admit women to degrees in medicine before it shall have considered the general question of their admission to the degrees of all the faculties'.[32] A supplementary charter admitting women was proposed and, despite opposition, the resolution went against the doctors. A new charter was introduced in 1878, but the decision to admit women to a medical course was left to the individual medical schools.[33] St Bartholomew's continued to refuse to admit women.

Jex-Blake's crusade for coeducation in Edinburgh 'left a bitter heritage in British medical circles that made further efforts at co-education nearly impossible'.[34] London's hospital schools resisted the admission of female students until the twentieth century; opposition that encouraged the foundation of the London School of Medicine for Women (LSMW) in 1874 to provide an alternative.[35] The licensing bodies were also opposed and the

[29] Cambridge Graduates Club, SC 1/1. This was not unusual: all-male student societies in provincial universities voted to exclude women: Carol Dyhouse, *No Distinction of Sex? Women in British Universities 1870–1939* (London, 1994), p. 200.

[30] Cited in Witz, *Professions and Patriarchy*, p. 83.

[31] *Lancet* i (1878), p. 687.

[32] Jex-Blake, *Medical Women*, pp. 216–18.

[33] Gillian Sutherland, 'The Plainest Principles of Justice: The University of London and the Higher Education of Women', in *University of London and the World of Learning, 1836–1986*, ed. F. M. L. Thompson (London, 1990), pp. 35–56.

[34] Bonner, *To the Ends of the Earth*, p. 129.

[35] Resistance on the part of colleges in Oxford and Cambridge to admit women saw similar moves to found all women colleges, such as Girton College.

London schools argued that there was no point in training female students when they could not be examined. Indeed, as middle-class families generally spent less money on their daughters' education, there was no economic incentive for medical schools to alter their misogynistic tendencies. Even in those universities that admitted women, mixed feelings existed. Separate teaching and accommodation for anatomy and dissection were often provided, which indirectly hampered women, while some feminist educational pioneers reinforced social and gender boundaries in a bid to confirm respectability.[36]

Conquest of the London schools

It was not until the First World War that seven of the twelve London hospital schools (led by St Mary's) accepted a limited number of women from the LSMW as clinical students. The *Daily Telegraph* noted that women's crusade to enter London's medical schools had 'finally secured its conquests'.[37] The decision was made against a background of falling student numbers and a shortage of staff, with students used to fill vacant posts. Under these wartime conditions, schools faced a marked fall in income and moved to admit female clinical students in an attempt to establish a 'durable source' of fees.[38] St Bartholomew's did not come to the same conclusion, despite pressure from the University, which, after investigation in 1915, found 'no valid objection' to the admission of female medical students.[39] Reconstruction of the University in 1900 had seen the recognition of Royal Holloway College for women, Westfield College and LSMW as university schools, and the success of coeducational classes in the Scottish and provincial universities had made the question less controversial. The Conjoint Board's decision to follow the Society of Apothecaries and open its examinations to women in 1910 only added to uncomfortable feelings in a university that otherwise prided itself on its early move to coeducation. Rising demand for places and pressure from women for access to London's teaching hospitals added to these concerns at a time when educational opportunities for women were widening.[40] These changes and the Haldane Commission's discussion of the role of women in

---

[36] Dyhouse, *No Distinction of Sex?*, pp. 157, 190–9; Sutherland, 'Plainest Principles of Justice', p. 39; Levine, *Feminist Lives*, pp. 143–4.

[37] Carol Dyhouse, 'Women Students and the London Medical Schools, 1914–39: The Anatomy of a Masculine Culture', *Gender and History* x (1998), pp. 113–14, 111.

[38] David Mitchell, *Women on the Warpath: The Story of the Women of the First World War* (London, 1966); James Stuart Garner, 'The Great Experiment: The Admission of Women Students to St Mary's Hospital Medical School, 1916–1925', *Medical History* xlii (1998), pp. 68–88.

[39] University of London, *Report of the Academic Council on Medical Education of Women in London*, Part i (London, 1916), p. 5.

[40] See Joyce Senders Pederson, *The Reform of Girls' Secondary and Higher Education in Victorian England. A Study of Elites and Educational Change* (New York, 1987).

the University of London created concern at St Bartholomew's. Although Victorian biological constructions of female inferiority had started to be eroded, the College, along with St Thomas's, Guy's and the Middlesex, opposed the University's assessment.[41] Their stance was extreme. However, even in those universities that admitted female students and employed women lecturers, prejudices persisted. Opposition, and a recognition of anxieties among male students who found women 'keener in their work' and 'unable to contribute to the athletic life of the school', ensured that the University decided not to force schools to cooperate given that wartime conditions were straining finance and leading to staffing problems. With several schools agreeing to train female students, the University decided that the situation had largely resolved itself.[42]

The move by the seven schools to admit female clinical students proved a temporary wartime expedient. Critics argued that these schools reversed their earlier decisions only because they were more concerned about women's impact on 'hospital games and sport' than about their contribution to, or suitability for medicine.[43] An influx of male students hardened by trench warfare after the war did create difficulties. At St Mary's it led to open hostility between male and female students in an emerging culture that favoured anti-intellectualism, team sports, duty and loyalty, encouraged by an intractable misogynist attitude among members of the teaching staff. Fears about institutional vitality were thought to be more important than financial stability, and it was decided in 1924 to stop admitting female clinical students.[44] St Bartholomew's and other schools voiced similar concerns. Many feared that they would establish reputations as almost entirely female schools at a time when men in other spheres were attempting to 'reclaim territory' they felt they had lost to women during wartime.[45] By 1928, only University College Hospital continued to admit a limited number of female students.[46] The BMJ concluded that London was in danger of reverting to 'the position it held before the war as the only great teaching centre in these islands without facilities for medical co-education'.[47] The press rushed to the conclusion that female students were being banned from London's medical schools and pointed to a sex war in medicine.[48] In response, the University decided in 1928 to appoint a committee to investigate.

[41] Agenda book, 30 November 1910, MS 16/2.
[42] *Report of the Academic Council on Medical Education of Women in London*, Part i, p. 5.
[43] *The Times*, 12 October 1942, p. 5.
[44] Garner, 'The Great Experiment', pp. 81–5; Dyhouse, 'Women Students', pp. 117–18; Wellcome: Medical Women's Federation council, 31 October 1924, SA/MWF/A.1/3.
[45] See Susan Kingsley Kent, *Making Peace: The Reconstruction of Gender in Interwar Britain* (Princeton, 1993).
[46] Dyhouse, 'Women Students', pp. 115–19.
[47] *BMJ* i (1928), p. 562.
[48] Wellcome: Medical Women's Federation press-cuttings, SA/MWF/D.9/5; Moberly Bell, *Storming the Citadel*, p. 174.

Elements in the University were becoming concerned about its role in training female clinical students at a time when 'the demand for Women Doctors is . . . increasing'. Educational provision for women was growing and opportunities for training female medical students had increased outside London, along with openings in general practice and local authorities. The work of the LSMW and the Medical Women's Federation highlighted divisions in training that ran counter to the University's policy of equality. Evidence suggested that with few educational opportunities in London, women were studying at the provincial universities.[49] Public opinion and the British Medical Association were reconciled to the need for female doctors in part because rising incomes removed some of the earlier financial threat female doctors were felt to represent. The University therefore concluded that there was no 'valid argument on the merits against the provision of co-education in medicine'. Although it deplored the feeling of antipathy towards women expressed by medical schools, the committee wanted to avoid recommending the universal admission of female students. It preferred voluntary arrangements and suggested that three types of school should be created: those for men, those for women, and those willing to offer clinical training on a coeducational basis.[50] When the report was forwarded, lecturers at St Bartholomew's replied that they were unwilling to admit women, having incorporated the idea of a single-sex male school in its 1923 Charter.[51] The opening of the professorial units had increased confidence in the College's position and with rising student numbers there was no financial incentive to admit female students. With only three schools willingly to admit female clinical students, the University decided not 'to compel a medical school to remain or become co-educational against its will'.[52] London's teaching hospitals remained unenthusiastic. Although Guy's, King's, The London, St George's, St Mary's and University College were reluctantly prepared to offer a limited number of places to women on their short postgraduate courses in the 1930s, only University College and King's adopted a guarded coeducational approach. For St Bartholomew's, even the admission of female doctors to postgraduate courses was going too far.[53]

While critics accused St Bartholomew's of harbouring anti-feminist feelings because of the 'traditional pride in . . . football', staff preferred to claim that male students, parents and large sections of the public were antipathetic to female students, fearing the impact of co-education on their

[49] Louisa Martindale, *The Woman Doctor and her Future* (London, 1922), p. 83; Wellcome: Medical Women's Federation Council, SA/MWF/A.1/3; Medical Women's Federation executive committee, 13 March 1929, SA/MWF/A.2/2.

[50] *Report of the Committee on the Medical Education of Women Undergraduates*, 28 October 1942, pp. 4–5.

[51] Charter of incorporation, MS 26/1.

[52] *Report of the Committee on the Medical Education of Women Undergraduates.*

[53] Wellcome: Medical Women's Federation council, 6 November 1931, SA/MWF/A.1/4.

sons. The First World War had served only to strengthen the masculine culture of the College. Many men considered the prospect of studying or working under female authority an unbearable affront to their dignity in a school and hospital environment that worked on gentlemanly codes and a patriarchal system.[54] Staff at St Bartholomew's shared a common belief 'that men, if they have a choice, prefer to go to schools that do not admit women'.[55] Students were certainly hostile to women using their educational and sporting facilities. The attitude concealed concerns about competition for appointments and women's impact on the athletic record of the College where 'rugby was almost a religion'.[56] With the income of the College dependent on student fees, staff literally could not afford to ignore student opinion. Alfred Franklin, lecturer in paediatrics, was clear that the future of women at St Bartholomew's was certain with the College an 'opponent of medical co-education'.[57] The few women who did work in the College were limited to research and, no matter what their qualifications, were confined to a purely technical role with many of the male staff seeing them as somewhat 'inferior'.[58] The Medical Women's Federation felt St Bartholomew's to be a lost cause. In 1936, it did not consider approaching the College as part of an attempt to increase the number of places for female students, preferring to focus on those hospitals that 'had at any time admitted women'.[59]

However, opinion was changing. The National Council for Equal Citizenship publicly deplored the exclusion of women from 'certain London medical schools' and condemned the principle of 'exclusion from professional training solely on account of sex', a view shared by many other women's organisations.[60] Even at St Bartholomew's the SU found it necessary in 1940 to relax its strict regulation and allow women to play tennis at their sports ground at Chislehurst.[61] By 1942, Dr Graham Little, MP for the University of London and an ardent supporter of women's medical education, felt that the public now recognised that 'the advantages which women would gain from being educated side by side with men would far outweigh any possible loss to the men'. Pressure was growing for the London medical schools to admit women 'on equal terms with men'. *The Times* thought 'the war has made it clearer than ever that the medical education of women must find ample

---

[54] Dyhouse, 'Women Students', p. 123.

[55] Cited in Bonner, *To the Ends of the Earth*, p. 163.

[56] Cited in Dyhouse, 'Women Students ', p. 125.

[57] 'A Bart's Women', p. 32.

[58] PRO: Memorandum, 18 November 1939, FD 1/3131.

[59] Wellcome: Notes re the work of the coeducation committee, February1936, SA/MWF/D.9/4.

[60] Wellcome: Medical Women's Federation Council, 8 May 1936, SA/MWF/A.1/4; *Daily Telegraph*, 27 March 1937.

[61] SU minutes, 26 June 1940, SU 11/2.

provision in the new hospital policy which is now in the making'.[62] Campaigners for coeducation, borrowing from the language of social medicine, argued that women were ideally suited to 'public health services, maternity and child welfare, school medical and dental services, the women's service'. They asserted that schools like St Bartholomew's were not rejecting female students on educational grounds 'but solely because they are women'.[63]

Coeducation, the University of London and Goodenough

Partly in response to these concerns, the University of London appointed another committee in 1943 to look into the question. Using statistics from the University Grants Committee (UGC), it showed that London, even during wartime, compared badly with the rest of the country, especially when 16 per cent of all registered medical practitioners were female. With a 237 per cent increase in female doctors between the 1930s and 1940s, and with all provincial schools admitting female students, London was falling behind.[64] Part of the problem lay with London itself. Bombing made the city dangerous, and the image of schools like St Bartholomew's as rowdy and coarse was believed to discourage parents. However, with more women applying to enter medicine, even those schools willing to educate women 'were obliged to refuse a large number of applicants they would have liked to admit'. The decision at University College and King's College to admit female medical students, bringing medicine into line with other subjects in the colleges, helped counter arguments that coeducation created problems for schools. Neither had been damaged. On these grounds, the committee felt that the issue could no longer be left to individual schools.[65]

This new feeling of cooperation may have been encouraged by the interdepartmental committee on medical education and discussions over the role of hospitals in a new national health service. At a time when the structure of medical education and healthcare in London was uncertain, many schools felt uncomfortable about being too strident. By 1944, Charing Cross, Guy's, the London, St Mary's, the Middlesex and the Westminster had all expressed a willingness to admit female students. Although St Bartholomew's remained opposed to the idea, it was prepared to consider the question.[66]

[62] *The Times*, 7 November 1942, p. 5.
[63] Ibid., 9 October 1942, p. 5.
[64] *Lancet* ii (1960), p. 1160.
[65] University of London, *Report of the Special Committee of the University of London to Consider the Medical Education of Women in London* (London, 1944).
[66] Ibid.

After weighing the evidence, the committee concluded that the University was not 'doing its share in the provision of facilities for women's medical education in comparison with the other English Universities'. It rejected the idea that more institutions should be opened for women only, and felt that 'it would be manifestly unfair to place the responsibility for the solution of the problem exclusively upon those Schools that already admit women'. On these grounds, the committee saw that the only solution was to make all medical schools in London coeducational; equality of opportunity rather than equality of numbers had to be the University's aim. However, the committee recognised that schools needed a degree of independence and therefore declared that 'it is not recommended that the University should prescribe any quota for the admission of women to the Schools'. Opposition was expected and problems of accommodation were recognised, with the committee concluding that until more facilities were provided, women could be admitted only by excluding a corresponding number of men.[67]

St Bartholomew's objected to the committee's recommendations. When the University had announced the investigation, a heated discussion had ensued in the College, with one contributor summing up the general opinion when he explained that 'the prospect of women entering the profession, and this Hospital' verged on a 'catastrophe'.[68] In preparing a minority report, William Girling Ball, as dean of the College, stressed that it was not the right time to discuss the issue when the future requirements of the profession were unknown. Girling Ball had been aware since 1942 that the College might be pressed to admit women and had suggested changing the 1923 Charter.[69] However, he wanted more time for discussion and warned of the consequences of a hasty decision. He was trying to avoid the issue. The minority report repeated familiar arguments about the lack of suitable accommodation. With St Bartholomew's facing extensive war damage, this reflected the difficult position of the College and uncertainties about its future. Girling Ball was convinced that there were simply not enough places for women, especially as priority was given to men returning from war. He saw in the admission of women to all medical schools a radical restructuring of medical education in London that went against the wishes of some schools. Girling Ball was adamant that in forcing all schools to admit women it would not *ipso facto* mean an increase in opportunities. He and his colleagues favoured the system suggested in 1929 whereby three types of school would be created. Girling Ball argued:

> that in this City with thirteen medical schools there should be schools for men only. We are not all CO-educationalists, and it is my experience, even at this date,

[67] Ibid.
[68] *St Bartholomew's Hospital Journal*, August 1943, p. 199.
[69] College Council, 27 January 1943, MS 28/2.

that many parents are against this system. Before they enter their sons the questions is still asked of the Dean as to whether his School takes women.

The minority report concluded that with lecturers at St Bartholomew's opposed to the admission of female students, it was unwise for the University to force the issue.[70]

However, Girling Ball's views carried little weight with the University. Shortly after the committee reported, the Goodenough committee, appointed to look into the whole system of medical education, came to the same conclusion. It recommended 'that the payment to any school of Exchequer Grants in aid of medical education should be conditional upon the school being co-educational and admitting a reasonable proportion of women students'. This 'reasonable proportion' was loosely defined as one-fifth of the annual student entry. It was not a new idea. The Medical Women's Federation had favoured a limited number of female places being made available in all schools since 1929.[71] The UGC accepted the Goodenough committee's recommendations and called for 15 per cent of students to be female, a figure below the average admission for universities outside London. It was not a target rigidly enforced.[72] The *Star* explained that 'only the Old Guard of medicine will frown upon the recommendation[s]', but the *BMJ* was critical of the decision, feeling that if women were to be admitted this should be done 'graciously and gallantly and not according to a quota so they did not feel unwelcome'.[73] The recommendations were part of a trend to increase educational opportunities for women. The 1944 Education Act had opened the possibility of an academic education for working-class girls, and three years later Cambridge finally agreed to allow women to become full graduates. A widespread distaste of single-sex education came to underpin provision as more schools became mixed. By the late 1940s the issue generated little public debate, although in some cases coeducation degenerated into running two schools under one roof and girls were discouraged from taking science subjects.[74]

Lecturers at St Bartholomew's expressed their 'disapproval' and stressed that they were 'very unwilling to admit women students because as experienced medical educationalists' they were 'of opinion that some Medical

---

[70] *Minority Report Special Committee of the University of London to Consider the Medical Education of Women in London.*

[71] *Report of the Interdepartmental Committee on Medical Education* (London, 1944); Wellcome: Medical Women's Federation Council, 12 May 1929, SA/MWF/A.1/3.

[72] Mary Anne Elston, 'Women Doctors in a Changing Profession: The Case of Britain', in *Gender, Work and Medicine: Women and the Medical Division of Labour*, ed. Elianne Riska and Katarina Wegar (London, 1993), p. 33.

[73] *Star*, 20 July 1944; *BMJ* ii (1947), p. 379.

[74] Sara Delamont, *Knowledgeable Women: Structuralism and the Reproduction of Elites* (London, 1989), pp. 163, 168–9.

College should be reserved for men'. However, it was realised that the College might be 'endangered by non-acceptance'. It was a consideration that forced the lecturers to accept proposals they otherwise deplored and felt to be impractical, arguing that this was 'government control of academic institutions'.[75] The recommendations contained in the Goodenough report, financial pressure from the UGC, and the University's decision, forced St Bartholomew's into accepting female undergraduate students. The College received a large number of applications and the first six women were admitted to the College in 1947. The initial group came from Oxford and it was felt that their maturity helped ease the transition. In 1948, the numbers admitted started to rise; many of the early female students being helped to cope with an all-male environment by those who had been in the Services.

The recommendations of the Goodenough committee and the University's decision were more important in ending sex segregation in medical education than for their immediate impact on the number of women who entered London's medical schools. They encouraged a system of 'quotas' in individual schools that persisted from the 1950s to the mid-1970s. Prewar differences remained, with provincial schools continuing to admit more female students than their London counterparts. It was not until the 1960s that this became a source of professional concern and an active effort was made to recruit more women.[76] Although 'training facilities in every branch of medicine . . . opened up for women proportionately', the Medical Women's Federation continued to find that women had to be better qualified than men to secure a place at one of Londons' medical schools.[77]

A coeducational school?

Pressure to admit women brought obvious changes to St Bartholomew's. A supplementary charter was prepared and efforts were made to 'provide the necessary accommodation' for female students.[78] A ladies' cloakroom was built once the problem of finding a suitable location was overcome. Arrangements reflected the College's attitude to women: the cloakroom contained 'a bed for the ladies to rest upon when exhausted by the day's work' and 'a supply of cups, saucers, teapots and the ingredients necessary for occasional refreshments'. This created a certain amount of indignation among the male students. The cloakroom was felt to be like a club and far superior to the discarded air-raid shelters the male students were forced to

[75] College committee, 10 January 1945, 10 February 1945, MS 29/2.
[76] *Report of the RC on Medical Education* (London, 1968), p. 274; Elston, 'Women Doctors', p. 33.
[77] Wellcome: Committee on medical education, 12 January 1956, SA/MWF/A.4/14.
[78] College Council, 24 January, 27 June, 24 October 1945, MS 28/2.

use.[79] At the sports ground in Chislehurst, less salubrious accommodation was provided by the SU, which was dominated by male students and was more hostile to the admission of women. A separate hut was built for women alongside the main pavilion. The constitution of the SU was altered to allow female students to elect a clinical and a pre-clinical representative, but female participation was otherwise kept to a minimum.[80] The Abernethian Room, however, remained for men only.[81] Women students in the College gradually formed their own societies.

Resistance and anxiety were expressed at the admission of women even though the number of women gaining places in the College remained small. One wag declared admitting women to the College to be worse than hell.[82] The Cambridge Graduates Club debated accepting women as members but decided that this would 'entirely alter its character'. The issue was discussed again at the 1950 dinner. Although those attending were adamant that neither women nor female guests should be allowed to attend, an informal meeting decided that women should be included. A compromise was reached: the dinner remained for men only and a separate sherry party was established to welcome 'the newcomers who had just come down from the University' whatever their gender.[83] The male students remained worried about the admission of women. Women were blamed for taking places away from men and for introducing the 'thin feminine edge of the wedge' into the hierarchy at St Bartholomew's. Some male students were alarmed by the additional level of competition which female students were felt to introduce, and they were also blamed for raising the standard of examinations.[84]

Tensions were not quickly resolved. Although efforts were made to ensure a 'more even distribution of women students throughout the surgical firms', the male students in 1957 were felt to be showing 'stoical tolerance' to the presence of women.[85] Attacks on women's suitability for medicine continued throughout the 1960s, as women were perceived to threaten traditional patterns of behaviour and experiences of medical school. When Harold Wykeham Balme retired as sub-dean in 1963, he told the St Bartholomew's Hospital Journal that the female students had added 'little to the hospital except decoration' and that one should not 'race a horse that is being used for breeding'. Many of the female students thought such attitudes were common and felt excluded.[86] It was only with rebuilding and an extension of the

[79] St Bartholomew's Hospital Journal, February 1948, p. 10.
[80] SU minutes, 26 June 1946, 26 February 1947, SU 11/2.
[81] AGM, 15 January 1964, MS 27/3.
[82] 'Hell Hath no Fury', St Bartholomew's Hospital Journal, April 1945, p. 38.
[83] Cambridge Graduates Club, SC 1/2–3.
[84] St Bartholomew's Hospital Journal, February 1950, p. 24.
[85] College committee, 2 February 1955, MS 29/4.
[86] St Bartholomew's Hospital Journal, July 1964, p. 294–6.

casualty department in 1964 that the Abernethian Room ceased to be all male.[87] The SU remained reluctant to improve conditions for female students. When the 'ladies' facilities' at Chislehurst were investigated in 1973, it was found that the women had been using two small rooms 'which are very cold', with one shower, 'three wash basins only providing cold water', and two toilets. It took nearly six months for the SU to be persuaded that improvements needed to be made.[88] Only in the late 1970s did female students at St Bartholomew's secure greater influence in the SU.

Despite moves by St Bartholomew's to admit more women students than the quota imposed by the UGC (see Table 9.1), only 20 per cent of the students in the College were women in 1972. According to *The Times*, 'a potential women student' at the College still 'had to have better A Levels than a man to obtain a place'. Only gradually did the number of female students rise in line with the number of women seeking places in medicine.[89] A similar disparity existed in appointments. Although attempts were made to resist the appointment of the first female professor in 1970, attitudes did slowly change and the male club atmosphere that had dominated the College since the nineteenth century was slowly eroded. A symbol of this changing attitude was perhaps the election in 1989 of Lesley Rees, a former student at St Bartholomew's, as the first female dean of a London medical school. Throughout the 1980s, female staff had played an increasing part in pushing through more innovative approaches to teaching in the College, and for the *Daily Telegraph* Rees's appointment was a sign of the College's desire to modernise.[90]

Table 9.1   Number of female students graduating, 1946–58

Year	Total
1946–7	5
1947–8	38
1948–9	40
1949–50	29
1950–1	22
1951–2	25
1952–3	23
1953–4	11
1954–5	18
1955–6	16
1956–7	15
1957–8	20

Source: UGC returns, DF 6

[87] AGM, 15 January 1964, MS 27/4.
[88] SU minutes, 11 December 1973, 11 June 1974, DF 318.
[89] Shooter to Pembleton, 9 January 1974, DF; *The Times*, 7 June 1972, p. 4.
[90] *Daily Telegraph*, 23 August 1988, p. 13.

10

'To produce a complete doctor'

Rebuilding and rethinking medical education

The end of the Second World War created a new mood of social expectation seemingly embodied in the National Health Service (NHS) and the renewed expansion of universities after the stagnation of the interwar years. The Goodenough report offered a blueprint for growth and marked a rediscovery of the pre-clinical sciences. It placed renewed emphasis on postgraduate training and initiated a discussion about pre- and post-registration that was to continue throughout the 1950s and 1960s. Institutional form was given to these ideas in 1945 with the creation of the British Postgraduate Medical School, to link together the work carried out in London's specialist hospitals. Looking back, Leslie Le Quesne, professor of surgery at the Middlesex, saw the 1950s as 'golden years, with a sense of ever-expanding horizons', a mood reflected across higher education.[1] Universities were deemed a source of national pride, academics treated with a degree of deference. In medicine, consultants secured considerable financial security under the NHS, and teaching hospitals formed a group of elite institutions that acted like a 'select club of mandarins' without responsibility.[2] The UGC, which had ceased to be a passive body, pressed for modernisation and expansion. London's teaching hospitals responded with new departments and research facilities, which committed them to more expense and a rapid growth in staff.

Le Quesne's optimistic assessment concealed problems. There was little effort to define a coherent role for higher education, and the UGC adopted a narrow conception of university activities. Little incentive was offered for change and many institutions remained complacent. It was not until the 1960s that a compromise was struck between 'liberal ideals and democratic expansion' following the 1963 Robbins report, which encouraged a shift from elite to mass higher education.[3] Medical education was slow to adapt and retained its elitist nature. Although the greater stress placed on technology and science by the 1946 Barlow committee on scientific manpower and the

---

[1] Leslie Le Quesne, 'Medicine', in *The University of London and the World of Learning, 1836–1986*, ed. F. M. L. Thompson (London, 1990), p. 142.
[2] Charles Webster, *The Health Service Since the War*, Vol. 1. *Problems of Health Care. The National Health Service before 1957* (London, 1988), p. 272.
[3] R. D. Anderson, *Universities and Elites in Britain since 1800* (Cambridge, 1992), p. 63.

UGC benefited London's medical schools, war damage and the need to adapt – culturally and financially – to the NHS slowed development. An emphasis on housing in the 1950s and the 'economic gale which blew around the Korean War' curtailed spending on health and education.[4] Although the financial restrictions of the 1950s were slight compared to later cuts successive governments pressed for economies as expenditure on hospitals rose. Teaching hospitals, despite their privileged position, resented the uniformity of the NHS and complained of financial restrictions made worse by inadequate funding for higher education. Medical schools coped as best they could and tried to implement the Goodenough report with varying degrees of success. Moves were made to appoint full-time clinical professors and to break with the vocational approach that characterised training. However, departments often remained understaffed and poorly equipped. By 1963, the Porritt report was clear that 'we cannot escape the conclusion that the medical facilities of British Universities are now lagging considerably behind those of many comparable countries in respect of research facilities, accommodation and available teachers'.[5]

Although stability proved elusive, the 1960s saw renewed debate over the structure of higher and medical education. Before 1939, discussion had been dominated by the value and position of science in training; postwar interest focused on achieving an integrated curriculum within an academic framework. How integration was to be reconciled with a curriculum still dominated by an apprenticeship-style approach and often compartmentalised, and with the nature of healthcare in London, was less certain. The appointment of a Royal Commission in 1965 under the Cambridge chemist Lord Todd sought to resolve some of these issues. Although the Todd report returned to the ideas expressed by the Goodenough committee in its vision for university medical education, it held important implications for London's teaching hospitals and remained influential for the next twenty-five years.

The legacy of war and the post-war problems in healthcare and education shaped the development of medical education at St Bartholomew's. The 1950s saw a drive to rebuild and adapt as the College moved closer to the University of London. It worked with the hospital to re-establish services and create new departments. Research facilities were extended and teaching was reorganised in the light of mounting debate on the medical curriculum. However, rebuilding disturbed teaching, delayed expansion and strained resources. Ambitious schemes adopted by other teaching hospitals, particularly in the delivery of teaching, were not attempted: the aim was to return the College to its prewar level. In comparison to other London teaching hospitals, facilities at St Bartholomew's remained overstretched; the situation

---

[4] Nicholas Timmins, *The Five Giants: A Biography of the Welfare State* (London, 1996), p. 197.
[5] *Review of Medical Services in Great Britain* (London, 1963).

was complicated by the limitations of the island site at West Smithfield. Tensions remained. Lecturers who had not trained at St Bartholomew's often found it difficult to break into what they saw as a closed establishment. Nor had war brought the professorial and non-professorial units together. A similar division existed between the pre-clinical and clinical departments, emphasised by Charterhouse's geographical distance from the hospital. Although the pre-clinical departments tended to be dominated by academics, the clinical staff continued to control the College. Difficulties were created by the competing demands of the region, the Ministry of Health, the General Medical Council (GMC), the UGC and the University. Pressure to absorb teaching hospitals into regional hospital boards provoked efforts to protect the College's independence. At the same time, the need to extend clinical teaching forced a closer association with non-teaching hospitals and the Northeast Metropolitan Regional Health Authority (NEMRHA). However, the creation of teaching links was not enough to solve the problems facing the College. By 1966, there was a growing feeling that St Bartholomew's needed to be reorganised to reflect changing patient, doctor and student needs. Meanwhile the recommendations outlined by the Todd report raised questions about the future of the College.

Peacetime dislocation

The damage sustained to Charterhouse during wartime left a legacy of problems. Under the secretive and manipulative Charles Harris, dean in the immediate postwar period, returning the College to its prewar position became 'a matter of great urgency'. With more students applying, staff felt frustrated by the lack of teaching accommodation. Damaged buildings were patched up to provide room for students returning from Cambridge before rebuilding started.[6] Labour disputes created additional delays and with little money for repairs teaching accommodation was at first often barely habitable.[7] Rooms were gradually rearranged and departments re-equipped. Other London hospitals faced similar, if not as extensive difficulties. To determine the extent to which the war had restricted teaching, the University conducted an investigation in 1950 into the state of London's teaching hospitals. It concluded that teaching faced grave problems across London. The situation at St Bartholomew's was perceived to be particularly severe.[8]

The University recognised that the College was 'undertaking the training of doctors under very difficult conditions'. Aware that the College had made strenuous attempts to meet the problems facing teaching, the University

---

[6] AGM, 21 January 1948, MS 27/2; 1945/6 annual report.
[7] 1949/50 annual report.
[8] Inspectors' report, 1950, DF 5.

noted that staff still 'endured many disappointments as a result of the makeshift conditions and the slow progress made to remedy them'. Pre-clinical lectures were held in the anatomy theatre (the only surviving lecture theatre) or in two temporary theatres 'built in the ruins of the Physiology and the Physics Blocks'. For clinical lectures, the old dissecting rooms filled the gap left by bomb damage to the hospital's lecture theatre.[9] Departments were jumbled together to make the best use of surviving facilities. Urgent improvements were needed to the pathology and pharmacology departments.[10] In the Department of Zoology, Denis Lacy remembered that when he joined the department in 1951 'all we had was half an optical microscope, an antique optical bench and a sheet of glass placed over a radiator to glaze prints'.[11]

Clinical teaching was also struggling. A shortage of beds at West Smithfield ensured that students continued to be sent to Hill End Hospital, St Albans for part of their training. Temporary measurers were introduced as the College was forced to wait until rebuilding in the hospital had started before any permanent solution could be discussed. Even though agreement had been reached in 1943 about which departments were desirable for 'a large Teaching Hospital', complaints were voiced that all the College's energies went into creating a 'sub-utopia' for the pre-clinical departments at Charterhouse. Facilities for clinical instruction were at first neglected. Huts sprang up around the hospital but could not relieve the 'acute shortage of facilities for clinical teaching'. The old lecture theatre, destroyed by bombing, was not replaced until the 1960s; many of the clinical laboratories were considered to be 'obsolete, dark and uncomfortable'.[12] Building work added an additional burden, and the rising clinical commitments entailed by the NHS demanded 'greater attention, longer time, more investigation and increased critical analysis' and took time away from teaching. It was only once the immediate problems had been dealt with that teaching accommodation received more attention.[13]

Throughout the early 1950s, the West Smithfield site rang 'to the tune of the builders' hammers' and posts went unfilled as the College struggled with rising expenditure.[14] Departments were gradually rebuilt and enlarged alongside a make-do-and-mend attitude when it came to equipment. Plans were put forward for the future but conflict arose with the Ministry of Health which tried to limit teaching hospitals to 800 beds, 200 fewer than

[9] Information furnished by the College, 1950, DF 5; *St Bartholomew's Hospital Journal*, March 1951, p. 48.

[10] Executive committee, 8 February 1950, 9 May 1951, MS 30/3.

[11] Lacy to Rotblat, 7 July 1976, DF 299.

[12] *St Bartholomew's Hospital Journal*, January 1958, p. 2.

[13] Medical development committee, 1966, DF.

[14] *St Bartholomew's Hospital Journal*, January 1951, p. 1.

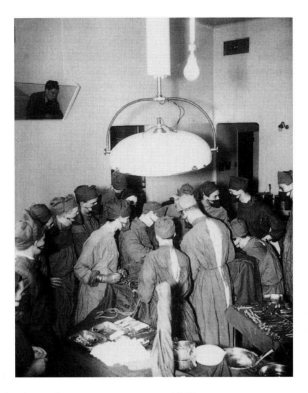

Plate 10.1 Students observing an operation, 1947

recommended in the Goodenough report. The College saw this as inadequate; part of a 'policy of despair' that did not match realities at St Bartholomew's at a time when new units were being established in cardiology, neurology, plastic surgery, thoracic surgery, genito-urinary medicine, endocrinology and diabetes.[15] A drive to specialisation, which had been resisted in the interwar period, reflected both advances in medicine and services established during wartime. Clinical services and personal interest rather than teaching now drove development. The Goodenough committee's emphasis on general practice was therefore often overlooked: physicians gradually came to think of themselves as specialists and felt less equipped to teach on subjects other than their own. Although a generalist ideology remained strong at undergraduate level, with attempts to shift specialist training to postgraduate study, this attitude looked increasingly out of place in the teaching hospital culture. At St Bartholomew's the strong faith in general medicine and surgery among older staff ensured that efforts were made to balance clinical services and specialist training, but even the 'most reactionary . . . was forced to bow

---

[15] Subcommittee, 8 September 1949, MC 1/13.

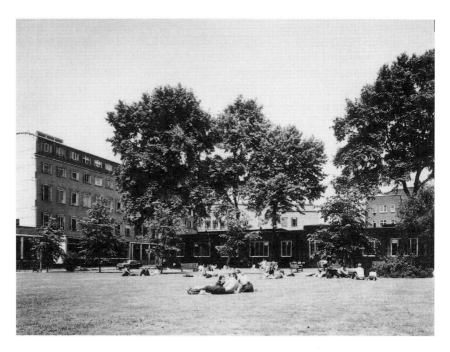

Plate 10.2 Charterhouse Square

before the storm and acknowledge the need for special departments'.[16] As the number of 'concealed' specialties grew, more teaching was conducted in the specialist departments and a concerted effort made to expand these subjects. The College believed that reorganisation was 'essential' to ensure high-quality care and 'the best training for undergraduates and ... Registrar[s]'. In 1959, it was decided that all students should be trained in 'complete' special departments (those with in- and outpatient facilities) with time allocated from the general firms.[17] Training in the 'concealed' specialties therefore tended to remain the function of the general units until more beds were found. Students were encouraged to take an interest in the emerging specialties, but were left on their own to organise the combined workload.

The expansion of clinical services throughout the 1950s was outstripped by rebuilding at Charterhouse. The Goodenough committee had stressed the importance of science to medicine and in the postwar period universities across Britain enlarged their science departments. With the College's pre-clinical buildings devastated by war, there was an opportunity for redevelopment. New accommodation for the physiology department was the

---

[16] Victor Medvei and John Thornton, *The Royal Hospital of Saint Bartholomew's, 1123–1973* (London, 1974), p. 200.
[17] Medical Council, 8 April 1959, MC 1/14.

first to be opened in 1954, followed by pharmacology in 1956 and biochemistry in 1957. The other pre-clinical departments were gradually housed in the new 'Science Block', which provided 'ample space and excellent laboratory and teaching facilities' along with a staff common-room 'to provide coffee . . . after lunch'. In 1962, the Science Block was extended to house the Wellcome Research Laboratory and a reference library. With more space and better facilities, more intercollegiate and graduate courses (especially in physics and biochemistry) were offered.[18]

The redevelopment of Charterhouse created resentment. Clinical departments were thought to take second place and interwar rivalries between pre-clinical and clinical lecturers remained strong. Although some departments were extended, such as endocrinology, bitterness had intensified by the mid-1960s when concerns were voiced about the hospital's encroachment on teaching space. Lecturers saw a 'whittl[ing] away' of facilities at a time when the College was being encouraged to increase its student intake by 15 per cent. What made matters worse was that St Bartholomew's had some of the poorest clinical teaching facilities in London, but among the largest number of students and lecturers. Staff accused the hospital's governors of failing to implement the 1946 National Health Act, which placed an explicit duty upon governors to supply the clinical facilities necessary for teaching and research.[19] The lecturers were not alone in their concerns. Conditions in London's teaching hospitals were coming to be seen as insufficient, the result of funding deficits over the preceding twenty years.[20] The governors at St Bartholomew's were compelled to increase the space available 'for the everyday life of the student' and to designate areas for teaching and research.[21] With the College seeking to redevelop the museum block, a fresh agreement over space was deemed essential. A concordat was reached recognising the College's position and future needs. Both sides acknowledged the importance of 'more elaborate' clinical facilities for teaching and care. Priority was given to the clinical departments. Blame was transferred from the governors to the Ministry of Health, which was accused of generating a climate in which 'excellent services' had become 'of . . . less political significance' than the need for economy.[22] However, the publication of the Todd report in 1968 redirected attention. Questions were raised about the future of Charterhouse, and planning shifted into creating joint clinical and academic departments with The London Hospital to solve some of the deficiencies facing the College.

---

[18] *College Calendar* (1960/1), p. 11; ibid. (1961/2), pp. 36–7.

[19] Memorandum, c.1965, HA 41.

[20] Wellcome: 'A Factual study of the Clinical Facilities Available for Medical Education in London' (1967), SA/CME/C.40.

[21] Memorandum, HA 41.

[22] Executive committee, 8 December 1965, 8 June 1966, 12 June 1968, MS 30/5.

'Expanding access': Forging teaching links

Rebuilding St Bartholomew's could not solve all the difficulties facing clinical teaching at the College. From the end of the war, there were problems about students' access to patients. With a change in the structure of population in London, the difficulty of gaining access to suitable cases for teaching became acute. The Goodenough committee had recognised that the uneven geographic distribution of London's medical schools would cause problems, and had argued for decentralisation, a policy endorsed by later investigations. Staff at St Bartholomew's were fully aware that the College 'would experience a problem in securing sufficient clinical material' for teaching. However, like other teaching hospitals in London, they were not prepared to move. Without a strategic authority to force decentralisation, there was little effective compulsion to force relocation. The only solution was for the hospital to 'extend its influence into a densely populated area'.[23] In planning the NHS, it had been hoped that teaching hospitals would be central to regional development and provide academic centres from which benefits in treatment would radiate. However, many teaching hospitals either remained aloof or tried to absorb regional beds to circumvent inadequate facilities for clinical teaching. In London, access to beds for teaching was a pressing issue and every medical school was forced to develop contacts with local non-teaching hospitals. Officials remained sceptical, worried that either teaching or care would suffer.[24] This did not stop the London teaching hospitals, and the idea that closer collaboration should be encouraged between teaching hospitals and regional boards gained ground. By the 1960s, this had become accepted policy in the NHS. Teaching hospitals were actively encouraged to establish regional services where the need to develop links had previously been driven by teaching.

The College had worked with the London County Council before 1939 to secure access to clinical services, but initially it was the wartime connections with Hill End that made it easier to send students to other hospitals. However, while Hill End had been tolerated during wartime, lecturers became frustrated by its 'primitive conditions' and 'geographical inaccessibility'. Hill End's position made consultation difficult and threatened the quality of teaching. As the number of beds was reduced at Hill End, its value declined.[25] New arrangements were therefore made, shaped by convenience and circumstances. After attempts to develop teaching at Hackney Hospital and Bethnal Green Hospital faltered, teaching links were established with the North Middlesex and Metropolitan hospitals. The latter was also used for clinical appointments and revision courses, because it was felt that the hospital offered

---

[23] Planning committee, 25 October 1948, HA 7/22.
[24] Christopher Ham, *Policy-Making in the National Health Service: A Case Study of the Leeds Regional Hospital Board* (London, 1981), p. 143; *BMJ* ii (1954), p. 516.
[25] Black to Carus Wilson, 29 April 1949, MC 5/14/5.

'considerable scope for expanding access to patients other than those at St Bartholomew's'.[26] Even with these links, other hospitals had to be used for instruction in obstetrics, psychiatry and plastic surgery.

By 1955, student concerns about teaching at the Metropolitan and North Middlesex began to attract attention. Efforts to increase the size of individual firms highlighted deteriorating conditions at the Metropolitan. Complaints were voiced that the clinical instruction offered was 'unsatisfactory' and confined to outpatients. In response, it was decided to stop sending students to the Metropolitan for surgery and in 1957 all teaching at the hospital was withdrawn. This added to pressure on already overworked firms at St Bartholomew's.

Despite problems and conflicts between the Board of Studies in medicine and in surgery – which had different views on the suitability of regional hospitals – it was felt that teaching in regional hospitals should be 'developed rather than abandoned'.[27] Students felt the experience of being sent to regional hospitals was of 'considerable value'. By working in other hospitals, students were able to see a wider variety of patients not normally admitted to teaching hospitals, and to work 'in a hospital that is not geared for teaching and to take on a degree of responsibility' than at St Bartholomew's.[28] One student remembered that he 'learnt more in a week working with the Houseman' in a regional hospital 'than I did in a month at the Hospital'.[29]

The University remained unhappy with the situation: it felt that 'the dispersal of teaching throughout so many regional hospitals' was undesirable.[30] Although the College was reluctant to concede these developments, the need to send students to other hospitals became a permanent feature; one the University was forced to accept. By the 1960s, the need to foster contacts between teaching and regional hospitals had become an accepted part of medical education. At St Bartholomew's links were motivated by necessity. The hospital had the second lowest level of outpatient admissions and inpatient beds in London but the largest clinical student entry. Because of this, the College was forced to use a greater number of regional hospitals for teaching than any other London medical school.[31] Further contacts with St Leonard's, Bethnal Green and Hackney were suggested by NEMRHB in 1963 to improve access to beds. NEMRHB was interested in postgraduate teaching and saw the presence of undergraduates in its hospitals as having 'a very stimulating effect'.[32] The scope for further cooperation had been recognised

[26] College committee, 2 March 1949, 6 July 1949, MS 29/3; 1945/6 annual report.
[27] College committee, 2 March 1955, 6 November 1957, 11 December 1957, MS 29/4.
[28] St Bartholomew's Hospital Journal, May 1962, p. 95.
[29] Ibid., December 1967, p. 444.
[30] Medical development committee, DF; Inspectors' report, DF 5.
[31] 'A Factual Study of the Clinical Facilities'.
[32] Wellcome: 'Proposed Evidence to Royal Commission on Medical Education', SA/CME/B.148 WE/24.

the year before and in 1964 a London-wide meeting was organised to talk about these issues. Subsequent deliberations expressed the necessity for teaching hospitals to play a larger role in meeting the capital's medical needs. The Ministry of Health pressed for the creation of regional joint consultative committees. The aim was to break down the fragmentation of services in London as part of a vogue for planning and efforts to initiate a hospital building programme. However, tension existed between these aims and the campaign for further economy. Greater emphasis was placed on district general hospitals, but at a metropolitan level the independence of London's teaching hospitals seemed threatened given the effort to extend regional services.[33]

An interest in closer cooperation and planning created an environment in which St Bartholomew's and NEMRHB started to discuss their relationship. To ease difficulties, and to promote a regional service, the need to 'ear-mark' regional hospitals 'for the concentrated attention of St Bartholomew's' was accepted through designation.[34] University College Hospital had moved towards such a system in 1961 and adopted a district responsibility in the same year, the first teaching hospital in London to do so. Designation and regional commitment became the accepted policies of the University and were favoured by the UGC and metropolitan regions. Both the hospital and College welcomed the idea and the governors agreed to supply district services for the City and Borough of Finsbury.[35]

The lecturers' support for greater cooperation was driven by necessity. The College's relationship with the hospital had become strained over the use of clinical space, which was considered to be 'quite inadequate' to cope with the increased student intake pressed for by the University. Although the hospital was willing to provide more beds in certain departments, the College saw the 'only remedy' to 'fulfil its teaching commitments . . . maintain its position and have the same clinical chances as the other Metropolitan Schools' was to make 'wider use of the facilities in the Region, where there is much first-rate clinical material'.[36] In the overstretched paediatrics department, Alfred Franklin was enthusiastic, prompting negotiations with Queen Elizabeth Hospital (QEH) in Hackney to meet the shortfall of beds for teaching. However, while QEH offered excellent facilities for paediatric teaching, the diagnostic services which students encountered in regional hospitals were often poor. The NHS had inherited many under-equipped hospitals and a

[33] Board of Governors, 10 September 1964, 9 September 1965, HA 1/35.

[34] Finance and general purposes committee, 20 June 1964, HA 6/4/2; 'Hospital Services in the NE Metropolitan Region', July 1965, HA 7/1/10.

[35] Geoffrey Rivett, *The Development of the London Hospital System, 1823–1982* (London, 1986), p. 299.

[36] Subcommittee on closer integration with NERB, 1963, HA 26/4/2; Meeting, 8 April 1964, HA 26/4/2; College committee, 4 March 1964, MS 29/5.

legacy of war damage. Resource starvation before 1939 and limited capital investment in the 1950s saw a large number of former local authority hospitals 'weighted down with anachronisms', and failing to adapt with 'sufficient alacrity to the needs of modern medicine'. In London, the northeast region had the lowest revenue and capital allocation: it was not until 1960 that capital allocation rose in real terms above its prewar level. Away from the teaching hospitals, conditions and services were often poor.[37]

If Enoch Powell's 1962 *Hospital Plan for England and Wales* saw an end to the 'make-do-and-mend' policy and was meant to remedy outmoded facilities improvement was slow. To raise standards, lecturers pressed for designation to gain control over provision. Designation had become the favoured solution of the teaching hospital community as a way of securing a well-balanced flow of patients for clinical instruction. At St Bartholomew's certain minimum criteria were stipulated so that the newly designated hospitals would be large enough to 'provide an adequate number of beds for those Departments which could not be adequately accommodated' at West Smithfield. To prevent a loss of identity and to ensure high standards, it was envisaged that consultants from St Bartholomew's would be 'scattered' throughout the designated hospitals.[38] As an interim measure, arrangements were made through the Central Group Hospital management committee for students to have access to seventy beds at St Leonard's, although the supporting services were initially so poor that the College was unable to send students there.[39] Negotiations with QEH proved less successful and the College turned its interest to Hackney.[40]

The appointment of Kenneth Robinson in 1964 as Labour's Minister of Health brought difficulties over designation. Robinson, the son of a general practitioner and a protégé of Bevan, had an open mind on the problems facing London's hospitals but was committed to the revised *Hospital Plan* and the need to cut patients' length of stay.[41] It was thought essential for teaching hospitals to extend their catchment areas as part of Robinson's attempts to promote 'maximum co-operation between the different branches of the Service'.[42] Robinson clung to a policy of coordination and envisaged that most hospital services would be met by teaching hospitals. To this end, plans were pushed for regional consultative committees, and Robinson imposed a

[37] Charles Webster, *The Health Service Since the War*, Vol. 2. *Government and Health Care: The British National Health Service 1958–1979* (London, 1996), pp. 216–20, 261, 292.

[38] Medical Council, 6 February 1963, 1 May 1963, 4 September 1963, MC 1/16.

[39] Executive and finance committee, 17 June 1965, HA 7/1/10.

[40] Medical advisory committee, 12 February 1965, DF.

[41] *The Hospital Building Programme: A Revision of the Hospital Plan for England and Wales* (London, 1966).

[42] Cited in Charles Webster, *The National Health Service: A Political History* (Oxford, 1998), p. 87.

selective moratorium on designation as he grappled with an examination of the administrative structure of the NHS. He feared that the 'independent and largely uncoordinated Boards of Governors' running London's teaching hospitals would use designation to serve their own interests and considered that this would be incompatible with efforts to promote greater unity.[43] As an interim measure, it was decided that designation would be accepted only if it was in line with regional policy.

In the face of Robinson's decision, the governors at St Bartholomew's dragged their feet, forcing new plans to be drawn up. Discussions with the Ministry of Health as part of talks on London hospital services saw Hackney, the Eastern and St Leonard's 'associated' with the College even though other medical schools had been designated hospitals.[44] It was a move dictated more by geography than by policy, and it engendered frustration. Despite encouragement from the Ministry, association was considered to be a temporary measure, especially after early attempts to make association work proved ineffective given the unwillingness of the UGC to spend money on associated hospitals. The University's desire to increase student numbers complicated the situation. By 1968, the acceptance of association over designation was believed by Michael Perrin, the treasurer at St Bartholomew's, to be a 'tactical mistake' after relations between St Bartholomew's and the associated hospitals had failed to work properly. Although the College was at pains to reassure the Ministry that it would embrace association, it continued to believe that designation 'was the best way to overcome the difficulties and provide . . . the greatest contribution to medical education'.[45] Interest now focused on Hackney.

A 'moving' curriculum

In the postwar period, contemporaries felt that medicine was undergoing a period of rapid advance and worried that training was either too narrow, too overburdened, or had failed to adapt. Although the *BMJ* recognised that 'periodic reshaping of the curriculum [was] inevitable', wartime discussions and the Goodenough report had resulted in pressure on the GMC to rethink its guidelines.[46] Existing teaching was criticised as stereotyped and shaped by qualifying examinations. Similar complaints had been voiced since the 1890s, but in the postwar period new concerns emerged. A temporary balance had been struck between science and the bedside, but the demands imposed by the NHS and the need to offer training more suited to general

---

[43] Board of Governors, 9 September 1965, Appendix b, HA 26/4/3.
[44] Medical Council, 7 February 1968, MC 1/17; *BMJ* ii (1967), p. 324.
[45] Executive and finance committee, 23 February 1968, HA 7/1/11.
[46] *BMJ* ii (1947), p. 374.

practice required a different approach. In addition, specialisation and medical advances had added a growing number of subjects to a curriculum that could not 'be materially lengthened' because of financial constraints.[47] When the GMC published its 1947 guidelines, medical education was caught between the need to produce good general practitioners and to provide the foundations for a medical career. Throughout the 1950s, questions continued to be raised about the purpose of medical education; about the type of doctors it was preparing. Reformers influenced by social medicine stressed the importance of 'an integrated and synoptic view' that took account of the 'whole' patient. Two strands existed: on the one hand a desire to make medical schools into mini universities; on the other to integrate teaching hospitals into the university system. The achievement of these goals was problematic: London's teaching hospitals were slow to adapt. They responded fitfully to the shift from vocational training to a general medical education suited to further training. Change was often opportunistic, with decisions to alter predominantly discipline-oriented courses frequently made at a departmental level. The result was a 'continual creaking and groaning over the over-all educational framework as local shifts and subsidences occurred with it'.[48]

The tenure of debate intensified in the 1960s. Ideas were borrowed from new methods being applied to other university disciplines, pointing to cross-fertilisation. Medicine absorbed a language of educational reform, stimulated by such works as *The Idea of a University*, which challenged traditional approaches to university teaching.[49] As doctors began to accept the notion that an undergraduate education could 'no longer [hope] to produce a complete doctor', the concept of a basic medical education as preparation for vocational training gained ground.[50] A pre-registration training component had been introduced by the 1950 Medical Act, but enthusiasm for basic medical education grew from an awareness that five years was insufficient to equip practitioners with a body of knowledge that was expanding rapidly. Encouraged by growing interest in social medicine, doctors saw a greater need for training in a non-hospital environment and general practice to equip students with an understanding of common illnesses. However, the survival of an apprenticeship mentality and hostility to an academic approach continued to curtail reform. While the Goodenough report and debates in the 1950s and 1960s had encouraged changes in how teaching in medical schools was organised, the Todd Commission still returned to ideals expressed over twenty years earlier.

---

[47] Harris to Molloy, 22 May 1947, DF 181.

[48] D. C. Sinclair, *Medical Students and Medical Science* (London, 1955), p. 130.

[49] *The Idea of a University* (London, 1963).

[50] *BMJ* iv (1967), p. 736; Wellcome: 'Survey of British medical students in 1966', SA/CME/C.31.

Efforts were made at St Bartholomew's to remodel teaching in the 1950s and 1960s. The appointment of new lecturers and professors, several of whom had not trained at St Bartholomew's, made the task easier and brought new blood to the College. In the physiology department, Kenneth Franklin set about reorganising teaching; John Blacklock in pathology undertook the same task. A spirit of reconstruction and a desire to implement the recommendations of the Goodenough report saw decisions pushed through, often with little consultation. Short courses were added that attempted to take account of emerging specialisms.[51] In general medicine, efforts were made to promote an understanding of the 'whole' patient. Research and follow-up clinics were offered in cardiology, endocrinology, diabetes and neurology to extend teaching. This created resentment. The Students' Union (SU) complained that the College had failed 'to give adequate and timely explanation or information of the various changes in the arrangements of firms and teaching appointments'.[52] Discipline was strict and students felt compelled to 'cram' in subjects. They complained that 'if the syllabus cannot be covered in the regulation number of hours allocated, then it should be curtailed'.[53] No satisfactory solution was found.

The main concern was to promote a more integrated curriculum. Here a continuing faith in a holistic approach was strongest and merged with the stress placed in social medicine on the importance of the whole patient. Although boundaries remained between subjects, staff from across the hospital were encouraged to attend ward rounds and post-mortems, and an attempt was made to promote greater continuity between the pre-clinical and clinical years. To further integration, a three-month introductory clinical course was started at Hill End. It helped bridge the gap between the pre-clinical and clinical course and avoided the concentration on too much systematic instruction characteristic of teaching at other schools.[54] Classes were given in 'methods in clinical examination', and students were encouraged to spend as much time in the wards and outpatient departments as possible when they were not in lectures.[55] Dissatisfaction quickly set in. Students argued that they began the course too soon after the second MB, and complained of the 'unusually heavy programme of lectures' that left little time for lunch.[56]

At the clinical level, Blacklock in the pathology department pressed for pathology to be integrated into medicine and surgery. Blacklock had come to St Bartholomew's from the Glasgow Royal Infirmary where he had built up teaching: in the College he attempted to apply the same ideas. Despite a

---

[51] Notice of lectures, DF 12.
[52] SU minutes, 26 September 1945, SU 11/2.
[53] Molloy to Harris, 21 May 1947, DF 181.
[54] Information furnished by the College, DF 5.
[55] Board of Studies in medicine, 18 December 1947, MS 103.
[56] Information furnished by the College, DF 5.

decision in 1946 to correlate lectures in 'Medicine, Surgery and Pathology, as far as this is feasible', his proposals were resisted until 1951 when a revised scheme was adopted.[57] The amount of pathology in the medical and surgical course was increased. Stress was placed on the desirability of students undertaking 'examinations which they might reasonably be expected to perform after qualification . . . and of seeing some more complex tests which they might be expected to ask for and interpret'.[58]

Social medicine provided an additional force in shaping the organisation of teaching. Although social medicine had been 'pushed . . . off the agenda and into the backwater from which it has never emerged' by the bitter debates that preceded the NHS, emphasis was placed on the importance of public health, epidemiology and medical sociology in an integrated curriculum.[59] At St Bartholomew's lecturers were asked to stress the principles of social medicine and the role of the ancillary social services. In most firms, this was achieved at an informal level.[60] A more ambitious scheme was organised in paediatrics. Child health had been identified by the Goodenough committee and the GMC as an area of concern. Teaching was improved at St Bartholomew's and 'practical instruction . . . in the proper use of the social services available for children' introduced. The course (the first of its kind in London) reflected efforts by Denis Ellison Nash to build up paediatric surgery in the hospital. As part of a new course on child health organised through University House in Bethnal Green, it required students to read sociology and undertake fieldwork as they learned about the social, medical and geographical structure of Bethnal Green. Students were introduced to family life in the community and offered practical demonstrations of local health services. Many considered the course a waste of time, or a poor substitute for experience gained by working with a general practitioner. In an attempt to meet these criticisms, a limited number of optional lectures on general practice were introduced in 1953.[61]

Postwar innovations in the structure of teaching were not enough to stem mounting debate on the medical curriculum. By the mid-1950s, the existing system of training had produced a 'congested' and unbalanced curriculum. The decision by the GMC in 1957 to revise the stringent regulations it had put forward ten years earlier and adopt a 'simpler and more elastic' curriculum designed to 'instruct less and educate more' focused debate. The hope was that the revised curriculum would remove the strait-jacket of the

[57] Board of Studies in medicine, 29 May 1946, MS 103.

[58] Board of Studies in pathology, 10 May 1951, 24 October 1951, MS 106/2.

[59] Nigel Oswald, 'Training Doctors for the National Health Service: Social Medicine, Medical Education and the GMC, 1936–48', in *Social Medicine and Medical Sociology in the Twentieth Century*, ed. Dorothy Porter (Amsterdam, 1997), p. 77.

[60] College committee, 1 October 1947, 5 November 1947, MS 29/2.

[61] *St Bartholomew's Hospital Journal*, January 1948, pp. 190–1.

pre-clinical/clinical split and promote an integrated course.[62] Encouraged, medical schools responded in a variety of ways. Experimental approaches to teaching were introduced as discussions on the curriculum focused on the difficulties of removing 'outworn' subjects and promoting integration.[63]

The emergence of new ideas spurred discussion at St Bartholomew's. Despite conservatism and an apparent reluctance by lecturers to become involved in national debates, there was an urgent need in the College for a 'comprehensive Teaching Curriculum' integrated with clinical work. In the face of mounting clinical commitments, many of the lecturers remained dissatisfied with how clinical teaching was organised. Students protested about the 'myriad of facts . . . drummed into [their] heads or forced down [their] throats'. They also complained that as they were expected to spend time away from West Smithfield during their first clinical year they frequently missed lectures and did not find suggestions that they should be more flexible helpful.[64] Radical restructuring was rejected in favour of a curriculum committee. Although the committee continued to think in evolutionary terms, it marked an effort to produce a more managed approach that took account of the less didactic teaching methods being implemented in a number of provincial medical schools.[65] The need for greater integration and a restructuring of examinations were at the centre of these changes.

Throughout the 1950s and 1960s, faith was placed in the promise of a new curriculum as the need for reform mounted. Concern was sharpened by the high failure rate in the first MB.[66] Other medical schools had also begun to rethink their examination system, but how this was to be achieved at St Bartholomew's and new subjects included proved problematic. In his 1961 annual report, Ellison Nash as dean reflected that 'to include in the clinical course an adequate amount of the ever growing fund of medical knowledge . . . is a problem incapable of an adequate solution'.[67] Individual courses were modified and teaching was extended to take account of new subjects, but this was not enough. Pressure to increase student intake by 15 per cent in 1966 made the need for a new clinical curriculum urgent. The year before the GMC had issued a further set of guidelines, and suggestions at St Bartholomew's that

---

[62] GMC, *Recommendations as to the Medical Curriculum* (London, 1957).

[63] See P. O. Williams and Mary J. Rowe, ed., *Undergraduate Medical Curricula Changes in Britain* (London, 1963).

[64] Board of Studies in medicine, 10 July 1952, MS 103; *St Bartholomew's Hospital Journal*, July 1957, p. 199.

[65] At Birmingham, plans were made to implement a horizontal integration of pre-clinical teaching whereby related subjects were taught together; at Aberdeen horizontal and vertical integration were tried so that students returned to pre-clinical subjects during their clinical years: S. Zuckerman and H. P. Gilding, ed., *Proceedings of the First World Conference on Medical Education* (London, 1954), p. 243.

[66] College committee, 7 February 1962, 1 October 1958, 1 July 1959, MS 29/4.

[67] 1960/1 annual report.

the College should adopt a single clinical entry after a six-term first MB added to demands for a new clinical course. As national debate on the structure of medical education intensified, the abolition of firms was canvassed in the College and proposals were made for students to be given greater responsibility for patient care. Small group teaching was called for against a background of dissatisfaction with existing arrangements, many of which were by now over fifty years old. Staff in the specialist departments hoped that a revised curriculum would combat the existing 'unbalanced apprenticeship'. Only in a few departments was it felt that the teaching worked well: most complained of inadequate facilities and lack of room.[68]

A revision of the curriculum was precipitated by a decision by the University of London to introduce a six-term second MB. The appointment of the Todd Commission and the introduction of new curriculum guidelines by the GMC encouraged the Faculty of Medicine to investigate the MB. Part of an effort to give constituent colleges in the University greater control over teaching, the faculty's appointment of an *ad hoc* subcommittee embraced the GMC's commitment to greater flexibility and academic medicine. It recognised that doctors must acquire 'knowledge and scientific understanding of human structure, function and behaviour in health and disease together with sound clinical method and an appreciation of the ethical and legal responsibilities of a medical practitioner'. With the MB seen as unsuitable for meeting these aims, and responsible for a 'potent cause of wastage', a degree of devolution was recommended. Examinations were split between the University and individual schools, with greater emphasis on summative examinations and regular course tests. The suggestions matched moves across the University. The faculty felt that the devolved course should be split between the traditional pre-clinical period and 'clinical studies and related science'. However, it repeated the now familiar assertion that a rigid distinction between the two should be avoided and pressed for integration. Although the faculty argued for greater attention to statistical methods, genetics, community health, medical ethics and pharmacology, its recommendation outlined a change in language rather than in substance.[69] The publication of the Todd report in 1968 saw these recommendations modified, initiating a period of further debate.

At St Bartholomew's modifications to the curriculum recognised the faculty's guidelines. However, with the impending report of the Todd Commission there was no radical departure from the existing structure of teaching. A six-term pre-clinical course had been introduced two years before to give students an opportunity 'for assimilating the material in the present course'.[70] This had placed an additional strain on the clinical years. In

[68] Medical development committee, 1966, DF.
[69] ULL: Faculty of Medicine, 'Outline Suggestions for Revised Regulations for the MB, BS degree', 10 March 1967.
[70] Board of Pre-clinical Studies, 16 October 1963, 3 June 1965, DF 201.

modifying teaching, the College welcomed the University's support for flexibility. After years of debate, it was finally decided that students should spend more time in the special departments.[71] The role of non-teaching hospitals in clinical training was accepted, so that students could escape from 'the artificial atmosphere of a teaching hospital'. At a practical level, further contact with regional hospitals was considered to be essential to meet increased student numbers. Calls for further integration saw an attempt to integrate medicine and surgery with some elements of pathology and psychiatry. In practice, this meant that pathology was taught at the same time as students attended the outpatient departments. Efforts were also made to introduce more group teaching and include examinations in the clinical course.[72]

It was hard for the College to break from didactic fact-laden teaching and an apprenticeship model that lacked a clearly defined philosophy. Complaints were made about compulsory attendance and the absence of effective contact between staff, students and patients. In many ways, the new curriculum was premature, with the publication of the Todd report in the following year forcing further change.

Modelling a research culture

As the College grappled with changes to the curriculum, attempts were also made to develop a research culture and infrastructure. In the list of priorities presented to the Guillebaud committee in 1956, research was seen as the third main function of a teaching hospital.[73] A dramatic increase in research funding from government and charitable bodies in the postwar period produced in medicine 'an explosion of new knowledge of physiological and pathological processes, and a proliferation of new laboratory-based diagnostic and therapeutic techniques'.[74] Although concerns were voiced that too few scientific researchers had a knowledge of clinical medicine, this did not stop teaching hospitals expanding their research facilities. At King's College Hospital, for example, a suite of research rooms was opened in 1954; and The London extended its laboratory accommodation in the mid-1950s.

St Bartholomew's was not so well placed. The two professorial units and the Dunn Laboratory did provide an academic environment for research, but accommodation in the College for research was limited. Support from the

---

[71] St Bartholomew's Hospital Journal, October 1967, pp. 371–2.

[72] Ibid., December 1966, pp. 456–7.

[73] Report of the Committee of Enquiry into the Cost of the National Health Service (London, 1956).

[74] Roger Cooter and Steve Sturdy, 'Science, Scientific Management, and the Transformation of Medicine in Britain, c. 1870–1950', History of Science xxxvi (1998), p. 445.

MRC had dwindled and remained concentrated in the war-damaged pre-clinical departments. It did not help that most of the research in the College remained outside the general trends in medical research. To overcome these problems, an attempt was made to build up a research culture. In doing so, the College had the support of the governors. This contrasted with the make-do-and-mend attitude apparent in other areas of the hospital. However, pressure for research raised questions about the role of the hospital and College and led to an awareness that without additional space St Bartholomew's ran 'the grave risk of becoming technically backward'.[75]

The formation of the research committee in 1948 marked the first move to create a more formal research culture at St Bartholomew's. Before 1939 cancer had provided the focus, but with the Goodenough report, and the importance attached to teaching hospitals as research centres in the NHS, the research committee had a wider remit. Taking advantage of the monies made available under the NHS Act, the Research Committee aimed to use funds from the hospital and College to promote and coordinate research, distribute apparatus, administer research funds and offer advice.[76] Guided by Arthur Wormall, professor of biochemistry, Joseph Rotblat in the physics department and Harris, a 'Research Endowment Fund' was established. It was anticipated that the fund would create a nucleus of funding, but it was not until 1951 that enough money was raised for grants to be awarded.[77] Preference was given to large or long-term projects. With comparatively few MRC grants – and most of those received by the biochemistry, physics and physiology departments – internal funding was vital in promoting the style of clinical research that had dominated before the war.[78] Money was found to employ a growing number of research assistants, many of whom were women. Although this reflected the low status that clinicians assigned to full-time researchers, it did see an increase in research staff. With Wormall playing a central role in the committee, his department benefited most, especially as clinical research came to favour a biochemical approach.[79]

Moves by the Ministry of Health and MRC to promote clinical research, and the role of research was assigned in the NHS, created tensions that were reflected at St Bartholomew's. Although both the College and hospital were committed to clinical research, for the governors research was subservient to clinical care, important in so much as 'advances may be made in the diagnosis and treatment of disease'.[80] The College had a different

[75] Meeting with representatives of the Ministry of Health, 1 June 1962, HA 26/4/1.

[76] Wormall to Harris, 8 October 1948, DF 189.

[77] Research committee, 24 February 1949, 19 March 1951, 1 May 1951, DF 189.

[78] Christopher Booth, 'Clinical Research', in *Historical Perspectives on the Role of the Medical Research Council: Essays in the History of the Medical Research Council*, ed. Joan Austoker and Linda Bryder (Oxford, 1989), pp. 232–3.

[79] Research committee, 24 February 1949, 28 April 1949, DF 189.

[80] Medical Council, 3 March 1954, MC 1/14; College committee, 6 October 1954, MS 29/4.

agenda: research staff were appointed only if they took 'part in the teaching or enhance[d] the reputation of the College'. An overlap was observed between teaching and research, a feature that became more pronounced as research-led departments were established. The strain that existed between these two conceptions of research led to periodic breakdowns in the management of research. A balance was struck in 1952 when it was decided that money from the governors would be used to support research of direct relevance to treatment.[81] By 1959, in the interest of promoting joint ventures, the research committee was reformulated as the joint research committee. By 1964 the committee was spending £99,000 annually and by 1969 £153,000, a rise that matched the rapid expansion of biomedical science in the 1960s.[82] The existence of internal funding removed the need to apply for outside support, creating a situation that would later prove damaging to the College.

Although the hospital was generally cautious about the research it supported, the governors retained their prewar commitment to cancer research. Heightened concern about cancer, particularly lung cancer and the link with smoking, encouraged further studies. Grants for research into this field were awarded by the MRC but it was the Imperial Cancer Research Fund (ICRF) under the chairmanship of Eric Scowen, reader of medicine in the College, that remained the principal source of funding.[83] When the ICRF failed to furnish support, the hospital was often willing to do so. Both emphasised the need to extend radiotherapy and cancer services. The favourable position of cancer research created jealousies, which were exacerbated by personal tensions surrounding the appointment of Rotblat in 1950.

Rotblat was a dynamic figure from a research background, having come to the College from Liverpool University where he had been director of nuclear physics. However, his public opposition to the Manhattan Project (on which he had worked at Los Alamos) earned him a reputation as a left-winger that jarred with the conservatism of St Bartholomew's.[84] That Rotblat was Polish, not a clinician, and had recently converted to medical physics out of a sense of horror of nuclear weapons, increased unease. With his appointment pressed for by the University, he was not initially popular and was frequently the butt of jibes in the research committee. However, under Rotblat the pioneering work on deep X-ray therapy developed at St Bartholomew's before 1939 was extended.

Although the College remained a prestigious centre for medical physics, research had declined during the war. To regain the lead, and to promote

---

[81] Research committee, 23 June 1952, DF 189.

[82] Ibid., 23 January 1968, 27 September 1966, DF 189.

[83] PRO: Kennaway to MRC, FD 1/1991.

[84] Rotbalt won the Nobel Prize for peace in 1955 for his anti-nuclear campaigning.

research, it was felt that a linear accelerator would not only offer better treatment but also a vehicle for further investigations. Rotblat approached the governors for funding, aware that the College would resist spending such a large amount during a period of rebuilding. Although some of the governors had doubts, support was promised.[85] External funding from the King's Fund eased the burden, but difficulties in securing a licence from the Ministry of Health, which was felt to be opposed to the idea 'of the Hospital having the apparatus', delayed development. It was not until 1955 that the linear accelerator was finally found a temporary home in Charterhouse.[86]

Two years after the linear accelerator was installed the machine was already in need of improvement, having failed to work properly. Tensions emerged over its use. The governors wanted to extend clinical research in radiotherapy and when the cancer committee suggested that the hospital's physics department should merge with the College's physics department under Rotblat, the treasure of the hospital, Sir George Aylwen, resisted.[87] The governors were also keen to use the accelerator for treatment. They encountered resistance from lecturers, who were more interested in research. Combined with problems of where to site the accelerator, it was not until 1961 that the 15 MeV machine was finally brought into clinical use.[88]

Under the cancer department committee, the linear accelerator was used for research into radiation physics, nuclear physics and the new field of radiobiology. Before 1939, Ronald Canti and Frank Hopwood had started work on the effects of radiation on cells. An early interest in radiobiology was an extension of this and Rotblat's interest in why radiation had an affect on cancer. Immediately after the war, the MRC had become interested in the 'biological aspects of atomic physics' and, with the MRC keen to encourage research, a number of departments began work on radiobiology.[89] St Bartholomew's was one of these organisations. Initially, studies looked at 'the primary effects of radiation and the method of their transmission from cell to cell'. Other projects investigated the effects of radiation on metabolism and the immune system. Links were developed with Wormall in biochemistry. He was interested in using radioactive isotopes as tracers (to determine immunity), and as diagnostic and therapeutic aids, particularly in thyroid disorders. A close association was also built up with the physiology department. Here Kenneth Franklin worked closely with Rotblat on the long-term effects of radiation on ageing. When funding was halved in 1954, research was given a clinical dimension and an application was made to the

[85] Executive committee, 20 July 1950, HA 7/1/2; Medical Council, 24 June 1953, MC 1/13.
[86] Board of Governors, 14 May 1953, HA 1/33.
[87] Executive and finance committee, 2 June 1955, HA 7/1/4.
[88] Executive committee, 12 April 1961, 10 May 1961, MS 30/4.
[89] PRO: MRC annual report, 1948–50, FD 2/28.

British Empire Cancer Campaign to cover the salary of Patricia Lindop who had worked with Franklin on the physiology of ageing.[90] Lindop wanted to use radioactive isotopes in her research, and to further this had started to collaborate with Rotblat. Proposals were put forward for the creation of a medical radiobiology department, and in 1960 the College secured a chair to which Lindop was appointed, despite opposition. Work in radiobiology expanded rapidly under Lindop, and classes in radiobiology were included in the curriculum.[91] Under Rotblat and Lindop, the College's work in radiobiology quickly acquired a national reputation.

Although work with the linear accelerator and interest in cancer formed a central component of the College's research culture, other areas were developed. Using funds from the hospital and College, major research projects on metabolism and isotopes, cardiovascular diseases and urology were supported. Money was found to encourage long-term research, for example, funding Reginald Shooter's investigation into infection, which helped promote more efficient sterilisation techniques.[92] However, the need for economy and restrictions on space in the late 1950s delayed work. Consequently, the College became more interested in attracting outside grants. Money from the Nuffield Foundation facilitated work on the physiology of ageing, and funding from the Wellcome Trust allowed the College to buy an electron microscope. Grants were also secured from drug companies to develop individual projects or to support research fellowships.[93] In 1962, a decision was made to attract external funding in a bid to discourage the public from thinking that 'there were considerable Hospital Endowment Funds available for research purposes'.[94]

By the 1960s, each department was actively trying to develop a research culture and build up its number of postgraduate students (see Table 10.1). Before 1939, the College had offered few formal courses beyond the Diploma in Public Health and a Diploma in Radiology. Limited and ineffectual teaching had been offered to general practitioners, and the College had provided opportunities for doctors to use the wards to gain additional experience for the FRCS. The College had cast itself primarily as an undergraduate institution, but with growing interest in post-registration training and in the value of science and research after 1945, a number of postgraduate courses were started, reflecting moves at other hospitals. B.Sc. courses were established in the 1950s (principally in physiology and anatomy). Initially, numbers on B.Sc. courses remained low, and attempts by Rotblat to encourage non-medical students to come to St Bartholomew's

90 Medical Council, 3 March 1954, MC 1/14.
91 College committee, 3 May 1961, MS 29/4.
92 Executive and finance committee, 4 April 1957, HA 7/1/5.
93 Executive committee, 11 September 1957, 10 June 1959, MS 30/4.
94 Medical council, 4 April 1962, MC 1/15.

Table 10.1   Postgraduate entry, 1957–67

Year	FRCS	MD	Ph.D./M.phil.	Clinical Practice	M.Sc.	Diploma
1957	28	–	4	1	1	8
1958	48	–	5	–	9	8
1959	50	–	5	7	11	18
1960	42	1	2	3	10	13
1961	45	1	6	2	7	10
1962	48	–	4	7	9	18
1963	45	–	13	3	8	12
1964	47	–	10	2	11	9
1965	50	–	16	3	11	6
1966	46	–	13	10	12	2
1967	42	1	–	–	1	12

Source: Postgraduate register, DF 148

were resisted for fear of diluting the College. More success, especially in physiology under Franklin, was achieved in promoting the B.Sc. for medical students.[95] By the 1960s, as the number using the College for postgraduate research had increased, the idea that non-medical and postgraduate students could contribute to the research culture had gained ground. In response to questions about the future of the College in 1966, a large proportion of staff commented that postgraduate teaching should be promoted. For some, this was necessary to prevent the College from becoming an educational 'factory'.[96]

Despite most postgraduates continuing to use St Bartholomew's to prepare for the FRCS, or to sit the diploma (particularly in medical electronics and radiation physics), a growing number of M.Phil. and Ph.D. students did begin to use the College. More students were also gaining research experience by studying for an M.Sc. Postgraduate teaching was undertaken mainly at Charterhouse, where efforts were made to develop a research framework. Although it was felt that 'there is ample accommodation . . . for research work' in the wards, new facilities were added and in 1964 a research library was opened.[97]

However, space remained problematic. Departments were confined to buildings opened in 1909, ensuring that research 'suffered badly'. In response to complaints from the UGC about the national shortage of research accommodation, plans were put forward in the College to enlarge the Dunn

[95] Franklin to Harris, 19 June 1951, DF 14.
[96] Board of Studies in intermediate subjects, 26 April 1956, MS 102; Medical development committee, 1966, DF.
[97] *College Calendar* (1964/5), p. 42.

Laboratories and ambitious schemes were suggested for a research institute.[98] It was realised that research was 'essential' if St Bartholomew's was not to 'fall behind in the race'.[99] Although more room was found, space remained limited by the need to solve overcrowding in the pathology department. Pressure was also created by the Royal College of Obstetricians and Gynaecologists, whose efforts to increase hospital births saw the hospital considering a new obstetric block. The solution was seen in a major investment programme and the development of special research departments. Perrin's appointment as treasurer of the hospital and president of the College in 1960 acted as a catalyst. Perrin had a background in industry: he had been chairman of the Wellcome Foundation and of the Postgraduate Institute of Cardiology as well as research adviser to ICI. He had also been deputy controller of Atomic Energy at the Ministry of Supply in the late 1940s, and had worked for the Department of Scientific and Industrial Research. Influenced by Rotblat, whom he knew through his work on atomic energy, he was interested in developing research in the College. As part of a rethinking of the hospital's financial policy, Perrin was able to push through proposals in 1963 in the face of opposition that permitted money from the Special Trustees for ward improvements to be used to make 'a substantial contribution to research work'.[100]

Interest had been shown in the need for research departments in the 1950s, particularly in connection to virology. Under Perrin, the idea was given a new lease of life. Perrin was assisted by a desire to strengthen research and by an influx of new staff, many of whom had not been trained at St Bartholomew's. Eric Crook in the biochemistry department brought a more dynamic approach from University College. Coupled with a UGC re-equipment grant and support from Scowen, Crook expanded the department and appointed a number of young lecturers all interested in research. In pathology, Walter Spector brought with him a basic philosophy that research was vital to the viability of his department. Research-active staff from other institutions were encouraged to come to St Bartholomew's. Plans to redevelop the West Smithfield site gave a framework in which efforts to extend research facilities and create new departments were made.[101] Special research departments were formed linked to the work in the wards and to research in the pre-clinical departments. Anthony (Tony) Dawson led one of the first of these departments. Having trained at Charing Cross and spent time at Harvard, he was part of a wave of appointments to bring new blood into the College. He quickly built up a research group in clinical gastroenterology in the biochemistry department. The success of clinical

---

[98] Draft memorandum, c.1966, HA 41; Development subcommittee, October 1964, HA 26/4/2; Executive and finance committee, 1 June 1961, HA 7/1/7.
[99] Medical Council, 7 March 1962, MC 1/15.
[100] Board of Governors, 10 March 1960, HA 1/33.
[101] Executive and finance committee, 17 November 1955, HA 7/1/5.

gastroenterology encouraged the formation of further special research departments in pathology and clinical pharmacology.[102]

Despite plans for extending research, a survey of departments in 1966 revealed that with the hospital taking on a greater clinical and regional commitment, 'research has suffered universally'. Lack of space was seen as the 'bottle-neck' of research in most medical schools, but with the College already worried about clinical facilities, and having just reached an agreement with the hospital over space, it was 'strongly against any further encroachment on teaching space'.[103] By 1969, the College recognised that a large clinical medical school with sufficient laboratory space on one site was no longer feasible. It was believed that the only way forward was to use buildings in Little Britain and Bartholomew Close to create 'viable nuclei for research activity in a number of specialities'.[104]

Students and apathy

A return to peace saw an immediate rise in student admissions. However, this trend did not continue. To balance war-damaged facilities with clinical teaching, a decision was made to reduce the clinical entry to one hundred.[105] To limit numbers, 'work and behaviour' of the first- and second-year students were carefully assessed, and a new committee was established to look at those students 'not guilty of serious idleness or other grave offence' but who produced unsatisfactory work. This was a return to a system of discipline established in the 1870s after the relative freedom of the war years. Those considered unsuitable, who showed signs of 'bad work' or who failed examinations were asked to leave. With a small number of students sent down, and with a high demand for places, it was not immediately possible to achieve the target clinical entry.[106]

Applications to medicine rose with demobilisation. The lure of professional status offered by medicine and the security of tenure promised by the NHS also served to inflate the numbers applying. Although applications rose, the College had to fit national and metropolitan targets. Before 1939 medical schools had been free to admit as many students as they wanted; with the outbreak of war admissions were regulated. This practice continued under the NHS, and national recruitment targets were set to meet the predicted

---

[102] *Dr Anthony Dawson: 21 Years at Bart's* (London, 1986); Nash to Carus Wilson, 21 July 1959, 19 January 1960, DF.

[103] Ronald Christie, *Medical Education and the State* (London, 1969), p. 9; Executive committee, 11 November 1964, MS 30/5.

[104] 'Organisation of Laboratory Facilities', January 1969, HA 26/3/2.

[105] 1946/7 annual report.

[106] Delayed qualification committee, May 1951, DF 202.

needs of the service. To control the supply of doctors, which was felt to be exceeding population growth, the 1957 Willink report proposed restrictions on student numbers. The report ran contrary to profession opinion. The College was forced to match undergraduate admissions to national and metropolitan targets. This had a stultifying effect.[107] Concerns about the emigration of doctors and a reliance on overseas practitioners in the 1960s encouraged the UGC to press for a departure from the figures adopted in the Willink report. It wanted medical schools to increase admissions, despite the problems this would create for teaching. The College was more sanguine than other schools about the UGC's efforts to bolster the pre-clinical intake 'without further capital expenditure'. Although dissenting voices were heard at St Bartholomew's, the College agreed to admit an additional fifty students and to enlarge the existing teaching accommodation.[108]

How these students were selected was attacked as 'dangerously amateur', a criticism that was levelled at every London teaching hospital.[109] Until the creation of University Central Council on Admissions in 1964, students could apply to any number of schools and accept or reject offers as they saw fit. The system was cumbersome, greatly increasing the work of individual schools. The College's reputation and links with the medical community encouraged a large number of applicants, matching a general trend towards rising applications. All applicants were expected to be of university standard with a broad general education and proof of versatility. In 1949, over 1000 students were interviewed and the problem of selecting the right candidates was considered to be a 'formidable task'. In 1950 the number had risen to 2100, making the 'work of the selection boards . . . as harrowing as it [is] exhausting'.[110] Numbers had dipped by 1962, but St Bartholomew's continued to receive more applicants than any other medical school in England.[111] Tensions existed between an interest in admitting students with a humanities background and the need for students to be versed in the 'language of science'. Mid-Victorian conceptions of the need for a liberal education remained. Complaints from the pre-clinical departments in 1953 that many students were 'inadequately prepared in the basic sciences' produced a tightening of the admission criteria. How much science was required by students, and how much training in science should be provided, remained problematic, pointing to an unease that had been present since the mid-nineteenth century.[112]

Fluctuations in admissions levels, and postwar changes in healthcare and

---

[107] *Report of the Committee to Consider the Future Numbers of Medical Practitioners and the Appropriate Intake of Medical Students* (London, 1957), pp. 31–3.
[108] College committee, 2 November 1966, 7 December 1966, MS 29/5.
[109] *THES*, 2 February 1962.
[110] Inspectors' report, DF 5; College committee, 1 February 1950, MS 29/3.
[111] BMA, *Recruitment to the Medical Profession* (London, 1962), p. 113.
[112] College committee, 4 February 1959, 6 May 1953, MS 29/3.

higher education, did not materially change the type of students admitted (See table 10.2). A survey in 1957 revealed that 34 per cent of those who had obtained a place at the College had come from a medical family, most having decided on a career in medicine by the age of 16. This was higher than the national average of 17 per cent. A public school background remained strong. The College also had a higher level of recruitment from professional families when compared to other London schools, second only to St Thomas's in London and to Oxbridge nationally. Although these generalisations were not rigid, Michael Besser remembered that when he entered the College in the 1950s, 'a medical background, a public school education and activities such as rugby and rowing were pre-requisites' for being accepted.[113] Students could be found throughout the College who resembled the parodies of Richard Gordon's *Doctor in the House*, especially as Gordon had trained at St Bartholomew's. It was only in the 1970s under Shooter that efforts were made to broaden the College's recruitment and achieve a greater parity between the sexes. Students claimed that they had chosen medicine for humanitarian reasons. An interest in science took second place, reflecting student attitudes elsewhere. About a quarter had chosen St Bartholomew's because they had a family connection with the hospital, 16 per cent coming to the College because of its reputation.[114] The College continued to favour students preparing for the University of London examinations; no student was accepted 'who is aiming solely at a Diploma qualification'.[115] The University of London now dominated the structure of teaching at the College, representing the culmination of a trend that stretched back to the 1840s.

Prewar traditions remained. Students at St Bartholomew's retained their hostility to the University of London Union, preferring to foster links with the London medical school community. Freshers' teas were resumed and societies that had been inactive during the war were revived. A new College Hall was opened at Charterhouse in 1952, providing student accommodation for the first time since 1923. A broadminded attitude, which remained in place until the mid-1960s, allowed students living in College Hall more freedom.

Despite attempts to return the SU and student services to a prewar footing, lecturers and activists in the SU worried about how a sense of community might be achieved. Although a corporate life had been fostered by sport and the activities of the SU, this appeared fragile after the war. Staff were aware that the separation of the pre-clinical from the clinical school presented 'some problems in building up the corporate life of the students'.[116] The continuation of wartime trends of sending students to different institutions

---

[113] *BLC*, autumn 1999, p. 3.
[114] Wellcome: 'Medical Students in Britain in 1961'.
[115] *St Bartholomew's Hospital Journal*, June 1960, pp. 169–70.
[116] Information furnished by the College, DF 5.

Table 10.2 Occupation background of students (fathers' occupation), 1961

	Medical	Other professional	Managerial/ official	Proprietor/ shop manager	Semi- professional	Clerical/ sales	Skilled manual	Semi- and un-skilled	No response
St Bartholomew's	27.9	20.1	19.2	11.9	7.7	4.9	4.4	1.5	2.4
All London schools	22.8	21.2	20.5	12.0	7.7	7.5	6.3	1.4	1.3
Oxbridge	28.5	24.7	20.5	7.9	8.7	4.3	4.5	0.4	0.4

Source: Wellcome: 'Medical Students in Britain in 1961', SA/CME/C.7

further strained feelings of solidarity, which was not helped by the evaporation of early sporting successes in inter-hospital competitions. Students were accused of apathy as a link was established between sporting success and the identity of the College. By 1953 the social life of the College was believed to be at a low ebb. Since the rebuilding of College Hall, there had been only one dance while other London teaching hospitals held them regularly. The Music Society had ceased to function, and the output of the Amateur Dramatic Society was desultory, due largely to problems in finding suitable venues.[117] The College's sporting achievements, apart from the women's hockey team, were believed to be even worse. Teams were difficult to field and the 'weekend-in-the-country bug' was considered to be crippling clubs.[118] It did not help that after the war facilities were overstretched: although the gymnasium and boxing room were unaffected, the squash courts needed repair, and the tennis courts had 'not recovered from their wartime use of a balloon anchorage'. A 'general apathy' was thought to be spreading, and the SU considered withdrawing from the British Medical Students Association because of lack of interest. Less critical observers saw the problem resting with inadequate funding or the demands placed on students by a curriculum that left 'little leisure time'.[119]

By the mid-1950s, a revival in the social and sporting life of the College had begun. Under Scowen's tenure as warden, a corporate spirit was encouraged in College Hall. This coincided with a return of the recreational facilities to a more normal footing and moves by sporting societies to employ coaches and organise regular training sessions. After protracted wrangling, the College agreed to take over the funding of the sports ground at Foxbury, which had proved an 'insuperable burden' for the SU, restricting development at the expense of 'recreational purposes other than outdoor sports'. The College's decision freed funds for the SU to use on other activities.[120] The closure of the rifle range under the medical records department in 1960 by the hospital, and disparaging comments from the UGC about 'the lack of extra-curricular activities and community life at St Bartholomew's' further encouraged the SU to focus more effort on sporting and social facilities.[121] In 1960, the annual smokers, which dated back to 1893 when smoking concerts were organised by the Cambridge Club, were revived. Greater attention was paid to organising balls, with the View Day Ball becoming an annual event. Individual clubs organised social events to

---

[117] *St Bartholomew's Hospital Journal*, October 1952, p. 514.
[118] Hockey Club, 4 June 1953, SU 71.
[119] SU minutes, 15 October 1958, DF 318; College Calendar (1949/50), p. 19; *St Bartholomew's Hospital Journal*, May 1953, p. 119.
[120] Silverston to Nash, 1 November 1957, DF; SU finance committee, 10 September 1958, DF 316.
[121] SU minutes, 24 January 1961, DF 318.

appeal to members and to raise money. With the opening of the new Abernethian Room, an agreement was reached with Whitbred, and a lunchtime bar was opened, despite reservations of the lecturers.[122] This was followed by a new College Hall bar in 1966. By the mid-1960s, the SU could claim thirty separate societies. However, it continued to complain of apathy: sporting success in inter-hospital and university competitions seemed elusive.

Redrawing the 'map of learning'

The 1960s saw attitudes to education shift with growing affluence and a rise in white-collar employment. Politicians on both sides pressed for expansion and an end to elitism to provide the skills deemed necessary for growth, and to meet social and demographic pressure for more university places. Divisions between the humanities and the sciences were called into question following Charles Snow's influential *Two Cultures and the Scientific Revolution* (1959), which attacked the rigid crystallisation in higher education.[123] The ensuing debate and the UGC's efforts to expand the university sector revived the concept of the university as a place of general and medical education. Faith was placed in interdisciplinary courses and the need to break down barriers.

These ideas have been closely associated with the 1963 Robbins report. The report embraced an interdisciplinary model and justified a policy of expansion already favoured by the UGC and the public. Although Robbins failed to outline radical restructuring, it did create a platform for growth. New universities were created (such as Sussex and East Anglia) which combined the liberal arts and the sciences. More interest was expressed in the need to promote equality, and to integrate different areas of study under a variety of coherent groupings to produce graduates of wider educational experience. For London, the Robbins Commission pressed for power to be transferred from the central bureaucracy, forcing a period of critical self-examination in the University under the threat of an independent inquiry.[124]

While the findings of the Robbins Commission raised questions about the structure of university education, a series of crises in the NHS, and the growing awareness that more doctors were required, highlighted the need to rethink medical education. Attempts to move from vocational training to a basic medical education highlighted the desired relationship between medical schools and universities. With a large number of doctors emigrating, and a growing reliance on overseas practitioners, studies suggested that there was an urgent need to rethink medical schools' intake. The media concentrated on a predicted crisis in the NHS, prompting the Ministry of

---

[122] Ibid., 20 June 1961, 12 March 1962, DF 318.
[123] C. P. Snow, *Two Cultures and the Scientific Revolution* (Cambridge, 1959).
[124] Negley Harte, *The University of London, 1836–1986* (London, 1986), p. 262.

Health to press for a review of medical school admissions.[125] A formal investigation was avoided, as it was felt that the Robbins Commission would deal with the issue. However, the Commission made only passing reference to medical schools, leaving the UGC, University and GMC to grapple with the problem.

The need for a rationalisation of undergraduate and postgraduate medical schools in London was long overdue by the mid-1960s. The London teaching hospitals had 'failed to implement some of the most important changes which the Goodenough Committee considered necessary'. The structure of health-care in London and the sheer number of medical schools complicated the situation.[126] In addition, an almost pathological opposition to too much academic direction combined with a strong sense of tradition to frustrate the UGC's efforts. The UGC had been forced to compromise and to concentrate on promoting academic medicine outside London. The need for more doctors refocused concern, and the appointment of the Royal Commission on Local Government fuelled criticism of the tripartite structure of healthcare in London.[127] The UGC thought 'a complete review and re-thinking of the role and the development of the London Schools is perhaps the most vital of all tasks'.[128] It had appointed a committee in 1961 to investigate a reorganisation of postgraduate training, and argued for closer association between medical schools and hospitals. At the Ministry of Health, a comprehensive review of teaching hospitals was also considered, and when the UGC sanctioned an increase in admissions, an investigation into medical education became crucial. Cuts in quinquennial estimates for universities created anxiety that medical schools would face a financial crisis, ensuring that they would be unable to meet the expansion in student numbers the UGC wanted. The need for a review was strengthened by calls for the closure of some of the London schools, amidst concerns that they were academically isolated and failing to provide an adequate number of patients for teaching. To resolve these issues and to discuss expansion, the UGC pressed for 'a sort of Robbins Committee' to investigate the nature and cost of medical education.[129] Support was found in government. Despite opposition from the GMC, which feared that an investigation would frustrate efforts to revise the curriculum, a Royal Commission under Lord Todd was appointed in 1965. It was charged with investigating undergraduate and postgraduate training in the light of national needs and resources.[130] Little time was given for the submission of evidence.

---

[125] Webster, *The Health Service Since the War*, Vol. 2, p. 284.

[126] Wellcome: London Hospital Academic Board, 25 January 1966, SA/CME/B.129 WE/48.

[127] PRO: Medical services review committee, MH 153/345.

[128] Wellcome: 'The London Medical Schools', SA/CME/B.211.

[129] PRO: UGC medical subcommittee, 13 February 1962, 9 October 1962, 1 December 1963, UGC 8/97.

[130] Harte, *University of London*, p. 272.

After some reticence, it was decided that the hospital and College should make a joint submission. Little of what was suggested was a departure from ideas already being voiced in the medical profession and implicitly accepted the need for a university-centred training. The College guided discussions, clear that 'the expansion of knowledge and the subsequent specialisation of medical practice demands a new formulation of the aims of medical education'. Building on earlier criticisms, the curriculum was criticised as too short, a 'disorderly jumble of short, specialised and vocational appointments with a multiplicity of teachers but no recognisable education plan'. It was believed to encourage passive learning, with the final MB 'a marathon of factual testing' that dictated students' learning experiences. To solve these problems, the College outlined proposals for a three-year undergraduate degree free from the 'shackles of the Medical Act 1886' to replace the first and second MB. A degree, it was felt, would promote the type of academic approach considered necessary by the Haldane Commission and by the Goodenough committee. Plans for an integrated three-year course had already been discussed as a solution to the perceived inadequacies of the A-level syllabus for medicine, and reflected a growing consensus that more critical study and independent learning was required. The College argued that a B.Med.Sci. would encourage the flexibility being demanded and offer a symbol that recognised the need for a university-focused education. Similar support for a B.Med.Sci. was expressed by The London and the Royal College of Physicians. The B.Med.Sci. was a compromise: one that suggested a continuation of the pre-clinical clinical split while recognising the importance of greater flexibility.[131]

The College was less clear on how the sense of isolation from the 'general stream of University scientific activity' might be reduced. The College reasserted its intentions to develop pre-clinical teaching, extend links with regional hospitals and broaden postgraduate training, points that had become central to debates on medical education in the 1950s and 1960s. In asserting plans for a revised pre-clinical course, the position of Charterhouse Square was defended. Of greater importance was the need to strengthen links with the University.[132] Despite a cooling of relations in the 1950s, and dissatisfaction about how the University was administered (a view echoed in the Robbins report), the College maintained its traditional support of the University. It reiterated the importance of academic medicine. The College was defending its professorial units and autonomy at the time when the Ministry of Health was suggesting that the administration of teaching hospitals should be transferred to regional boards.[133] It believed that this

---

[131] Memorandum, HA 44/1/1; Board of Governors, 11 November 1965, HA 1/15; Executive committee, 13 April 1966, MS 30/5; College committee, 1 July 1964, MS 29/5.
[132] Evidence to the Royal Commission on Medical Education, HA 26/4/3.
[133] Draft memorandum, November 1966, HA 26/4/3.

could be prevented and closer collaboration achieved with the University through the creation of links with a multi-faculty institution. A strong case existed for this as the curriculum became less vocational. University College, and the new medical school at Nottingham, had gone some way in promoting this idea, and the need to establish links between the sciences and the humanities had been central to Robbins and UGC policy.[134]

While the submission presented by St Bartholomew's reflected debate in medicine and higher education, it did not echo attitudes at other London teaching hospitals. Medical schools agreed on the problems facing medical education, but remained divided over the solutions. Widespread support was expressed for the need for teaching hospitals to adopt a district role and for doctors to follow a scientific training within a flexible curriculum. Innovation was welcomed. However, while St Bartholomew's pressed for stronger links with the University, most schools tentatively endorsed the idea of a federal structure.[135] Attitudes to working with multi-faculty institutions ranged from sceptical to hostile. More enthusiasm was shown in the idea of a fully integrated curriculum.[136] The suggestions put forward by St Bartholomew's were considered a way of protecting the College, and of promoting further expansion. It many ways, it pre-empted the Todd report.

When the Commission delivered its report in 1968, it reaffirmed many of the principles outlined in 1944 by Goodenough. The *British Journal of Medical Education* explained that the report embodied an 'accurate reflection on existing trends' and built on debates that favoured an interdisciplinary, university-centred approach.[137] Because of this, the bulk of the report was uncontroversial, consolidating a number of changes that had evolved from 1940s onwards. Only minor alterations to the curriculum were suggested and the Commission pressed for a defined educational and career structure to remove the multiplicity of diplomas and memberships. Greater integration was called for and the need for training to equip graduates with an 'understanding of medicine as an evolving science and art, and to provide the basis for future vocational training'. It was widely accepted that it was no longer possible for a medical student to learn everything in five years, and both the GMC and the Todd Commission saw continuing education as vital.[138] The Todd Commission also argued that restrictions on student numbers imposed by the Willink report should be removed and four new university medical schools created outside London. In its support for academic medicine, it

---

[134] Evidence, HA 26/4/3.

[135] Wellcome: University of London, note by the secretary, SA/CME/B.131 WE/84.

[136] Wellcome: Evidence submitted by King's, SA/CME/B.121 WE/76; The London, SA/CME/B.129 WE/48; Guy's, SA/CME/B.96 WE/68.

[137] *British Journal of Medical Education* ii (1968).

[138] *Report of the RC on Medical Education* (London, 1968); GMC, *Recommendations as to Basic Medical Education* (London, 1967), p. 4.

reiterated the principles of the Goodenough report 'that every modern medical school worthy of that description should have academic departments, with professorial heads'. However, it recognised that teaching hospitals now had to be managed as part of a regional framework, a model adopted in Scotland. In a challenge to the traditional structure of medical education, the Todd Commission asserted the need for an educational approach to break the stranglehold of anatomy. To achieve this, the Todd Commission suggested the abolition of the first MB and the creation of a three-year pre-clinical course to strengthen the university element.[139]

Although much of the report was uncontroversial, proposals for the future of the London teaching hospitals were. The Commission wished an end to the haphazard system that had evolved. At an administrative level, it recommended that Boards of Governors be abolished and University Teaching Boards created in each region. This recognised in part that the existing system had weakened regional boards. To compensate for the loss of autonomy, universities were to have a greater say in how regions were run. The Commission went on to stress that if the London teaching hospitals wished to retain their prominent position reform was essential. In outlining the need to extend scientific training and keep abreast of scientific developments, the Commission asserted that most London schools lacked the staff to deliver the scientific training it envisaged. To overcome this, and to meet the clinical entry proposed by the UGC, a series of mergers were proposed to end the academic isolation of London's teaching hospital. The aim was to reduce the number of schools from twelve to six and to associate these with a multi-faculty institution. Since the 1910s, those concerned with medical education had found it hard to break with the ideal represented by University College Hospital and its association with University College, as it appeared to embody a style of university education that was being sought for doctors. Support for medical schools as part of multi-faculty institutions reflected this and concerns which had emerged in the 1960s about the importance of building bridges between science and the arts.[140] Links with multi-faculty institutions were also believed to promote interdisciplinary teaching.

The pairing of St Bartholomew's and The London linked in a new medical faculty as part of Queen Mary College (QMC) was just one of the six proposed mergers outlined in the report. St Bartholomew's and The London were considered comparable institutions and were the only two teaching hospitals in NEMRHB. QMC also had links with medical education. It had provided first MB classes for students from The London in 1917, and although numbers taking the course declined, it was still being offered in the 1950s. A joint lectureship in engineering physics was created after the war;

[139] *RC on Medical Education.*
[140] Ibid.

part of the lecturer's duties were in The London's radiotherapeutic department.[141] QMC was also the only University college in London's East End.

The Todd Commission felt that the policy of mergers and the inclusion of medical schools in multi-faculty colleges not only made financial sense when university funding was under pressure, but was also compatible with 'a continuation of the highest standards in medical education' that the existing haphazard system was believed to frustrate. The Commission was convinced that the proposals represented a 'logical and practicable reorganisation' that would produce a more integrated system of medical education in London.[142]

Many contemporaries believed that the Todd report marked a shift in emphasis in medical education from a primarily vocational to an essentially educational course 'so as to produce graduates equipped to cope with a professional life characterised by continual change'.[143] The London schools were among the first to criticise the report. Plans for an increase in student intake were quickly made, but how the report's proposals for the future of London's medical schools should be implemented required detailed consultation. The future was uncertain.

---

[141] Ibid., pp. 50, 84, 97.
[142] Ibid., pp. 24–5, 178–82.
[143] British Journal of Medical Education ii (1968).

Part IV

After Todd 1968–95

11

'The way forward'?

The publication of the Todd report in 1968, with its support for twinned medical schools and amalgamation with multi-faculty institutions, outlined an agenda that shaped debates on medical education into the mid-1990s. The report was essentially utopian, however. If a consensus was reached over the need for rationalisation and reform, how these were to be achieved created conflict. As issues had to be discussed at college, university and state level, planning was slow. It was only after the 1980 Flowers report, designed to solve the deadlock over amalgamation and the structure of medical education in London, that pressure on teaching hospitals to merge with multi-faculty institutions increased, encouraged by changes in the NHS and higher education. Debates over NHS reform and funding cuts forced the pace and resulted in a series of unhappy marriages between medical schools. St Bartholomew's inevitably became caught up in these debates and felt keenly pressures exerted on the NHS and university sector. The result was a blurring of the relationship between the hospital and College, and an often circular, drawn-out debate over a merger with The London Hospital in Whitechapel and Queen Mary College (QMC) – later Queen Mary and Westfield College (QMW) – in Mile End.

The history of the events surrounding the collaboration and the eventual creation of a confederation between St Bartholomew's, The London and QMC in 1986 is a complicated, often unhappy one, compounded as it was by the intervention of the University of London, University Grants Committee (UGC) and NHS. St Bartholomew's periodically felt bullied, not least by a UGC that was determined to push ahead with the ideas expressed in the Todd report. Whereas the UGC had originally worked to preserve university autonomy and minimise its intervention in how funds were allocated, it had evolved into a powerful body that expected to shape university development. Having lost control over a number of financial issues, the UGC was determined to become more 'dirigiste'.[1] However, the College was unprepared to accept the UGC's model. Conflict with the UGC, and the fluctuating debates over amalgamation, resulted in a planning blight that limited development in the College. Throughout, despite internal divisions, a united front was presented, and the need to discuss issues fully slowed decisions, engendering frustration outside St Bartholomew's. The positions of the

---

[1] Michael Shattock, *The UGC and the Management of British Universities* (Bristol, 1994), p. 20.

351

pre-clinical departments at Charterhouse Square and QMC emerged as sticking points, and relations between the institutions involved in negotiations over amalgamation became acrimonious, leading to the threat of a judicial review in 1985.

The College's position was based not so much on tradition, as from the 1970s there was an influx of staff who had not trained at St Bartholomew's, but on a view of academic medicine and the role of the College not shared by the other institutions involved. QMC and the College presented two different cultures; neither side fully understood the other. Relations with The London were better, but it was often The London that was felt to force the situation by moving closer to QMC. Perceptions of the College as a closed, traditional institution further damaged its position, especially in the University of London. Hospital and College were conflated, and the impression of the two as arrogant institutions persisted, ensuring that those outside the College were not always sympathetic. It did not help that from the 1980s most London teaching hospitals felt under threat and willing to endorse any scheme if it meant saving their own institutions.

'The end of excellence'?

To understand the debates surrounding the protracted moves to merge St Bartholomew's, The London and QMC it is important to realise the pressures on the NHS and universities in this period. Although the University of London and the UGC agreed that medical education had to be conducted in a university atmosphere, the policy had to be matched to the realities of a cash-strapped NHS.[2] Despite the popularity of the NHS, doubts about its ability to deliver had emerged in the 1950s. Until the mid-1980s successive governments focused on managerial reorganisation, regional inequalities and the anomalous position of London's teaching hospitals and healthcare in their attempt to deal with issues of cost and access to beds.

The NHS underwent its first major reorganisation in 1974. The Ministry of Health sought better lines of communication and closer links between teaching and regional hospitals. Reorganisation placed community services and hospitals under district management and planning was transferred to Area Health Authorities (AHA), with teaching hospitals losing their independent boards of governors as recommended in the Todd report. Considerable effort was devoted to filling gaps in healthcare and to provide a more equitable service.[3] However, it was acknowledged by the late 1970s that reorganisation had not been a success.

---

[2] See *The University and Health Care in London* (London, 1976).
[3] See Charles Webster, *The Health Service since the War*, Vol. 2. *Government and Health Care: The British National Health Service 1958–1979* (London, 1996).

In the reorganised NHS, teaching hospitals were actively encouraged by the General Medical Council (GMC) to experiment with the curriculum and the Department of Health and Social Security (DHSS) to make greater use of region services for teaching. In London, attempts were made to remodel services and match clinical needs to educational and research activity. Initially, with the Board of Governors gone, and responsibility for managing the hospital divided, St Bartholomew's felt lost. However, the district health authority in which the College was located quickly proved beneficial: close collaboration and academic links were established first with Hackney, then with the Homerton Hospital. High expenditure on healthcare between 1974 and 1976 encouraged optimism, but with the subsequent oil crisis and a contraction of funding dissatisfaction grew. Plans for expansion were shelved, and the creation of the Resource Allocation Working Party (RAWP) in 1976 redirected resources. The formula adopted by RAWP aimed to correct geographical inequalities by directing resources from well-endowed regions in London and the Southeast to poorer areas, mainly in the North.[4] The hope was that this would allow the rest of the country to catch up. The formula was not well received in London, where it contributed to a growing sense of despondency. Although healthcare expenditure continued to rise, the UGC and University of London were in the unfavourable position of having to fight 'to safeguard the costs of teaching hospitals'.[5] RAWP had proposed little protection for teaching hospitals other than the Service Increment for Teaching (SIFT) allowance paid for clinical facilities used in teaching. Health authorities involved in teaching required money to remain centres of excellence, but this was not always compatible with RAWP. The North East Thames Regional Health Authority (NETRHA), of which St Bartholomew's was a part, sought to safeguard teaching beds. However, with the region inheriting dilapidated hospitals in need of redevelopment, this could be achieved only by cutting money for general services. Beds for teaching remained 'a little thin', and the health authority struggled on with less money and a wider range of responsibilities.[6] A funding crisis produced by a mismatch of expenditure to demand in the 1980s led to further unplanned bed closures.

While the RAWP model strained resources and threatened teaching, the College was also affected by further changes made to the NHS in the 1980s. A new NHS management structure was introduced in 1982 following the consultation document *Patients First* (1979), which endorsed a patient-

---

[4] Julian Le Grand, David Winter and Francis Woolley, 'The National Health Service: Safe in Whose Hands?', in *The State of Welfare: The Welfare State in Britain since 1974*, ed. John Hills (Oxford, 1990), p. 89.

[5] Cost of teaching working party, 13 May 1977, DF 307.

[6] Report of the teaching hospital costs working party, 1977, DF 307.

centred and local approach that borrowed from a radical critique of institutional medicine.[7] The administrative structure was simplified: AHAs were abolished and greater responsibility was transferred to districts. The resulting reforms left the service unsettled. The University of London welcomed greater local authority participation, but was unprepared for Margaret Thatcher's Conservative government's enthusiasm for making the NHS more businesslike to cut expenditure on welfare. Consultation with hospitals quickly stopped and more managers were appointed. All these developments generated a general sense of crisis in the NHS. Underfunding deepened, beds closed and nurses went on strike. Public dissatisfaction increased as suspicions mounted that Thatcher's government sought to privatise healthcare.[8] For St Bartholomew's, underfunding and a reallocation and reduction in NHS resources represented a fundamental threat to teaching. The future seemed 'fragile'.[9]

The discussions over the structure of medical education at St Bartholomew's also occurred against a background of reform and cuts in higher education. In the decades after the Todd report, the London medical schools and the University faced a deepening financial crisis. University policy became 'tentative, even apologetic', losing the vibrancy of the Robbins era.[10] Despite an economic recovery and efforts to expand access in the 1980s, Conservative governments under Thatcher were determined to hold back public sector expenditure. Higher education joined healthcare as a prime target, an attack on two fronts for the College. If the NHS experienced financial anxiety, universities suffered the same unrelenting pressure for economy and efficiency and competition for scarce resources. Having lost control over a number of financial issues, the UGC found itself having to react to government policy. It became determined to press ahead with innovation and was prepared to make significant reductions in funding allocations and take the lead in making what it felt to be the tough decisions necessary to cope with cuts.[11] Capital spending was slashed and universities were encouraged to seek non-governmental sources of income. Early retirements and redundancies rose as universities struggled to deal with cuts while retaining academic excellence. In the University of London, moves to amalgamate medical schools were added to these policies in a bid to reduce spending, given the high cost of medical education, and to prevent further financial damage. Under the guise of encouraging competition, selectivity was imposed across the higher education

[7] DHSS, *Patients First. Consultative Paper on the Structure and Management of the National Health Service in England and Wales* (London, 1979).

[8] Nick Bosanquet, 'The Ailing State of the National Health', in *British Social Attitudes*, ed. R. Jowell, S. Witherspoon and L. Brook (Aldershot, 1988), pp. 93–108.

[9] *Barts Journal*, December 1988, p. 19.

[10] John Carswell, *Government and Universities in Britain: Programme and Performance, 1960–1980* (Cambridge, 1985), p. 156.

[11] Shattock, *UGC and the Management of British Universities*, p. 20.

sector – a move the Committee of Vice-chancellors and Principals (CVCP) saw as a 'sharing out of misery' – just at the time that universities were expected to expand access.[12] Universities found that they were being 'made accountable in new and sometimes painful ways', assessed for their research, and encouraged to find other ways to enhance their income. The CVCP defended the role which universities played. In medicine, the special relationship between universities and the NHS was stressed in an attempt to protect both.[13]

In this new financial climate, the College had to turn its attention to resource allocation and cost saving. By 1982 the University admitted that the College had become 'the cheapest and most cost-effective Medical School' in London at the expense of staffing reductions and restrictions on development.[14] Greater efforts were made to secure outside funding and attract money from the Special Trustees. Increasingly, decisions were dominated by financial concerns. Ultimately the post-Todd period had brought about circumstances that could not have been foreseen when the report was published. Twinning and amalgamation became driven by financial not academic concerns. It was in this climate that the amalgamation of St Bartholomew's, The London and QMC was discussed.

The way forward?

The publication of the Todd report in 1968 produced a flurry of activity. Although the ambition to include medical schools in a university framework and develop academic medicine had been voiced since the 1900s, no consensus existed on how this should be achieved. With several reports due on the structure of the NHS and local government, discussions were frequently confused. Fearful of having an outside solution imposed on London, the University was at pains to show that it was 'willing to carry out the recommended changes if they were given the necessary tools'.[15] Teaching hospitals were less enthusiastic. For the Teaching Hospitals Association, 'the frying pan of the present structure may not be completely suitable, but the fire of a hastily accepted new system could be less so'.[16] Most teaching hospitals were unhappy with the principle of twinning and opposed amalgamation with multi-faculty institutions. Mergers insulted traditions of independence and each proposed set of twins regarded the prospect with little enthusiasm.

---

[12] CVCP press information, 21 May 1986, DF 288.
[13] Nicholas Timmins, *The Five Giants: A Biography of the Welfare State* (London, 1996), pp. 483–5.
[14] University to College, 23 May 1982, DF 286.
[15] 1968/9 annual report.
[16] Teaching Hospital Association draft memorandum, 10 September 1968, HA 44/1/2.

At St Bartholomew's opinion on the Todd report was divided. Because the publication of a Green Paper on the NHS was expected imminently, the governors of the hospital felt they could not comment, especially as they were already embroiled with the Ministry of Health over the designation of district hospitals for teaching. When the Green Paper was published in 1968, comparisons were drawn with the Todd report and the two became conflated. Despite reservations, the governors decided it was important to 'take the lead in the bold experiment' and not fight 'an emotional rearguard action'.[17] Reactions in the College to the Todd report were less confident. Some feared that if it was implemented the College would lose its identity, others that the report's findings were misguided. It was clear that the report could not be discussed in a leisurely manner, and many wondered if the University's haste was a reaction to the threat of intervention rather than a desire for reform. Staff felt rushed into giving an opinion and the educational issues raised by the report were pushed into the background.

Attempts to promote cooperation between St Bartholomew's and The London had been made at a regional level throughout the 1950s.[18] By 1963, as part of schemes to develop closer ties between teaching hospitals and regional boards, St Bartholomew's and The London had joined the Northeast Metropolitan Regional Health Authority in forming a joint advisory committee. The government's Green Paper equally favoured greater cooperation between the two hospitals as an offshoot of the creation of new area authorities. The College welcomed 'the opportunity which such a scheme would offer for collaboration with The London ... in the organisation of medical and related care in a defined area which included their existing districts'. Cooperation was seen as a way of rationalising specialist services, which had interested both hospitals since the early 1950s. Because the 1968 Green Paper ascribed an important role to teaching hospitals, St Bartholomew's and The London believed they could play a central role in shaping regional services to suit their teaching needs.[19]

While minor disagreements emerged over the extent of cooperation between the hospital authorities at St Bartholomew's and The London, the College's attitude to QMC was more hostile. Staff resented the implications of the Todd report over amalgamation and did not see the College as a small school with inadequately staffed academic departments. In the triumvirate recommended in the Todd report, QMC was the junior partner.[20] With its

[17] Board of Governors, 9 May 1968, 19 November 1968, HA 1/35.
[18] Medical Council, 16 December 1953, MC 1/13; ibid., 3 March 1954, MC 1/14.
[19] Ibid., 4 September 1968, MC 1/17; Board of Governors, 14 April 1966, 14 July 1966, 8 June 1967, HA 1/35.
[20] For origins of QMC, see Anne J. Kershen, 'Higher Education in the London Community', in London Higher, ed. Roderick Floud and Sean Glynn (London, 1998), pp. 82–3.

origins in the desire to improve workers' and technical education in the East End in the 1880s, QMC had become a school of the University in 1915. In the 1930s, emphasis in the college shifted from a technical to a liberal education, and new buildings and departments for science and engineering as QMC grew. Expansion continued in the postwar period. In the 1960s 'scarcely a year went by without . . . [QMC] starting or finishing a large building scheme'.[21] Although the strength of the medical school at St Bartholomew's was on the clinical side, staff in the College felt that the teaching and laboratory facilities at Charterhouse were at least the equal of those at QMC, if not better. They did not view the academic record of QMC favourably and feared that the distance between Mile End and West Smithfield would create barriers. If staff recognised the need for a drastic overhaul of medical education in London, it rejected as impracticable the fusion of The London's and the College's pre-clinical schools at QMC. Instead, it was felt that either St Bartholomew's should be enlarged or, if a merger became national policy, that Charterhouse should house new departments for the applied sciences. The preferred solution reflected the ambivalence that existed between the clinical and pre-clinical departments.

Divisions between the pre-clinical lecturers (who were mainly academics) and the clinical staff were both geographic and intellectual. The clinicians retained the upper hand in how the College was managed, and often appeared to undervalue the work of their pre-clinical colleagues. They believed that the basic medical sciences at St Bartholomew's were competent but not a strength. They were therefore prepared to sacrifice some pre-clinical teaching to free Charterhouse from 'its present purely "pre-clinical" departments', so that new departments for basic science applied to medicine integrated with a number of postgraduate institutes could be developed. For this to be achieved, the clinical staff envisaged developing links with one or more multi-faculty colleges. QMC was not high on their list of choices. With QMC having no biological side comparable to other multi-faculty institutions in London, the College could afford to delay.[22]

These suggestions were put to the Todd report steering committee established by the University to implement the report. The committee called for informal discussions between St Bartholomew's, QMC and The London, but the publication of a joint statement by the UGC and the University in 1969 accelerated the pace of reform. Although problems with finance and geography were recognised, the statement argued that twinning would advance the formation of more specialist academic departments than was feasible in existing schools. It was also anticipated that amalgamation with multi-faculty institutions 'would develop co-operation between the medical,

[21] G. P. Moss and M. V. Saville, *From Palace to College: An Illustrated Account of Queen Mary College* (London, 1985), pp. 61–3, 74, 97.
[22] Executive committee, 4 September 1968, MS 30/5.

the natural and the social sciences in both teaching and research', facilitating the 'introduction of new subjects into the medical curriculum'. Twinning was to be the first step in the creation of the multi-faculty institutions envisaged by the Robbins (1963) and Todd (1968) reports to give expression to the perceived need to bridge the gap between science and the Arts. The principle of twinning was easily subsumed into the University's policy of encouraging greater cooperation between constituent colleges.[23]

The UGC and the University recognised that twinning and amalgamation would not be possible for some teaching hospitals, but decided to press ahead where it was deemed 'practicable', even if this meant separating pre-clinical and clinical departments. Plans to unite the Royal Free with University College were supported, along with suggestions to amalgamate the pre-clinical departments at St Bartholomew's and The London as part of an enlarged biological science complex at QMC. What had previously been exploratory talks between St Bartholomew's, The London and QMC now took on a new dimension. John Ellis, dean at The London, was particularly keen, having sat on the Todd Commission. The College was in agreement, aware that money for any scheme was unlikely to be forthcoming for some time. A merger became the central policy of the University and UGC, with the arrangements between St Bartholomew's, The London and QMC becoming abbreviated to 'BLQ'.

'A great flexibility of mind, great generosity of spirit': 1968–75

Two years after the Todd report, the governors of the hospital optimistically claimed that 'we are entirely happy to be associated with The London and are trying to develop this association beyond the starting point of a joint pre-clinical school by considering what further steps can be taken in the direction of rationalisation'. Encouraged by the region, which accepted the dual role which teaching hospitals played in education and treatment, St Bartholomew's and The London worked together to promote regional ties and the use of non-teaching hospitals for clinical training. Although opposition was encountered, the College and John Dickinson, professor of medicine, became actively involved in developing Hackney District Hospital to provide a teaching environment. In planning access to regional services, The London was consulted since the various twinning arrangements 'induce us willy-nilly to take account of our relationship with them'.[24] However, because the College felt that BLQ was unlikely to be implemented 'until the

---

[23] UGC and University of London joint statement, 1969, HA 44/1/1; Logan to College, 27 September 1968, DF 298.
[24] Brook to Crossman, 17 October 1969, HA 44/1/2.

end of the present decade', it was half-hearted when it came to planning with QMC.[25] An association with The London was seen to be far more realistic.

Early reassurances from the UGC that Charterhouse would be maintained enabled plans to develop the site as an 'academic complex serving the research and postgraduate needs of the twinned schools'.[26] The London, keen to extend the academic content of its teaching, welcomed collaboration. Its existing pre-clinical and clinical facilities were scattered and in danger of becoming overstretched. Many at The London predicted that collaboration would solve these problems and meet the predicted difficulties facing teaching hospitals as the curriculum grew.[27] Common ground was found over para-clinical and clinical needs and the desire to increase student entry. With neither school able to fill the gaps identified in the Todd report, several joint academic departments were proposed. Negotiations were slow. While appointments were often accepted in principle, uncertainty over funding created delays. Financial cuts, however, helped to overcome reservations. Joint departments (in virology, community health, immunology, obstetrics, reproductive physiology and rheumatology) were established in the 1970s, encouraged by Reginald (Reggie) Shooter, dean of the College, and Ellis, who held weekly lunchtime meetings. Yet links were not as extensive as initially envisaged. Funding restrictions caused by rising service costs and large pay awards ensured the shelving of plans for some joint departments. Often departments were joint only in name, the result of political manoeuvring.

Although lecturers in the College remained suspicious of The London, moves towards twinning were more advanced at these two hospitals than were those between other medical schools, which were either geographically isolated or reluctant to give up their autonomy. Both St Bartholomew's and The London recognised the advantages of twinning. The London was able to use links with the College to strengthen existing departments and develop the academic component of its teaching.[28] At St Bartholomew's, joint departments presented a solution to deficiencies in clinical teaching and research.

Planning for joint clinical services and a division of regional responsibility was one thing; plans to fulfil the educational aims of the Todd report and to merge medical schools with multi-faculty institutions were another. Although the Board of Pre-clinical Studies welcomed the idea of a flexible course structure and tentatively planned a new curriculum with The London, the College was less enthusiastic about a merger with QMC.[29] Neither was QMC always positive: in 1980 the Flowers report recognised that QMC could

[25] *St Bartholomew's Hospital Journal* (1970), p. 388.
[26] 1971/2 annual report.
[27] Development plan 1977/82, DF 298.
[28] College Council, 16 January 1974, MS 28/3.
[29] Board of Pre-clinical Studies, 22 May 1968, DF 201.

have done more 'to engender inter-faculty co-operation'.[30] Clashes occurred over the new curriculum. With the UGC determined to locate further expansion in the provinces and with uncertainties over student numbers problems were foreseen. The purchase of land in 1971 along the eastern boarder of QMC (which covered the Jewish burial ground) for the new basic medical science faculty temporarily boosted hopes about BLQ. However, when planning was halted by capital restrictions, the pre-clinical staff at St Bartholomew's voiced their dissatisfaction. In a letter to *The Times*, staff protested that the merger was a 'token gesture towards concepts that obviously are not being followed in toto'. They argued that the two schools were little more than 'expensive "guinea-pigs"'.[31] While staff at St Bartholomew's felt that to abandon BLQ would be disastrous, the future of the pre-clinical departments and Charterhouse continued to be sticking points. Staff were resolute that they would agree to BLQ only if 'the facilities at [QMC] should be equal to the current facilities at Charterhouse'. Determined to press ahead with the merger, the UGC was equally forthright. It implied that if the Todd report was not implemented none of the schools concerned would receive funding.[32]

A new framework for London: 1975–85

Uncertainty over BLQ depressed morale among the pre-clinical lecturers at St Bartholomew's, who felt isolated and complained of insufficient consultation. With the question of where to site the pre-clinical departments 'unresolved', pre-clinical staff at St Bartholomew's and The London expressed their reservations. In 1975, the Board of Pre-clinical Studies asserted that 'the proposed development at QMC was undesirable on academic grounds'. Fears were expressed that BLQ would segregate teaching when the opposite was needed.[33] Cuts in DHSS and UGC funding had strained resources and threatened teaching, forcing the College to economise. The pre-clinical departments were hardest hit, especially as a decision by the University to end the first MB in 1981 reduced teaching in some departments and merged others. The crisis was not limited to St Bartholomew's. By the 1980s teaching hospitals were generally encountering difficulties in recruiting and retaining pre-clinical staff. A wider problem existed in the University where a reduction in recurrent grants forced departments to scale down. In the College, cuts meant that some of the pre-clinical departments encountered problems

[30] *London Medical Education – A New Framework* (London, 1980), p. 62.
[31] *The Times*, 22 July 1971, p. 15.
[32] Joint policy committee, 4 November 1971, DF, 1C7.
[33] Board of Pre-clinical Studies, 11 June 1975, DF 201.

meeting their teaching commitments. Research suffered and Charterhouse began to be neglected.

The clinical departments were in a better position however. Efforts were made to extend clinical medicine and work began on an 'educational and social complex'. The new building, which opened as the Robin Brook Centre in 1980, greatly improved facilities and provided a much needed, and widely applauded, environment for clinical teaching.[34] In terms of research, the College pressed forward: several departments had developed a strong research profile, attracting substantial funding from non-government bodies. Building on trends established in the 1960s, the appointment of new staff such as John Landon, professor of chemical pathology, and Tony Dawson, attracted young researchers and contributed to the drive to extend research. The new emphasis on clinical science and the radioimmunoassay techniques – the latter pioneered by Landon – rather than surgical techniques helped shift the power-base in the College. This was encouraged by Eric Scowen, professor of medicine, Shooter, and Walter Spector, professor of pathology, to boost research. One member of staff remembered that it was an exciting period, which stimulated research across the College and brought new technology into laboratories. Although cuts created frustration and delayed development, a number of new departments with a clear research bias emerged. Although oncology remained important, endocrinology, immunology and gastroenterology attracted increased attention. New professorships followed after a dearth of appointments in the 1960s. The new departments quickly established themselves as leading centres, often with national or international reputations, that attracted researchers and staff to the College.

If staff in the College continued to support the 'sharing of facilities' with The London, uncertainty about funding for BLQ made them hesitant. While the UGC strove to maintain the credibility of the 'BLQ concept', it was overstretched. The redevelopment of the former colleges of advanced technology as universities strained funding, and the UGC was forced to admit in 1978 that money for BLQ would not be available 'for some time'.[35] After plans to site institutes for gastroenterology and ophthalmology at Charterhouse fell through, and discussions over a Medical Research Council statistics unit collapsed, the College became more reticent about BLQ as pressure from The London and QMC mounted. QMC wanted to establish new departments, and with the AHA scaling down redevelopment at Whitechapel, The London was keen to press on with BLQ and develop Mile End Hospital for clinical teaching. The pre-clinical departments were overcrowded at The London, confined to buildings opened in 1887. For The London, BLQ offered the expansion and modernisation it desired. The College thought differently. Although the fruitful cooperation established

---

[34] College committee, 2 November 1977, MS 29/6.
[35] College Council, 18 October 1978, MS 28/3.

with The London was acknowledged, the College remained unwilling to commit itself on the pre-clinical side. It pressed for an urgent re-evaluation of BLQ that same year.[36]

In the University of London, the question of how to implement the Todd report and rationalise teaching hospitals remained unresolved. After all, the Todd report had been published at a time when money was available to fuel expansion. St Bartholomew's and The London were virtually alone in moving towards twinning: most teaching hospitals feared closure or a drastic reduction in facilities. Increasing specialisation and a reduction in the population of inner London were markedly affecting acute bed needs, creating further problems for how the NHS should be organised. By the mid-1970s,

> so many pressures, including those of resource constraint and the predictable interest of the Royal Commission on the NHS in London's problems, were combining to lay fresh emphasis on the need for making the best use of all available resources, and for resolving as quickly as practicable those problems which stood in the way of that objective.[37]

To overcome this, and to encourage supra-regional services, the DHSS pressed for links between regional health authorities, AHAs and universities. In London, discussions focused on rationalisation and on how to make teaching hospitals function as district general hospitals. London-wide plans for rationalisation were put forward to match population to services. NETRHA argued that teaching practices would have to change to rely 'to a greater extent on outpatient services or possibly on community hospital practice' in response to these changes in the NHS.[38] Attempts to match educational and service needs at a metropolitan level either faltered or alarmed London's teaching hospitals. Staff at St Bartholomew's were clear that advances in medicine made rationalisation a 'sterile exercise' of demography and geography. However, they recognised the need for reform. In a climate where the 'financial support for medical teaching in London has been so reduced', they feared that 'a stage may be reached when the total revenue available will be insufficient to enable . . . existing Medical and Dental Schools and Postgraduate Institutes to continue as viable units'.[39] The UGC was equally concerned. It wanted educational needs to play a significant role in shaping the NHS, arguing that distribution 'optimised strictly from the service point of view . . . resulted in reduced, less effective and more expensive medical education'.[40]

---

[36] Board of Pre-clinical Studies, 3 October 1978, DF 201; Joint policy committee, 1 December 1978, DF 314.
[37] London coordinating committee, 27 January 1976, DF 309.
[38] 'Rationalisation of Services' (1975), DF 277.
[39] College committee, 6 December 1978, 7 February 1979, MS 29/6.
[40] 'Rationalisation of services' (1975), DF 277.

To solve these problems, and provide a forum for discussion, the London Health Planning Consortium was established in 1977 to reconcile teaching needs with NHS services. This had been recommended in 1968 by the Todd report, but had been initially rejected by the University, fearing a threat to academic independence.[41] By 1977, a downturn in the financial fortunes of the University made the policy less objectionable. The University encouraged the Conference of Metropolitan Deans to appoint a working party to consider rationalisation just as the Labour government established a Royal Commission to look into the 'complex and cumbersome administration' of the NHS. The Conference of Metropolitan Deans recognised that major savings were needed and that these could be achieved only through a review of medical education and the closure of a medical school. However, they were unable to produce firm recommendations, or make the difficult decision as to which school should close. With the Royal Commission recommending a simplified administrative structure for the NHS, a stance supported by the 1979 White Paper *Patients First*, proposals were needed for medical education that took account of financial restrictions and demographic trends. In response, the vice-chancellor of the University, Noel Annan, appointed a working party under Brian Flowers, rector of Imperial College London, to investigate the redeployment of medical teaching resources.[42]

Annan was strongly influenced by the Noble prize-winner Alan Hodgkin, professor of biophysics at Cambridge, who was convinced that the London pre-clinical departments were too small to produce significant research. Annan was therefore convinced that the existing pre-clinical departments were a waste of resources. He charged the working party with considering 'what redevelopment . . . should be adopted even if this were to lead to the phasing out or radical reconstruction of one or more Schools or Institutes'. In the decade following the Todd report, the problems it had sought to solve had been complicated by financial cuts. Although the University was clear that 'the whole question is at bottom purely a financial one', Flowers resisted pressure. He was determined to evaluate the problems facing medical education without any preconceptions, and was willing to make the difficult decisions deemed necessary. However, while the working party realised that some of the recommendations contained in the Todd report were no longer appropriate, interest was shown in BLQ and plans to merge University College Hospital with the Royal Free.[43]

The reports of the Flowers working party and London Health Planning Consortium appeared simultaneously. The Consortium argued that 'the level of clinical facilities needed to support medical schools concentrated in the

[41] ULL: Minutes of Senate, July 1969, ST.

[42] Geoffrey Rivett, *The Development of the London Hospital System, 1823–1982* (London, 1986), p. 333.

[43] *London Medical Education*, p. 65; College Council, 17 January 1979, MS 28/3.

centre' could no longer be justified. It called for a reduction in the number of acute beds in central London, and for regional hospitals to be linked with medical schools to provide core teaching, reviving ideas voiced by the Ministry of Health in the 1960s.[44] The working party under Flowers adopted a different approach. Determined only to make recommendations that were practicable in the existing financial climate, the report pointed to the over-capacity of pre-clinical provision. Like the Consortium, it adopted a language of rationalisation, arguing that fewer, larger schools made academic and financial sense. Although Flowers was clear that his report was not a regurgitation of the Todd report, the two embraced a similar ethos and aimed to promote 'integrated and inter-disciplinary teaching'. For Flowers, the starting point was that clinical medicine could not be divorced from science. This attitude was combined with an awareness that cuts would deepen, thus making rationalisation vital.[45]

The Flowers working party outlined several schemes that it hoped would protect medical education in London. It supported the need for a moratorium on appointments and the possibility of redundancies to save money. Major savings were also to be made through the twinning of medical schools. For Flowers, 'the time has come to look closely at the London medical and dental scene and not . . . be influenced to any extreme degree by . . . traditions and understandably fierce loyalties'.[46] Collaboration was widely accepted as the best way of reducing the impact of cuts at a time when the CVCP feared that Thatcher's Conservative government was determined to run down the British university system.[47] In response to these concerns, Flowers proposed that thirty-four separate academic institutions be grouped into six schools. Aware that not every teaching hospital could or should be associated with a multi-faculty institution, Flowers was impressed by the progress made towards twinning at St Bartholomew's and The London. However, although the College had informed the working party that severing links between pre-clinical departments and hospitals in favour of amalgamation with a multi-faculty institution was educationally redundant, the weight of opinion was against the College. Flowers saw a merger of St Bartholomew's and The London (and including Newham, Homerton, QEH, and the Institutes of Urology and Ophthalmology) to form the 'Harvey School of Medicine and Dentistry' as feasible and desirable. Concern about the use of acute beds and distribution of specialist services had been growing, and a number of health authorities had begun to rationalise smaller hospitals. NETRHA had followed this trend and built large district general hospitals at Newham and Homerton. St Bartholomew's had already transferred the teaching links

---

[44] *Towards a Balance* (London, 1980).
[45] *London Medical Education.*
[46] Ibid.
[47] Press information from CVCP, 12 March 1981, DF 300.

forged with Hackney to the Homerton, and had worked with The London to create links with Newham.[48] The Flowers report recognised this in its proposals for the 'Harvey School' and recommended that pre-clinical departments should be gradually concentrated at Charterhouse until resources became available to move them to QMC.[49]

Caught up in the uncertainty surrounding the future shape of the NHS and the furore caused by the London Health Planning Consortium, the Flowers report created unease and attracted more opposition than the Todd report. Medical schools dug in and defended their independence. Although there was widespread agreement on the need for a new educational framework for medicine, a difference of perception separated the London teaching hospitals from the University and Flowers. Reactions ranged from anger to resignation. In a poor financial climate, and with little possibility of obtaining finance for new buildings, it was hard to convince medical schools of the merits of the report.

While students from the Westminster medical school paraded with coffins outside Senate when it received the report, staff in the College discussed it in depth. During the debate, it was felt that the report would arouse so much opposition that no medical school would implement it. Some staff therefore suggested that it should be rejected; others counselled that this might be dangerous. Compromises were made and broad agreement expressed in the need for rationalisation. However, staff, already unsympathetic to Annan and the University over the end of the first MB, noted their 'grave misgivings' that an evolutionary model had been ignored. They expressed anxiety that the size of the projected schools would threaten personal contact and efficiency. Staff outlined their support for shared government with The London on a federal basis – a move that would allow all constituent parts to retain their identity – but were clear this should not be rushed. They saw the future of the College in 'sharing facilities in the East End of London and beyond into Essex, with the London Hospital Medical College'.[50] Having felt under 'considerable external pressure' to merge with QMC, staff welcomed Flowers' support for Charterhouse. They were heartened 'because it seemed to us that this was the first occasion that a University Committee had looked at Charterhouse and its facilities'.[51]

The London was equally concerned about Flowers, but by now it was already developing strong links with QMC. The London's pre-clinical accommodation remained inadequate and it was under pressure from the health authority, which wanted the space to develop clinical services. The

[48] Newham health district DMT, 21 May 1974, DF 254; Healthcare in Newham, September 1975, DF 254.
[49] London Medical Education.
[50] College committee, 21 April 1980, MS 29/6; College Council, 20 May 1980, MS 28/3.
[51] AGM, 21 January 1981, MS 27/5.

building of a new Alexandra Wing highlighted problems, and to provide further teaching accommodation the Whitechapel site had been in a permanent state of 'demolition and reconstruction' throughout the 1970s.[52] The pre-clinical departments were moved to what was hoped would be a temporary home in an austere building. BLQ represented a solution to these problems. Aware that medical education would continue to become more expensive, and that a concentration of resources was necessary, staff at The London accepted the need for the pre-clinical departments to be based in multi-faculty institutions. They argued that QMC was ideal for this and plans to move pre-clinical departments to Charterhouse were rejected. Although staff in The London were clear that 'it would be tragic if the opportunity now existing to develop the Harvey School on the basis of the BLQ project were to be lost', they also welcomed an evolutionary approach.[53]

Although attitudes to Flowers were different in the two schools, informal ties were strengthened. A number of joint research seminars were organised in the biochemistry department, where staff were more sympathetic to a merger, and in 1981 a committee was established to help promote liaison. Original plans to create a biomedical faculty, with the possibility of incorporating the pre-clinical departments, were rejected in favour of a faculty of basic medical sciences. This was more palatable to St Bartholomew's.[54] However, little time was available for discussion and QMC wanted to move quickly.

Those planning medical education in London appeared not to be 'sufficiently aware of each others plans'.[55] If the University's joint medical advisory committee supported a joint school along the lines proposed by St Bartholomew's, Senate did not. Faced with cuts and bitter opposition, it failed to accept the Flowers report. This created confusion in the University, where morale was already low because of cutbacks, and hampered attempts to devise a new regional structure in the NHS. As David Richtie, dean of The London, noted, 'for a couple of days it looked as though all was lost'.[56] Senate accepted the need to look into the situation. A new committee was appointed under Leslie Le Quesne, deputy vice-chancellor and dean of the medical faculty, to investigate the financial costs of undergraduate medical education and the possible closure of one of the London schools. The study made a number of assumptions – some of which were open to challenge – and confirmed the high cost of running newly built medical schools. A decision by the UGC in December 1981 to reduce the University's grant over the next three years pushed discussions forward. The seriousness of the cuts made

[52] John Ellis, *LHMC 1785–1985* (London, 1986), p. 147.
[53] Comments by the London hospital medical school on the Flowers report, 1980, DF.
[54] Board of Pre-clinical Studies, 22 October 1980, 25 February 1981, DF 200.
[55] Ibid., 26 May 1982, DF 200.
[56] Cited in Ellis, *LHMC*, p. 181.

reorganisation vital 'if the University is to remain solvent'.[57] Avoiding contentious plans to close one of the London schools, the working party followed Flowers and accepted a reduced staff to student ratio and the policy of merging medical schools as the most cost-effective solutions. Although Annan later admitted that St Bartholomew's had a strong case for locating the joint pre-clinical school at Charterhouse, BLQ was supported as 'academically the most desirable way forward', given the University's commitment to developing education in the East End.[58]

The UGC's unwillingness to find additional funding to maintain BLQ led to rumours that The London or QMC might close to save money. Staff at The London rallied to BLQ and Senate agreed to look more closely at the pre-clinical arrangements in East London. Another working party was appointed under L. C. B. Gower, vice-chancellor of the University of Southampton, to investigate the financial implications of siting the pre-clinical departments at QMC or Charterhouse.[59] Senate also insisted that joint planning with QMC should be abandoned in favour of a consortium between St Bartholomew's and The London. For The London this was a step backwards. Collaboration between the two schools broke down, encouraged by a change in deans who had very different styles and were under more pressure from the University.

The conclusions of the 1981 Gower working party had disturbing implications for the College. From the start, it was aware that BLQ was the University's preferred solution. Economy and collaboration between teaching hospitals were constructed as the only feasible way the University could meet a reduction in its recurrent grant.[60] It was also felt that BLQ had clear benefits, providing an 'invaluable asset to QMC, enhancing both its academic reputation and its relations with the public and local community', an important concern for the University. The Gower working party recognised that if the Todd report was accepted, 'it also has to be accepted' that implementation 'demands something more than collaboration, however cordial, between medical schools with different traditions and methods, miles apart from each other and divorced from any multifaculty institution'. In supporting BLQ, it admitted that development at QMC or Charterhouse would result in the same savings. However, with the UGC only prepared to fund pre-clinical departments at QMC, the working party concluded that BLQ represented a '"better buy" for the University'. The working party also argued that a move to QMC would offer a better start for the venture; one that would prevent staff at The London from feeling that they were being taken over by St Bartholomew's. In response, the University asked the UGC to implement BLQ.[61]

[57] Committee on academic organisation, January 1982, DF 257.

[58] AGM, 20 January 1982, MS 27/5.

[59] Ibid.

[60] Committee on academic organisation, DF 257.

[61] Working party on the siting of the joint pre-clinical school, June 1981, DF.

Attitudes at the three institutions remained mixed. QMC and The London were eager to press ahead. The London had 'denounced' Charterhouse as a viable location for a pre-clinical school. Throughout the 1970s, it had seen BLQ as 'the light at the end of the tunnel'.[62] Although relations between the College and The London had deteriorated, the College continued to accept a merger with The London. It claimed it was keeping an open mind, but felt that neither The London nor QMC were interested in a partnership and wanted to asset strip St Bartholomew's. The College remained committed to retaining Charterhouse and in the light of the Gower working party pushed for a study of the options.

Claims by the UGC that money was now no longer available for BLQ forced the University to rethink. The UGC suggested that the pre-clinical schools could move into existing space at QMC, but on investigation the College found the accommodation 'a far cry from the originally proposed purpose-built BLQ building' and inferior to existing facilities at Charterhouse. With the University and UGC anxious for a solution, The London and QMC informed the University of their support for the transfer of The London's pre-clinical departments to QMC, and explained that St Bartholomew's now opposed BLQ. The College repudiated the claims and repeated recommendations made by Flowers that if money was not available for BLQ, then a joint school should be established at Charterhouse. The University agreed, having lost faith in QMC and the UGC for trying to push through a 'botched-up job'.[63]

By now staff were frustrated that fourteen years of planning 'had achieved nothing, and has wasted much money and energy'. If anything, the College had come under increased pressure. The end of the first MB had seen further reductions in staffing and soured relations with the University. Individual departments were threatened, and the pre-clinical departments were 'beginning to rattle around in Charterhouse'. Clinical staff were accused either of being powerless or too indifferent. Disillusionment was widespread, especially with low staffing levels and rumours of further cuts.

As the College was forced to make economies, and with further restrictions being predicted, it was decided that if funding for BLQ was not forthcoming by 1983, the College would no longer be bound to support the scheme. Such a move had been discussed in 1979, but by 1981 staff in the College were adamant that they should do so. Concern had grown in the intervening period about facilities at QMC and the suitability and future of Mile End Hospital (located near QMC and used by The London) for clinical training. To overcome these problems, fresh submissions for BLQ (including necessary improvements to the infrastructure of QMC) were presented to the

---

[62] Ellis, LHMC, p. 187.
[63] College Council, 21 October 1981, MS 28/3; AGM, 19 January 1983, MS 27/5; Meeting, 28 May 1982, DF 286.

UGC. Compromises were suggested, and the UGC outlined a staggered development, a policy the College considered to be 'potentially disastrous educationally'.[64] When the UGC rejected further submissions, the University appointed a further committee in 1983 under Frederick Dainton, former chairman of the UGC and vice-chancellor of Nottingham University, to consider all aspects of medical education in the City and East London. Dainton had been responsible for starting a new medical school at Nottingham and had clear ideas on the importance of integrating universities with NHS services to limit the effects of funding cuts on both. He was convinced that only in universities could doctors be equipped with the scientific knowledge they needed.[65] The creation of the committee was designed to 'bring matters to a head' and Dainton saw his remit as finding a way to establish BLQ.[66] For the College, the committee marked the 'final attempt' to develop BLQ, but explained that because 'there was still no confirmation of . . . funding' the College felt no 'longer bound' to its original commitment to BLQ.[67] At the same time, it tried to convince Dainton of the merits of Charterhouse.

While the University and UGC vacillated, 'fruitful' links continued to be developed with The London and NETRHA. Several joint committees were established and plans were submitted for a joint department of general practice, which was established in 1984. Joint academic units, such as in human psychopharmacology under John Silverstone, were also created.[68] Nevertheless, the College remained preoccupied with funding restraints and attempts to implement University policies. The need to reduce staff to student ratios in order to trim expenditure fostered a climate of anxiety. The student intake was cut, departments were restructured and the number of staff was reduced. Continued doubt about the future of the pre-clinical departments complicated the issue, but, despite cuts, it was felt that the quality of teaching and research had been maintained.

Despite this background of cuts, there were advances, especially in research. Between 1979 and 1984, research funding rose from £1.2 million to £3.6 million, a testimony to the College's skill in securing grants. The problems of space that had dogged the development of a research infrastructure in the 1960s were addressed. After a successful research appeal, Dominion House was gradually opened, helping to redress the difficulties created by the overcrowded Dunn Laboratories and the 'higgledy-piggledy mass of laboratories' in Bartholomew Close. Dominion House created a

---

[64] 1981/2 annual report.
[65] Frederick Dainton, *Reflections on the Universities and the National Health Service* (London, 1983), pp. xv-xvi, 94.
[66] College committee, 2 February 1983, MS 29/7.
[67] 1982/3 annual report.
[68] AGM, 19 January 1983, MS 27/5.

research complex that made it easier to obtain grants for new posts.[69] Dominion House brought additional benefits. It freed up space for research-active departments to expand, allowing new units to emerge, the first of which being the recombinant hormone unit. New departments were also created. For example, a multidisciplinary department of environmental and preventive medicine was established around Nicholas Wald, who had come to St Bartholomew's from Oxford. Collaborative work with other institutions was extended and by 1984 the College was turning out 'twice as many postgraduate degrees as any other London . . . medical school'.[70] Closer cooperation was also built up with the City and Hackney health authority. The College took advantage of the opening of the Homerton in 1986 and the government's drive towards 'Care in the Community'. Links with the Homerton did much to improve and democratise opportunities for clinical teaching, with the Homerton benefiting from linked academic appointments.

'BLQ is dead, long live the Confederation'

By the mid-1980s, as pressure mounted to merge the three institutions, the College had become worried that BLQ had departed from educational issues to focus on buildings and the benefits to QMC. The ground had shifted throughout the 1970s as frames of reference changed, and the College pointed to inconsistencies in University policy. While the University pressed for BLQ to be implemented, three medical schools had recently been built on new sites but had not been linked to a multi-faculty environment. The College's belief was that BLQ was only being pursued to bolster QMC, subordinating the needs of medical education in the City and East End. Although St Bartholomew's and The London had made headway in promoting 'joint-ness', by the mid-1980s their situation was beginning to appear anomalous. London's regional and district structure was undergoing reorganisation following the 1982 NHS reforms and a period of resource starvation. Medical schools, which had resisted mergers in the 1970s, now started to amalgamate as spending cuts bit and the University became less able to offer clinical medicine the protection it had previously enjoyed. Most of the marriages were strained. Health authorities in London were experiencing the same process, 'huddling together for strength and warmth'.[71] This was the very solution advocated by the Dainton working party when it delivered its report in 1984.

Dainton called for a single phased development and was determined to press ahead with BLQ. Threats were made and the College was informed that

[69] 1984 annual report, p. 33; Research plans, DF 283.
[70] 1984 annual report, p. 33; Research plans, DF 283.
[71] Cited in Geoffrey Rivett, *From Cradle to Grave: Fifty Years of the NHS* (London, 1998), p. 336.

if it did not toe the line, 'not even your Royal charter will save you'.[72] The College ignored the intimidation. It insisted that it would support BLQ only if St Bartholomew's and The London remained independent. A new proposal was delivered to the UGC, which, after so many false starts, finally agreed to fund BLQ. The UGC recommended using the chemistry building at QMC for the pre-clinical schools as the cheapest option, but this was unacceptable to the College. Instead, it submitted a proposal for a joint pre-clinical school based at Charterhouse but linked to QMC, arguing that this would have some of the advantages of BLQ at a fraction of the cost. However, the future of Mile End Hospital presented problems as rumour circulated that its future role might change. Without any long-term plans to develop acute medicine and surgery at Mile End, the College thought that it would be difficult to integrate pre-clinical and clinical teaching at QMC.[73] Distrust mounted on both sides and the College became more reticent.

In the University, however, elements were already convinced that a joint medical school as part of a faculty of medicine at QMC would be established sooner or later. The University regarded BLQ as a cost-cutting exercise, a way of limiting the damage caused by cuts to recurrent grants.[74] Impatient with the progress made, the UGC became interested in how the Flowers report was being implemented. Funding cuts had made the UGC more assertive, and with further reductions in the recurrent grant predicted for 1984/5, it wanted decisions made, especially in the expensive sector of medicine. Since 1980, the UGC had been convinced that without retrenchment universities would cease to control their future. To prevent this, it pressed for greater selectivity in the allocation of resources. Medicine in London was a prime target. Facing mounting criticism from all sides, the UGC told the University that if BLQ was rejected it was 'accepting that the replaced capacity was not needed and that therefore its medical numbers might eventually be reduced'. Attempts were made to convince the University that St Bartholomew's could be left intact only if funding to other London schools was reduced. The University felt constrained; under pressure to resolve the problem presented by medical education in London. It did not want to reject BLQ for fear that it would be 'tantamount to an offer to accept a reduction in clinical numbers for the university as a whole'.[75] The situation was confused by the fact that different parts of the University's administration were saying different things about BLQ.

A crisis was reached in 1985, precipitating a train of events that led the College to press for a judicial review. In July of that year, the UGC finally decided to award £10 million to BLQ using money from the medical sub-head

[72] THES, 25 May 1986, p. 12.
[73] Ibid., 13 December 1985, p. 3.
[74] Board of Pre-clinical Studies, 13 February 1985, DF 200.
[75] College Council, 16 October 1985, MS 28/3.

on the grounds that clinical teaching would be developed at Mile End. Funding was conditional on St Bartholomew's and The London moving their pre-clinical schools to QMC. Any resulting benefits to medical education were considered to be of secondary importance to the 'strong economic, social and political factors' of consolidating education in the East End.[76] As the dean of the College, Ian Kelsey Fry, told the *Bart's Journal*, 'having gone this far down the line towards marriage, [there is] no doubt whatsoever that we should and will join with the London'.[77] But QMC was still the problem. For the College, a merger with QMC had profound disadvantages, especially as staff continued to see QMC as a second ranking institution in the University. Efforts to integrate the curriculum had also encouraged the belief that separating 'basic medical sciences from clinical sciences, was not the way forward to the 1990s'. Fears were expressed that splitting the pre-clinical from the clinical school would put the College at risk and threaten the hospital. The position of Mile End further complicated the situation after NETRHA warned the University that 'Mile End is an old hospital and as renovation or replacement of old buildings becomes necessary, decisions will have to be taken as to whether the facilities houses therein should remain'.[78] Although some (especially in the biochemistry department) felt that BLQ would result in a stronger school, a majority voted to withdraw from BLQ. It was explained that this 'result should not inhibit the enthusiasm of Bart's for joining with the London Hospital Medical College'. The College's attitude reflected the opposition of London medical schools to rationalisation.[79]

Attempts were made to win the College over. The University agreed to a review and the College was asked to make alternative suggestions. However, although the UGC continued to recognise that the College had considerable reservations, it was determined to press ahead. Both QMC and The London had accepted the possibility of a bilateral merger (LQ) and had prepared proposals along these lines. Committed to developing QMC and expanding educational provision in the East End, the UGC saw a merger of The London and QMC as the best alternative to BLQ. Given the funding limitations, the UGC was clear that LQ could be implemented only if future grants to the University omitted provision for pre-clinical teaching at Charterhouse.[80] Therefore, the College's withdrawal from BLQ was not greeted favourably.

The College continued to argue its case through the academic committees of the University. In Senate, the views of the College were misrepresented, and the University voted to move forward with a London/QMC merger.[81]

[76] College committee, 26 September 1985, MS 29/7.
[77] *Bart's Journal*, summer 1985, p 7.
[78] Ibid., summer 1986, p. 23.
[79] College committee, 6 November 1985, MS 29/7.
[80] *THES*, 11 April 1986, p. 3.
[81] ULL: Minutes of Senate, 21 May 1986.

Concerned about funding and the future of medical education in London, the University believed that it had little choice but to follow the UGC. Both appeared to rely on the longevity of BLQ as an argument for its academic merit, and having made a substantial investment in planning both were unwilling to back down. The College felt marginalised and accused the University of uncritically accepting the UGC's decision, despite the promise of a review. The College was now faced with the situation that if it failed to join BLQ grants for its pre-clinical departments would cease and The London and QMC would merge. At a meeting at the College in October 1985 Flowers told staff that 'in these circumstances the future of Bart's in its present form and occupying its present buildings' was more 'seriously at risk than it has ever been before'. He strove to convince staff that BLQ was the least damaging solution for St Bartholomew's and for 'London's medicine as a whole'. Although Flowers was adamant that he had not come 'to bully or brow beat', this was not how his address was interpreted by staff.[82] Lesley Rees, the sub-dean, resigned her post as public orator of University in protest. Not everyone was as forthright. Some of the pre-clinical lecturers began to feel uneasy about opposing the University. They argued that with The London obviously planning to merge with QMC, efforts should be made to negotiate a better position.[83]

Feeling under threat, the College decided to seek a judicial review, arguing that crucial decisions had been made about its future outside the normal process of consultation. The University was accused of withholding consideration of alternative proposals put forward by the College and of blindly accepting UGC policy. It was argued that those involved in discussing BLQ had not appreciated the changes that had taken place in medical education since 1970. Frustrated that the University had apparently failed to reappraise BLQ or given serious thought to alternative schemes, the College pressed for a judicial review. At the same time, it continued to develop links with The London and began fitful discussions with City University in a bid to protect Charterhouse. City University was keen to expand. With the reorganisation of higher education in London, it felt left out and wanted to establish links with other institutions to raise its standing and develop vocational courses. Discussions were never serious, mainly because the College was unprepared to give up the University of London degree. Negotiations with City University were therefore designed to put pressure on the University of London and quickly stalled.

The turn to a judicial review sent 'shivers through the academic medical world'.[84] The UGC was attacked in the press. The *Times Higher Education Supplement* thought the College's decision was neither 'hasty nor

---

[82] College Council, 16 October 1985, MS 28/3.

[83] *Evening Standard*, 21 May 1986.

[84] *Hansard*, 19 April 1995, p. 286.

ill-considered', merely the turning point in a seventeen-year debate.[85] The College was accused of stalling and of going along with BLQ only because it believed that funding would never be forthcoming. However, the threat of legal action was enough to stimulate discussions in the University about alternative options. Talks were started between St Bartholomew's, The London and QMC, but the College remained dubious about the possibility of reaching a decision. The result was the document 'The Way Forward'.

'The Way Forward' represented the 'maximum concessions' the College was able to extract, much to the annoyance of QMC, which had been obstructive during discussions. Charterhouse was to be protected and used for pre-clinical teaching. Some of the arguments in favour of BLQ were accepted and 'The Way Forward' outlined the creation of a faculty of basic medical sciences at QMC formed from the two existing pre-clinical facilities. However, instead of a merger it proposed a confederation (the City and East London Confederation (CELC)) whereby the three colleges would keep their existing governing bodies and university grants. A federal structure had been suggested in 1981 and discussed as a way of uniting University College Hospital and the Middlesex. Roy Duckworth, dean of The London, felt that under such a scheme 'tribal loyalties' would be maintained. For Kelsey Fry, 'The Way Forward' represented 'the most exciting medical development in this country and potentially the most powerful', giving the three organisations more influence in the University.[86]

At St Bartholomew's, the concessions were seen as an opportunity to extend into the East End and to start work on a new curriculum. Attitudes ranged from enthusiasm to reservation. Despite some suggestion that St Bartholomew's should 'fight on', the College accepted 'The Way Forward' on the proviso that legally binding assurances were secured and a commitment made that a significant proportion of pre-clinical teaching and research would continue at Charterhouse.[87] CELC, although a disappointment, was at least seen as an end to the BLQ dilemma.

CELC

Under the confederation, the College remained an autonomous institution in the University, which agreed to retain all the existing buildings at Charterhouse. The University fully supported the move, admitting that the policy of restructuring and rationalisation adopted since 1981 had sacrificed 'worthwhile aspects of the University's work' and that 'something of value in the broader educational sense has inevitably been lost'. The vice-chancellor

---

[85] THES, 25 May 1986, p. 12.
[86] Barts Journal, spring 1997, pp. 20–1.
[87] College Council, 2 October 1986, 11 October 1985, MS 28/3.

promised to seek adequate funding to ensure that CELC proceeded smoothly. Considerable hope was placed in the venture, which was to come into being in 1990. It was expected 'that the creation of the Confederation will provide a framework within which the present fruitful relationship between the two clinical schools will be . . . further developed' with academic medicine extended. In a period of uncertainty about the nature of medical education, the pooling of medical and scientific teaching resources entailed in CELC offered, in St Bartholomew's view, 'the best guarantee of maintaining . . . operations within one of the strongest and best resourced centres in the University'.[88] However, delays occurred in planning and local grievances continued to emerge with The London, especially over teaching and financial arrangements. While the initial agreement had stipulated that a 'significant' proportion of teaching should be undertaken at Charterhouse, some courses refused to transfer their teaching.[89]

Although the College had exploited Charterhouse to house new departments, including the London Sports Medicine Institute and the William Harvey Research Institute, the general feeling was that BLQ had resulted in a planning blight, complicated by under-funding. Uncertainties about the future and the possible transfer of pre-clinical departments had seen the College concentrating on the clinical school.[90] New departments were established in clinical subjects, with a number funded from outside sources or through 'new blood' lectureships supported by the DHSS and Wellcome Trust. The pre-clinical departments had consequently suffered. They had endured the brunt of redundancies imposed by cuts, which had been exacerbated by the end of the first MB. Departments with the smallest teaching loads were hardest hit. Physics and radiology departments, despite their academic status, were threatened and had to seek outside funding to prevent 'severe cuts'. The physiology department was demoralised while the Department of Zoology was hampered by personal rivalries. On the other hand, the biochemistry department, despite being spilt between ten separate sites, had developed teaching and research in the 1970s and early 1980s, benefiting from the clinical orientation of its research.[91] Overall, however, the position of the pre-clinical departments was poor. When lectureships became vacant, there was serious soul-searching to see if departments could be restructured to save money. Often this was not the case, leaving posts vacant and reducing the efficiency of teaching and research. To make room for new units, some of the pre-clinical departments had been forced to give up part of their accommodation. The 1989 review by UFC revealed the

---

[88] Statement on the policies and objectives for the University of London, 29 November 1985, DF 283; Finance and estates committee, 24 January 1990, DF.

[89] College committee, 3 May 1989, MS 28/4.

[90] Summary of development proposals, DF 298.

[91] Space allocation, 1984, DF 264.

damaging effect BLQ had had. While the clinical departments had a dynamic research profile, attracting £5.8 million in research income, the pre-clinical schools at St Bartholomew's and The London received low grades.[92] The implications for the basic medical sciences caused apprehension, and both schools blamed the University and UGC for making a major policy decision without making sufficient funds available. This, it was felt, had damaged the pre-clinical departments at both schools.

After nearly twenty years of debate, turmoil and fighting, a compromise had been reached that allowed a workable confederation. The judicial review had given the College a strong hand and a determination to press on with development after years of planning blight. CELC was to bring a period of peace, allowing the College to address curriculum reform and the delivery of medical education. However, at the time, how to take the College forward and work with The London and QMC in the new confederation was fraught with difficulties. Charterhouse had been protected and a full merger with QMC avoided. In the rapidly changing NHS, how long this was to be the case remained uncertain.

[92] There were exceptions with the departments of biochemistry, endocrinology and medical oncology receiving commendations: College committee, 4 October 1989, MS 2/8.

12

Training tomorrow's doctors

In an article in the *BMJ* in 1993, the assistant editor confidently claimed that 'after years of stagnation medical education in Britain is changing'.[1] Although it appeared that the pace of reform had accelerated in the 1990s, many of the changes had been debated since the 1960s. A gradual shift from vocational training to the concept of a basic medical education as preparation for future practice had left the structure of the curriculum undecided. How to integrate the curriculum and amalgamate London's medical schools with multi-faculty institutions became the new goals. If the 1968 Todd report outlined a broad consensus on how medical education should be remodelled, the means by which the university-based training it envisaged was to be achieved proved elusive. By the 1990s, the focus had altered again. In the National Health Service (NHS), fresh criteria came to shape care, with greater stress on evidence-based and community medicine. New forms of treatment and diagnostic technology altered the nature of hospital care. New diseases such as AIDS emerged; old ones became resistant to antibiotics. Advances in genetic medicine, organ replacement, endocrinology and radioimmunoassay launched different avenues of research and fresh ways of approaching ill-health. While the number of cases treated increased, length of stay fell, making it difficult for students to see patients. These changes required educationists to rethink how medical students gained clinical experience. Although the need to include medical education in a multi-faculty environment remained important, the extension of community-oriented learning was constructed as the way forward and reflected a shift in the NHS and a growing critique of hospital-based medicine. Greater stress was placed on the value of primary care to training, and teaching hospitals were encouraged to extend links with community services. When *Tomorrow's Doctors* was published by the General Medical Council (GMC) in 1993 it marked the consolidation of educational debates that had their roots in the 1950s.

The late 1950s witnessed a blossoming of interest in medical education. Often discussions went round in circles: fashions in learning and teaching came and went, and were frequently misunderstood or overestimated. As more disciplines were added, new ways of learning were suggested to cope with an overloaded curriculum. Greater attention was paid to the technology of learning and medical schools attempted to break away from didactic

---

[1] *BMJ* cccvi (1993), p. 258.

lectures. However, teaching remained firmly under the control of individual departments (or boards), and medical schools adapted the GMC's guidelines to local circumstances. Students' experiences often remained haphazard and uncoordinated.

By the late 1980s, some feared that 'the health of academic medicine is in serious jeopardy'.[2] Others thought this encouraged 'a revolution in attitudes towards the quality of education'.[3] Studies in the USA, Australia, The Netherlands and Canada proved influential. Methods of teaching were revised as medical schools sought to reappraise their undergraduate arrangements in response to recommendations from the GMC and to changes advocated by various professional bodies. More thought was given to constructing systems-based courses to promote closer integration between the basic medical sciences and clinical teaching. Those concerned with medical education came to favour the need to equip students with an ability to analyse, and not merely to absorb facts. Interest in self-directed learning (SDL) and problem-based learning (PBL) to stimulate students grew, inspired by practices at McMaster University in Canada and Newcastle in New South Wales. The new modes of teaching were linked to the need for a core curriculum to resolve the apparent conflicts in the undergraduate course. Yet how these changes were to be achieved remained problematic.

It should be emphasised that innovation was often difficult for medical schools. Although the GMC sponsored experimentation and new approaches to training, most medical schools were bound by the functions of a teaching hospital, its services and regional commitments. The value attached to individual subjects was invariably determined by bed allocation in the specialisms concerned. Radical change was not easy: modifications in teaching were frequently made in response to alterations to the structure of healthcare. Although the Todd report recommended that primary care should play a larger role in teaching and called for a better-planned curriculum, change was slow. In individual schools, debates revolved around the difficulties presented by an overcrowded curriculum – heavily biased towards factual knowledge – and the need for an integrated and community-oriented approach. Teaching hospitals were reluctant to change for fear of 'getting it wrong'. SDL and PBL were not easy to introduce in schools that had relied on traditional methods. Frequently these concepts represented a 'thin . . . veneer' on teaching.[4] New methods were all too often embraced because they appeared to be an end in themselves, and were introduced without full consideration of the educational or curricula aims. By the early

[2] *BMJ* ccxcviii (1998), pp. 573–9.

[3] Lesley Rees and Brian Jolly, 'Medical Education into the Next Century', in *Medical Education in the Millennium*, ed. Lesley Rees and Brian Jolly (Oxford, 1998), p. 267.

[4] R. M. Harden, Susette Sowden and W. R. Dunn, 'Educational Strategies in Curriculum Development', *Medical Education* xviii (1984), p. 284.

1990s it appeared that 'something was seriously wrong with medical education in Britain'.[5]

St Bartholomew's image as a conservative institution and its reputation for tradition concealed changes to the structure of teaching and assessment. The curriculum had been revised throughout the 1950s and 1960s, and while it was recognised that radical change was not possible, the Todd report stimulated further reforms. Curriculum restructuring was initially piecemeal, and it was not until the early 1980s that more ambitious schemes were attempted. A concerted effort was made after the 'planning blight' of the BLQ period (see Chapter 11) to reorganise teaching and extend educational provision to take advantage of the opportunities offered by the City and East London Confederation (CELC). There was also an emphasis on developing community-oriented teaching and a new curriculum in conjunction with The London. Staff were frequently divided and reforms were pushed through by a number of key individuals. After a series of leaps and bounds, the outcome of over thirty years of reforming initiatives was a curriculum that was seen as one of the most modern in England.

Tomorrow's doctors

The Todd report and the protracted discussions surrounding BLQ involved the need to plan a new curriculum at College and University level. Todd was clear that the existing apprenticeship system was an 'obsolete concept'. It called for students to acquire 'a knowledge of the medical and behavioural sciences', the latter marking an attempt to reintroduce the ideal of a liberal education that had been central to discussions in the mid-Victorian period. Although the Todd report did not challenge the pre-clinical/clinical divide, it did identify the need for integration and a more flexible course. To achieve this, the report called for the adoption of new teaching methods and less emphasis on didactic learning. Although the proposals outlined in the report had been adopted by the GMC the year before, a number of issues were left unresolved. How best to 'equip those entering the profession to go on learning until . . . they retire', and how to match training to spiralling medical costs in a health service undergoing almost permanent revolution were problematic.[6] With NHS services given priority over teaching, it was not easy to unravel these tensions, especially as higher education was also facing funding problems. Numerous schemes were outlined, including systems-based courses and topic teaching. Experiences were mixed: some institutions were better than others at devising and implementing change. If Newcastle, Leicester and Southampton were often pioneering, other schools

---

[5] Stella Lowry, *Medical Education* (London, 1993).
[6] M. M. Webb-Peploe, *Challenge of Medical Education* (London, 1976), p. 3.

like Oxford retained a traditional approach. However, all recognised the need for reform and were encouraged in this direction by the GMC. All too often the result was a 'teachers' curriculum'; only gradually were students included in the debate.

Even before the Todd report was published, the University of London had pressed for revisions to the MB. In the revised regulations, the basic science component was broadened through the introduction of sociology, ethics, statistics, genetics and community medicine, reviving the concept of social medicine that underlaid the 1944 Goodenough report on medical education. Medical schools were given the freedom to choose between a University-based course and a school-based course approved by the University. While flexibility was welcomed and imaginative new courses (as at St George's and the Royal Free) were encouraged, the speed at which the revised regulations were introduced created anxiety. Joining with other London teaching hospitals, St Bartholomew's resisted the University's attempts to modify admission criteria and condense clinical training, fearing that this would lower standards. Efforts to win concessions were resisted: in some cases, suggestions from the College met with derisive laughter in part because St Bartholomew's was considered to be 'conservative'.[7] However, if the College remained traditional in its approach, this did not mean that it was resistant to reform. Teaching had been modified throughout the 1960s and lecturers broadly accepted that the pre-clinical course required a drastic overhaul. This awareness, combined with attempts to develop closer ties between the College and The London and devise a curriculum to suit the two institutions, ensured that the College was already discussing reform when the Todd report was published. The University's decision to revise the MB complicated an already changing situation.

To encourage integration, the Board of Pre-clinical Studies at St Bartholomew's welcomed the idea of a flexible course and modular system embraced by Todd and adopted by the University.[8] To combat student perceptions of pre-clinical teaching as dull or unrelated to medicine, attempts were made to merge the teaching interests and experiences present at The London and at St Bartholomew's into a joint curriculum.[9] However, with staff unable to decide on the structure of clinical teaching, it was resolved to opt for a University-based course. In doing so, greater harmony was secured between the courses offered by the two schools.[10] While this created a basis for joint planning, disagreements emerged among the clinical staff, and although attempts were made to promote integration and implement the

---

[7] Crook to Shooter, 26 November 1971, DF 278.
[8] Board of Pre-clinical Studies, 22 May 1968, DF 201.
[9] *St Bartholomew's Hospital Journal* (1970), p. 353; ibid. (1973), p. 42; Pre-clinical staff–student committee, 21 March 1973, DF 183.
[10] Joint developments, c.1974, DF 298.

revised MB, a strong emphasis on teaching clinical skills through apprentice-ship was maintained. It was recognised by Joseph Rotblat, professor of physics, that 'any radical re-appraisal would take a long time' given the divisions between the clinical and pre-clinical departments.[11] Departments competed for time. Students criticised the academic workload, which was thought to damage 'many student activities and clubs'. It was claimed that much of this burden was caused by unnecessary repetition, necessitating a better-planned curriculum.[12]

If the College and students were sceptical about fully integrated teaching, citing problems in Nottingham where students found an integrated course restrictive, a reduction was made in formal teaching and new subjects were added. To compensate, more weight was given to the merits of SDL. Lectures in sociology, psychology and statistics were included to make students aware of 'why patients and their families behave as they do' and of the 'social and cultural factors which influence patients' expectations and responses'.[13] Modularisation was adopted and the clinical content of teaching was empha-sised, as recommended by the GMC. Closer contacts with The London – notably in gynaecology, venereology and urology – were established and a greater proportion of clinical teaching was transferred to the district general hospitals, with Hackney Hospital playing a leading role.[14] Fewer alterations were made to pre-clinical teaching which 'by choice' remained conventional. The new arrangements were considered to be 'workable' and compared favourably with models presented to the Association for the Study of Medical Education.[15]

Many (including the students) remained disappointed. Teaching was still largely traditional in style and contact between staff and students decreased as funding cuts forced the College to reduce the number of teaching staff. Students also spent less time sharing in the work of the clinical units. New subjects had been introduced without a sufficient reduction in existing subjects, so that students felt under pressure. There were timetabling clashes too, and staff in the pathology department struggling with clinical lecturers over the allocation of teaching time.

Criticisms at St Bartholomew's were part of a growing awareness that the medical curriculum had serious shortcomings. Changes in the NHS and the growing emphasis on primary care had important implications for how medical schools arranged their teaching. Although critics felt that a 'singular disinterest' existed in how the 'educational experience might be managed' there was a growth in the literature on medical education. New methods of

---

[11] Board of Pre-clinical Studies, 10 October 1973, DF 201.
[12] Ibid., 10 October 1973, 25 February 1974, 8 October 1975, DF 201.
[13] *Bart's Journal*, summer 1977, p. 40; 1978/9 annual report.
[14] College committee, 3 March 1971, 5 May 1971, 3 July 1974, MS 29/6.
[15] Board of Pre-clinical Studies, 17 November 1976, DF 201.

learning were discussed. Ideas involving a problem-based approach were borrowed from North America and The Netherlands.[16] The question of how to teach medical students to develop clinical reasoning had attracted increasing attention since the mid-1970s. The concern was that students acquired knowledge only to be unable to apply it. In this climate, PBL became a panacea to answer the 'chronic maladies' believed to exist in medical education. It offered one mechanism through which students' critical thinking could be extended and an integrated body of knowledge melded. However, opinion on the value of PBL was divided, and its nature remained fluid. Difficulties were encountered in its implementation, but PBL's supporters saw it as a means of breaking from the traditional framework in which clinical skills had been taught through a 'complete' history and physical examination.[17] Despite problems, both SDL and PBL became the new educational catch-phrases, a perceived solution to why students often forgot what they had been taught.

Poor examination results at St Bartholomew's – particularly in surgery – highlighted deficiencies and forced change, a move welcomed by the University, which was dissatisfied with clinical teaching in the College. Modularisation had limited students' sense of belonging, and the curriculum was seen as too prescriptive. Fragmentation of clinical teaching between a number of district general hospitals also made it problematic for students to return to St Bartholomew's for midday lectures. Students criticised the lack of scheduled teaching in some firms, calling for more bedside instruction in others. Teaching in cardiology, obstetrics and gynaecology fared particularly badly.[18]

Under the guidance of Ian Kelsey Fry, the dean, and Lesley Rees, the sub-dean, a teaching committee was formed. Kelsey Fry was interested in creating a comprehensive curriculum that emphasised conventional medicine and at the same time incorporated new elements like medical ethics and primary care. Open to new ideas, he wanted pre-clinical students to be more closely involved in hospital life and pressed for integration.[19] Lesley Rees, after devoting her efforts to endocrine research, was encouraged by Kelsey Fry to develop medical education at St Bartholomew's. She regarded reform as essential if the University of London wanted to compete with the provincial schools in obtaining high-calibre medical students. Questionnaires were issued and revisions made. Although the College appeared receptive to students' criticisms, pre-clinical staff complained of being marginalised and

---

[16] *BMJ* ii (1976), pp. 26–7; *Medical Education* xxi (1987), pp. 92–8; ibid., xxiii (1989), pp. 108–17.
[17] *Undergraduate Medical Education in General Practice* (Exeter, 1984), p. 2; *Surgery* cii (1987), pp. 291–6.
[18] *Bart's Journal*, spring 1991, pp. 16–17.
[19] Ibid., summer 1995, p. 5.

argued that their clinical colleagues lacked comprehension of the pre-clinical course. Others pointed to the autocratic way in which decisions were sometimes made.[20] To aid reform, a Joint Medical Education Research Group (JMERG) was established with The London, which undertook a number of studies that emphasised the failure of the curriculum to keep pace with the growth in medical knowledge. JMERG found that teaching invariably concentrated on rote learning, with assessment geared to the retention of information. These approaches were incompatible with the new stress on community medicine and SDL. A reduction in factual information was considered to be vital if new topics were to be incorporated. Investigations also revealed that clinical teaching was at times perfunctory and that students were humiliated on the wards.[21] Studies suggested that undergraduate preparation was deficient in exposing students to practical procedures, common conditions and communication skills.[22] The same set of criticisms was voiced by other institutions, as teaching hospitals were slow to overcome their traditional culture of learning.

To meet some of the perceived problems facing the undergraduate course, longer general medical and surgical firms were introduced to increase students' sense of involvement. Under Gerald Slavin, the new professor of histopathology, pathology was reorganised into blocks to break down fragmentation. Working with The London, several new courses, such as on medical ethics, were added, building on the critique of a biomedical approach that stressed the need for doctors to take greater account of social and psychological factors. Following the University's extensive review of clinical teaching in 1985 – forced by a reduction of acute beds in central London – the use of district general hospitals for teaching was extended. Although the new arrangements were not ideal, it was felt that 'the advantages outweighed the difficulties and the latter were in the process of being ironed out'.[23]

It was moves to establish CELC in 1990 that provided the opportunity to implement sweeping changes to teaching. Despite previous attempts to reform teaching at both schools, the curriculum was still seen as somewhat staid. Desire for curriculum reform at St Bartholomew's was mirrored at The London, helping the two colleges to work together. As Kelsey Fry realised, planning for CELC was like creating a new school. The major challenge was in planning a course to 'minimise the disadvantage of having the Basic Medical Science Departments separate from the clinical school'.[24]

It was recognised by the late 1980s that undergraduate teaching in London

[20] Horst Noack, ed., *Medical Education and Primary Health Care* (London, 1980), p. 308.

[21] Brian Jolly and Lesley Rees, *Room for Improvement* (London, 1984).

[22] Brian Jolly and Margaret Macdonald, 'Education for Practice', *Medical Education* xxiii (1989), pp. 189–95.

[23] College committee, 5 June 1985, MS 29/7.

[24] 1987 annual report, p. 8.

was 'uneven in quality, variable in commitment and lacking in co-ordinated objectives'. It was believed that medical schools were boring students with courses overloaded with information that was 'neither retained nor useful'. Teaching in the basic medical sciences was divorced from a clinical context, encouraging students to compartmentalise their knowledge. Further pressure to realign how and where medicine was taught was added to by the emphasis on primary care in the NHS.[25] It was not just a London problem: concern in Britain was reflected at a world level as calls mounted for a global reorientation of medical education. In response, medical schools produced a spate of curriculum reforms.

Building on the growing critique of how doctors were trained, and on apprehension about the state of medical education in Britain, questions were raised at St Bartholomew's and The London about the scope of the curriculum. Guided by the educational objectives voiced in the Todd report, and by studies made by the JMERG, the aim was to create a core curriculum between the three colleges. Staff from St Bartholomew's and The London interested in innovation were brought together through the work of the curriculum review group. 'International experts' were consulted and ideas from other institutions incorporated. The main innovation was not the ideas adopted – which although sometimes controversial were being implemented elsewhere – but in the overall structure.

Opposition was encountered, especially from the surgeons and from the pathology department at St Bartholomew's. Elements at St Bartholomew's and The London were bitter about the confederation and this complicated a process that relied on the willingness of departments to relinquish some of their autonomy and teaching time. Sacrifices were made in the time devoted to individual subjects, and some ideas such as a compulsory B.Med.Sci. (see Chapter 11) were rejected along the way. Four main principles were adopted: a defined core curriculum, a reduction in rote learning, an integration of basic medical sciences, and the introduction of new assessment methods. It was also seen as essential to create a compatible clinical course between the two schools. In the pre-clinical curriculum, the hope was to achieve these aims through a systems-based approach, with the time allocated to basic medical science reduced to five terms. Change was deemed necessary in part because the existing course was too fragmented. However, the CELC wished to go further. Using money from the Enterprise in Higher Education initiative under the Training Agency, it wanted to make greater use of SDL, increase community teaching and develop communication skills. It envisaged links across the curriculum, combined with student projects and a staff development programme. The Training Agency viewed the reforms outlined by the CELC as unusual and exciting, while enterprise money allowed the CELC to develop and extend the curriculum into new areas.

---

[25] *BMJ* ccxcvi (1988), pp. 1278–9; ibid., ccciii (1991), pp. 41–3.

Despite enthusiasm about integration, some staff were anxious about the 'increased encroachment of clinical material into the already overcrowded pre-clinical course'.[26] Others had to be bullied into accepting change. Gradually a blueprint was produced for a new curriculum. In the CELC curriculum, the apprentice-style approach was reduced. Teaching was arranged into three phases organised into coherent blocks, the final phase being a clinical period that was left to the individual colleges to plan. Only the first two phases, which covered the traditional pre-clinical subjects, were integrated between St Bartholomew's and The London. Traditional pre-clinical teaching was abandoned in favour of a systems-based approach that had been implemented elsewhere since the 1970s. Boundaries between anatomy, biochemistry and pharmacology were dissolved and the subjects approached as integrated aspects of whole body systems. Demonstrations and clinical histories were introduced at an early stage, although time on individual firms was shortened, challenging the culture of medical education as personal contact between staff and students was reduced.[27] The London went further in its adoption of a new curriculum than St Bartholomew's, where attention was directed at the pre-clinical course. Although modifications were made, essentially clinical teaching in the College remained unaltered.

To ensure that subjects were incorporated without detriment, new teaching methods were adopted, encouraged by the JMERG and the Department of General Practice. Less stress was placed on didactic lectures to combat the overload of factual information associated with the traditional curriculum. Lectures continued to be used throughout the course, but more stress was placed on SDL, PBL and group teaching through interdisciplinary modules. Some departments had already moved towards seminar-based work and SDL, with medical ethics and general practice playing an important role in developing these modes of teaching. The CELC was designed to extend this. By the early 1990s, SDL had become a key part of the course's philosophy, if not always its teaching practice.

In Phase 1 students were based at Queen Mary and Westfield College in Mile End. Here they received an interdisciplinary training in the basic medical sciences. A community health component was added to introduce students to health and social services outside a hospital setting. Throughout, considerable emphasis was placed on communication skills. But it was Phase 2, split between the behavioural sciences and a clinical component, that was considered unique. It aimed to equip students 'with the necessary clinical and communication skills' for the clinical component. Project work was introduced to promote the critical thinking that educationists and critics of science-based medicine were calling for. Rather than replacing the

---

[26] Pre-clinical curriculum committee, 29 March 1984, 17 May 1984, 3 June 1985, DF 199.
[27] College committee, 9 November 1988, MS 29/8.

pre-clinical/clinical split, the two-term Phase 2 bridged the gap, giving students a focus on core clinical skills such as history-taking and the technique of examining patients.

For some years there had been growing professional concern about doctors' communication skills, their lack of empathy and their failure to provide patients with information. In the late 1970s, students and staff at St Bartholomew's had started to voice unease about the 'disappointing lack of attention to anything other than the . . . medical aspects' of patient management.[28] Studies began to show that with students' educational experience dominated by history-taking, less attention was given to how this information was obtained.[29] Systematic teaching of communication skills was started in the 1980s at other institutions (encouraged by the Nuffield Provincial Hospitals Trust), but investigations at St Bartholomew's and The London revealed that students continued to receive little training in this area.[30] The publication of the 1989 White Paper *Working for Patients* also emphasised the importance of training doctors to communicate with patients, their families and the public. The GMC added its support. If St Bartholomew's was more reticent than other teaching hospitals, the CELC made communication skills central to Phase 2. Under Annie Cushing's encouragement, use was made of small-group teaching, role-play and video playback in an attempt to break from passive learning, incorporating ideas already adopted in some departments, in particular pathology and radiology.

Fewer changes were made to the clinical course that formed Phase 3. Under the guidance of John Wass, the sub-dean following Rees's appointment as dean, the importance of clinical skills was emphasised. Tutorials and workbooks were introduced and new modes of assessment added. Academic half-days were to provide integrated teaching alongside work on the wards, although moves to establish them were not made until 1992. Greater stress was placed on teaching in the community. Optional courses were designed to overcome the perceived reduction in 'the coverage of the clinical specialties'. It was anticipated that this would create the choice that had been initially desired.[31]

Funding problems in the basic medical sciences raised questions about implementing the new curriculum, and unplanned bed closures in the NHS forced new teaching methods. Each firm was encouraged to develop clearer learning objectives and greater importance was attached to student feedback. However, students continued to grumble about the lack of hands-on experience. Despite these difficulties, the new curriculum was implemented

[28] *Bart's Journal*, autumn 1977, p. 28.
[29] *Medical Education* xi (1977), pp. 175–82; *Proceedings of the Twenty-fifth Annual Conference on Research in Medical Education* (Washington, 1986), pp. 171–6.
[30] Jolly and Macdonald, 'Education for Practice', p. 192.
[31] College committee, 9 November 1988, MS 29/8.

in 1990 before all the details had been finalised.[32] Money from the Enterprise scheme was used to make appointments to deliver new components. In 1991, a communication skills coordinator was appointed, and a breaking bad news course was established after questionnaires found that this was seldom done in clinical training.[33] Lesley Rees felt that students and staff responded well to the new ethic and SDL, although there were problems because students initially avoided SDL when they found it was optional and not assessed. This was resolved by making all aspects of the course examinable. Other problems were encountered: some lecturers tried to cram their unchanged lectures into the shorter time slots.[34] However, higher examination results suggested that the new curriculum worked well.

Although the CELC curriculum aimed to resolve some of the problems facing medicine at a local level, the medical curriculum and its delivery came under increasing attack in the late 1980s. Restrictions on funding made it difficult to maintain teaching quality, and in London the perennial problems posed by the structure of healthcare and access to teaching beds placed medical schools under increasing pressure. The situation was compounded by NHS reforms. Teaching hospitals suffered under the internal market (see Epilogue), and the broad clinical base necessary for teaching was threatened. To investigate, the College joined with the King's Fund to examine the implications of changes in healthcare to undergraduate teaching. It was admitted that medical schools were struggling to deliver 'the right quality and quantity of clinical experience' and had failed to respond to the reorganised NHS. There was a return to concerns reminiscent of debates that had surrounded the curriculum in the early twentieth century. A balance was sought between the need to avoid factual overloading and to offer training that accounted for the rapidly changing nature of medicine. The concept of PBL and the need to deliver a 'core' curriculum were approached with greater vigour as those interested in curriculum development attempted to produce an 'undifferentiated doctor' ready for further training.[35]

The principles adopted by the investigation and the curriculum implemented in the CELC influenced the GMC. It welcomed the findings of the curriculum review group and visited the CELC as part of a wider review. When the GMC came to prepare a consultation document in 1991 to explore possible revisions to its curriculum guidelines, many of its suggestions 'corresponded with . . . the ideas forming the basis of the new CELC curriculum'.[36] St Bartholomew's and the CELC could not claim all the credit.

---

[32] Ibid., 1 November 1989, 3 May 1990, 1 May 1991, MS 29/8.

[33] Ibid., 1 May 1991, MS 29/8; Jolly and Macdonald, 'Education for Practice', p. 192.

[34] Changes in Medical Education xiv (1995), p. 3; Barts Journal, spring 1991, p. 4.

[35] See Angela Towle, Undergraduate Medical Education: London and the Future (London, 1992).

[36] College committee, 3 July 1991, MS 29/8.

In spite of the introduction of the pre-registration year and the gradual relaxation since the 1950s in statutory requirements imposed on the curriculum, it was still felt that there was 'a persisting drive towards an unrealistic degree of completeness in the curriculum'. This was reinforced by the widespread reluctance in individual departments to give up teaching time. By the 1990s, the GMC felt that medical schools were determined to 'break the mould'.[37] Pressure from students and teachers, from professional bodies, and from changes in the way healthcare was organised, all forced a rethink of how medical students were taught. Many of the ideas adopted by the CELC, and later by the GMC, had been expressed in the late 1970s and 1980s and were being implemented elsewhere. The study by the King's Fund (published in 1992) pointed to a consensus about the problems facing teaching, the need for new methods of learning and assessment, and a better balance between hospital and community experience.[38] Changes in the NHS added pressure. Tomorrow's Doctors produced by the GMC in 1993 recognised this, building on work in the CELC.

Tomorrow's Doctors sought to 'facilitate the changes widely accepted as desirable' to produce a curriculum that differed substantially from the traditional approach.[39] The GMC admitted that the criticisms levelled at the curriculum were the same in 1993 as they had been in 1980. Stress was placed on the importance of a core curriculum that encouraged student-centred learning through a systems-based approach. It was anticipated that this would equip students with practical clinical skills, a scientific foundation and the ethical, financial and professional tools deemed necessary for work as pre-registration house officers. Integration and cooperation between disciplines continued to be thought vital. A national core curriculum was rejected in favour of local experimentation. The GMC was also keen to develop communication skills, with special study modules (SSM) providing additional educational opportunities outside of the core curriculum to allow students to explore areas of interest in depth and develop a self-critical approach to medicine. As in 1980, the GMC argued that students should gain greater experience of primary care and community medicine. Some at St Bartholomew's feared that the effort demanded for reorganising London's teaching hospitals along the lines suggested by the 1992 Tomlinson report (see Epilogue) would leave medical schools with little energy for the innovations outlined in Tomorrow's Doctors.[40]

[37] GMC, Tomorrow's Doctors: Recommendations on Undergraduate Medical Education (London, 1993), p. 6.
[38] Towle, Medical Education.
[39] GMC, Tomorrow's Doctors, p. 6.
[40] BMJ cccvi (1993), pp. 258–61.

Into the community

Tomorrow's Doctors placed a premium on community medicine, but the need to promote better training in general practice had already been heralded by the Goodenough report in 1944. Although postgraduate provision had been made before 1939, most medical schools had failed to provide training at an undergraduate level.[41] During the war, medical academics inspired by an ideology of social medicine had 'hoped to reform medical practice and education . . . increasing doctors' sensitivity to the social and environmental causes of ill health'.[42] However, the NHS offered little to general practitioners, and while the Goodenough report stirred enthusiasm, it brought no immediate action. It was only with the formation of the Royal College of General Practitioners in 1952 that progress was made. It stimulated medical schools to develop attachment schemes: by 1953, fourteen of the twenty-eight teaching hospitals in England and Wales sent students on a one- to four-week attachment with a general practitioner. Only in two was an attachment compulsory, and most schemes owed a considerable debt to the idea of an apprenticeship.[43]

Despite growing interest in the role of general practice, attitudes were slow to alter at St Bartholomew's. Some of the senior clinical staff had opposed the formation of the College of General Practitioners and resisted the idea of general practice as a discipline. Opinion was divided over the importance of requiring students to spend time with a general practitioner, but as a conciliatory gesture it was decided to offer final-year students a series of lectures by local general practitioners. Students were also advised to 'go out and observe it [general practice] by visiting . . . practices for a week or two' but no room was made available in the timetable. The promise of external funding permitted the College to appoint G. F. Abercrombie in 1957 as adviser on general practice.[44] A student-attachment scheme was started in the following year. However, students who took advantage of the scheme tended to sandwich attendance between finals and the start of their pre-registration posts as a way of filling time.[45]

By the mid-1960s, just at the time that general practice was emerging as a discipline, greater attention turned to the need to offer training. Although over 50 per cent of students ended up in general practice, general practitioners continued to be considered as 'failed specialist[s]'. In the mid-

---

[41] Ibid., ii (1952), pp. 490–1.

[42] Mark Perry, 'Academic General Practice in Manchester under the Early NHS: A Failed Experiment in Social Medicine', *SHM* xiii (2000), p. 111.

[43] See C. M. Harris, *General Practice Teaching of Undergraduates in British Medical Schools* (London, 1961).

[44] Executive committee, 13 November 1957, MS 30/4.

[45] *St Bartholomew's Hospital Journal*, July 1957, p. 206.

1960s, there was a move to break from this feeling by bolstering the academic element of general practice.[46] Under the 1966 Family Doctors' Charter, the importance of training was stressed as the 'boundaries between hospital and general practice altered as GPs reclaimed some aspects of medical work from hospitals'.[47] Under pressure from the GMC, medical schools forged closer links with local practitioners; a trend strengthened by a 'renaissance' in general practice.[48] Most courses remained vocational however.

The Todd report reiterated the GMC's recommendations and suggested that general practitioners become actively involved in undergraduate teaching through senior academic appointments. Todd's support for primary care became linked with growing concern about the discontinuities between medical education and practice.[49] In response, medical schools established departments of general practice, with Edinburgh taking the lead. Most were comparatively small and inadequately funded, and encountered resistance. Few were 'practice linked' and the great majority were only able to develop 'practice-based' programmes in which students were attached for short periods to general practices. Objectives were often poorly defined beyond a need to offer students some experience.[50] St Bartholomew's adopted a different, more successful approach.

Changes in the regulations for the University of London's MB in 1976 to ensure that students spent some time in general practice encouraged the College to develop its general practice teaching. Under the new regulations, medical schools in London were required to offer training 'with particular reference to health and disease in the home and the community, the influence of social and emotional factors on health, early diagnosis and the long-term management of chronic health and disability'.[51] The College and The London had been approached by two Newham medical officers of health interested in developing teaching in primary care. A Northeast Thames Regional Health Authority (NETRHA) working party had also concluded that because teaching hospitals had neglected 'general practice', it was vital for St Bartholomew's and The London to expand community medicine. Following the reorganisation of the NHS in 1974, the region wanted to promote cooperation between hospital and community services,

---

[46] John Anderson and Frederick John Roberts, *A New Look at Medical Education* (London, 1965), p. 20.

[47] D. Pereira Gray, 'The Emergence of the Disciplines of General Practice', *Journal of the Royal College of General Practitioners* xxxix (1989), pp. 228–33; Virginia Berridge, *Health and Society in Britain since 1939* (Cambridge, 1999), pp. 42–3.

[48] GMC, *Recommendations as to Basic Medical Education* (London, 1967).

[49] *Medical Education* x (1976), pp. 339–40.

[50] David Hannay, 'University Medical Education and General Practice', in *General Practice under the National Health Service, 1848–1997*, ed. Irvine Loudon, John Horder and Charles Webster (Oxford, 1998), p. 168.

[51] College committee, 7 February 1973, MS 29/6.

and develop primary care training to increase the role of the general practitioner and community services.[52] Interest was not limited to England: in the Alma Ata declaration the World Health Organisation asserted the importance of developing primary healthcare. Several medical schools, principally in The Netherlands, Canada and New South Wales, had become famous for their emphasis on preparing students with a primary healthcare focus, and in Britain, Nottingham and Southampton were moving in this direction. Progress was slower in London, where support for a traditional hospital-based course remained strongly entrenched.

Reggie Shooter, dean at St Bartholomew's in the 1970s, was keen to give students the opportunity 'to spend time in general practices situated in various parts of the country'. He worked to place students with general practitioners and pressed for an extension of general practice teaching. Lessons were learned from the course run at University College, and negotiations were started with the London School of Hygiene and Tropical Medicine to develop community medicine. To further this, and in face of pressure from the NETRHA, a general practice teaching unit was established under Mal Salkind in 1977.[53] Using money from the Inter City Partnership, the unit had a nucleus of four general practitioners working in three local practices and developed links with other practitioners. Training began in earnest. Students spent a month in the unit, comprising an introductory period and a two-week attachment. Even so, attitudes to the course were mixed; the four weeks spent on general practice were criticised by some as being too long.[54]

By the 1980s interest in primary care had grown further. Illnesses previously treated in hospital were now being managed in general practice, and with greater longevity, chronic, degenerative diseases of old age and multiple pathologies started to be predominant. Resources available in the community and through general practitioners had consequently risen. Doctors were also beginning to pay more attention to social and psychological factors in illness. In response, primary care was constructed – somewhat idealistically – as a 'new comprehensive approach to health and health care' as it became almost 'fashionable' to criticise hospital-based practice.[55] But there were practical reasons, too. In a cash-strapped NHS, it was thought that strengthening primary care would be cost-effective, as it could prevent the onset of serious illness.

These changes inevitably had an impact on medical education. With a larger number of patients being treated outside a hospital setting, and with

---

[52] Primary medical care in Newham, February 1974, DF 255; Planning for primary healthcare, July 1978, DF 255.
[53] Staff–student committee, 23 May 1973, DF 182; Working party on social medicine, 15 January 1974, DF 170.
[54] *Bart's Journal*, spring 1991, p. 16.
[55] Noack, *Medical Education*, p. 318.

a reduction in length of stay, opportunities for students to observe patients had fallen. Even in hospitals the focus was altering, with a greater reliance on outpatients and day surgery. In 1980, the GMC made it clear that the overall objective of basic medical education was to produce a doctor who had been 'introduced to the concept of illness and its range, variations and consequences in order to acquire an understanding of disease'. General practice became one of the channels through which this was to be achieved.[56] Leading figures in medical education began to assert the need to 'identify the community dimension more explicitly as part of the total structure of the curriculum' at the same time as educational orthodoxy asserted the need for students to spend more time in general practice.[57] However, development was slow. The tensions created by the demands of a hospital-based course were an obstacle, and although advances were made in general practice teaching, often individual departments were not well placed to implement change. Although medical schools were encouraged to re-evaluate their teaching to include more general practice training, they did not always adapt quickly, especially as few individuals involved in primary care were incorporated into their management. As the introduction of primary care into undergraduate training required 'significant changes in the traditional medical school curriculum', resistance was perhaps inevitable.[58]

Following the 1981 Acheson report on Inner London general practitioners, which showed that standards were low, the University Grants Committee (UGC) made money available for the creation of two academic departments in general practice. St Bartholomew's submitted a proposal, which the UGC accepted, and a joint Department of General Practice and Primary Care with The London was established at Charterhouse. With The London reticent, the new department built on work carried out by Salkind and his department at St Bartholomew's. It endeavoured to teach medicine to undergraduates from the perspective of primary care, but also offered courses to general practitioners. Central teaching was augmented by access to over 250 general practices, most concentrated in the City and East End. Students had a ten-day training session after which they were sent to a general practice before returning to Charterhouse for a week-long academic component. Revisions to the curriculum in 1985, pressed for by Lesley Southgate, the senior lecturer in general practice, led to greater emphasis on primary care. This reflected growing criticism of the comparative neglect of primary healthcare and the prevention of disease in undergraduate teaching. The publication of the 1987 White Paper *Promoting Better Health*, which placed general practitioners firmly at the centre of primary care, and *Working for Patients*, which appeared in 1989, added further pressure to give students a

---

[56] GMC, *Recommendations on Basic Medical Education* (London, 1967).
[57] *Medical Education* xvii (1983), p. 70.
[58] Noack, *Medical Education*, p. 227.

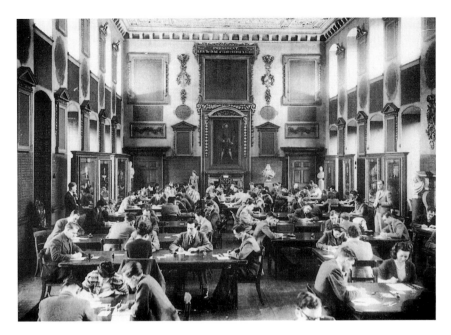

Plate 12.1 Examinations in the Great Hall

'much deeper knowledge of the way in which the health service operated within the community'.[59] A number of reports had also stressed the need to train students in a variety of skills in diverse settings. It was felt that community-based activities and primary care offered these opportunities.[60]

At St Bartholomew's, the new CELC curriculum aimed to make students more aware of community medicine and general practice. The general practice module was revamped. Like many schemes, it was included in a public health context.[61] Students were required to do an introductory week with a local practice, and a two-week stint with general practitioners scattered across the country. Despite initial scepticism, a community module was introduced in 1991 using money from the Enterprise scheme. Teaching in community medicine with a strong emphasis on epidemiology had been organised since 1978, but the new module was seen as a fresh departure,

[59] *Promoting Better Health. The Government's Programme for Improving Primary Health Care* (London, 1987); *Working for Patients. The Health Service Caring for the 1990s* (London, 1989).
[60] See *'Physicians for the Twenty First Century'*, *Report of the Panel on the General Professional Education of the Physician and College Preparation for Medicine*, (s.n., 1984); *Edinburgh Declaration, World Conference on Medical Education* (s.n., 1988).
[61] David Hannay and P. D. Campion, 'University Departments of General Practice', *British Journal of General Practice* xlvi (1996), pp. 35–6.

and the most innovative aspect of the CELC curriculum. It relied on support from the City and Hackney Community Health Council, which had pressed for the extension of community-based opportunities for students. 'Clusters' of twelve students were sent in small groups to Tower Hamlets, City and Hackney and Newham health authorities to undertake a variety of activities. Fifty tutors were recruited to help with the module, many of whom were drawn from community organisations in East London, and were given the freedom to interpret the module according to local circumstances. As a result, students became involved in activities ranging from walking the beat with police officers to attending local schools, old people's clubs and centres for the homeless.[62] The aim was to expose them to what life was like in the City and Hackney.

Building links with local practitioners was 'painstakingly slow and difficult'.[63] Neither was the module welcomed by all staff teaching the basic sciences and was perceived by some 'as something imposed on the curriculum that threatens the teaching time of other subjects'.[64] Overall, however, the module was considered to be a success and formed one of the most comprehensive schemes developed in London at the time. One student felt the community module gave 'an insight into the conditions and problems of people in an environment very different from my own'; another that it made students think about 'a patient as a whole person and as part of a community'. Others found the process more daunting given the lack of formal teaching.[65]

The publication of the Tomlinson report in 1992 heralded the demand for investment in primary care in London, shaking up the structure of metropolitan healthcare and threatening the future of St Bartholomew's (see Epilogue). In the following year, the NETRHA outlined plans to strip responsibility for midwifery, psychiatric care and many services for children and the elderly from hospitals in East London as a way of meeting this.[66] Similar moves were being made elsewhere that fragmented the traditional role of the hospital. These changes emphasised the importance of primary care and the need to transfer teaching to the community where patients lived and worked. Although Tomlinson's report did not address the educational implications of its drive to primary care, medical schools developed an unprecedented interest in community medicine as it became clear that teaching requirements would no longer dictate bed numbers. Fears were aroused that some of these initiatives were merely a 'rapid response to external pressure and not part of any overall curriculum philosophy'.[67]

---

[62] L. Babaei-Mahani, 'Evaluation of a Health Advocate's Training Course', *Medical Education* xxvi (1992), pp. 71–2.

[63] *BMJ* cccvi (1993), p. 259.

[64] Angela Towle, *Community-Based Teaching* (London, 1992), pp. 9–19.

[65] 1991 annual report, pp. 5–6; *Bart's Journal*, September 1991, p. 21.

[66] 1994 annual report, p. 26; *Guardian*, 5 August 1993, p. 19.

[67] Towle, *Community-Based Teaching*, p. v.

An extension of community-oriented teaching often entailed more than a change in the location of teaching. By the 1990s, in the context of medical education the 'community' had developed beyond general practice attachments.[68] It came to be seen by some as a solution to the perceived problems facing undergraduate training, a way of fostering PBL and educational self-reliance, ideas the GMC argued should be central to training. The World Health Organisation was equally keen to support these developments, arguing that community-based education helped students learn a sense of social responsibility.[69] Medical educationists were strongly influenced by these ideas and suggested that learning medicine in a general practice setting offered students opportunities missing from a hospital-based course, playing on concerns about hospital training that had been present since the late nineteenth century. Experimentation was called for and general practitioners were keen to assume a higher profile in undergraduate teaching.[70] Several experimental schemes began in the mid-1990s and the approach was endorsed by the GMC in *Tomorrow's Doctors*. Despite this enthusiasm, a large number of community-based initiatives were solutions to local problems brought about by changes in the health service rather than a sea change in the educational orthodoxy at most medical schools.[71]

While it was recognised at St Bartholomew's that general practitioners had much to teach medical schools about effective ways of learning, the College was aware that incentives for teaching in general practice were low, and that organising such training was difficult. It was also thought that whereas students valued experience in local communities, the effort demanded of public health and community organisations was considerable at a time when they were under pressure.[72] Teaching in the College reflected these competing forces, as efforts were made to extend the primary care element in the curriculum. Group project work was undertaken and in 1994 a 'Patients as Partners' scheme was started with funding from the King's Fund. It linked students with patients 'to gain insights into the experience and perspective of individual health service users regarding their health and access to services in a community context'.[73]

Community-oriented teaching was not limited to the community module and general practice. In obstetrics and gynaecology greater use was made of

---

[68] B. Hamad, 'Community-oriented Medical Education: What is it?', *Medical Education* xxv (1991), p. 16–22.

[69] World Health Organisation, *Community-based Education of Health Personnel* (1987).

[70] S. Iliffe, 'All That is Solid Melts in Air: The Implications of Community Based Undergraduate Medical Education', *British Journal of General Practice* xlii (1992), pp. 390–3.

[71] See Nigel Oswald, 'Long-term Community-Based Attachments', *Medical Education* xxix (1995), pp. 72–6; Peter McCrorie, F. Lefford and F. Perrin, *Medical Undergraduate Community-Based Teaching* (Dundee, 1991).

[72] *BMJ* cccvi (1993), pp. 258–61.

[73] 1994 annual report, p. 26.

the Well Street clinic, although an initial pilot scheme to send students to work in a well-woman clinic was not a success. In the paediatric module, efforts were made to increase the primary care element, with students spending an eighth of their time on the module in the community.[74] Students were felt to be enthusiastic about their experiences of community medicine, but many staff remained to be convinced. Introducing a community element created considerable organisational problems, and resources to develop community teaching were strained.

Assessment and the search for objectivity

The investigations made by the JMERG and the thinking behind the CELC stressed the need to match assessment criteria to curricula aims. The philosophy and practice of assessment had undergone a gradual process of change since the 1950s, with attempts to introduce more objective examination criteria to break from a system whereby students were felt to learn merely to pass tests. St Bartholomew's was slow to respond. A move to objective examinations was first taken in the biochemistry department in 1957 by Eric Wills, professor of biochemistry. Wills had brought back a system of multiple choice questions (MCQs) from the United States, having spent a year at the University of Vermont. Always interested in teaching methods, he participated in discussions at the Institute of Education on medical education and felt that MCQs offered an objective yardstick. By the mid-1960s, objective examinations were included in final-year clinical papers. The new academic unit in the Department of Obstetrics and Gynaecology devised a research programme to investigate teaching and assessment, and seized on the use of a bank of objective questions to assess the breadth and depth of students' knowledge. Monthly MCQs were introduced in 1968. The idea was to test teaching rather than students' learning, but moves in the unit suggested a new approach to assessment.[75]

As MCQs came to monopolise examinations in the 1970s, they were introduced throughout the College. Structured answered questions to replace unstructured essays in finals followed in turn, and considerable discussion was generated by the merits of continuous assessment and regular examinations. However, long cases, involving use of a real clinical setting and face-to-face basic examinations, continued to dominate. Not everyone welcomed the change. New assessment techniques were criticised and considerable support was voiced for viva voce examinations.

While long cases continued to dominate assessment at St Bartholomew's, a few medical schools in the late 1970s and 1980s started to import a new

---

[74] Towle, *Community-Based Teaching*, pp. 52, 51.
[75] *St Bartholomew's Hospital Journal*, June 1969, pp. 229–30.

type of assessment based on multiple short cases from the USA and The Netherlands.[76] Doubts had emerged about the reliability of long cases. As experience was gained of existing objective-type tests dissatisfaction mounted. Studies in the 1970s revealed the limitations of MCQs, which tested only a body of factual knowledge and not a wide range of competencies. With assessment theory moving towards the need to achieve fidelity with real situations, MCQs failed to test an overlap of skills. There was also suspicion that a range of answers gave students too many prompts. Alternatives that sought to test the application of knowledge in a clinical context were proposed, but many of these encountered difficulties regarding scoring. Studies argued that problem-solving was highly dependent on the context and that a modification of case content often yielded very different results. Interest thus focused on the need for more reliable methods to test core clinical skills. The objective structured clinical examination (OSCE) appeared to solve some of these problems. OSCE was not really a single method, rather a flexible mode of assessment that allowed a range of skills and clinical tasks to be incorporated. In an OSCE students followed a circuit of stations. At each station they are tested on a different clinical skill against set criteria, so that all students were examined on the same content with standardised marking. OSCEs challenged existing modes of assessment and studies began to suggest that in some fields it was 'a more appropriate [examination] . . . than any tried so far'.[77]

Despite the interest shown in assessment, most British academics were initially sceptical of OSCEs given the difficulties inherent in assessing clinical competence and in standard setting. A few schools took the lead, among them Cambridge. Its initiatives found support in the JMERG, which was interested in the examination because of the encouragement to student-centred education given by Peter Cull in the department of Medical Illustration. Initially there continued to be a heavy reliance on objective paper-and-pencil measures of clinical competence, and questions were raised about the reliability of an OSCE. However, it was widely acknowledged by 1994 that conventional techniques for assessing the knowledge and clinical competence of undergraduates were unsatisfactory.[78] The extent to which these could be replaced by an OSCE remained open to considerable doubt.

At St Bartholomew's interest in OSCEs first manifested itself in surgery, where it built on links with the JMERG and a sense that students regarded

[76] R. M. Harden and F. A. Glesson, 'Assessment of Clinical Competence using an Objective Structured Clinical Examination', *Medical Education* xiii (1979), pp. 41–54.

[77] W. Hall-Turner, 'An Experimental Assessment Carried out in an Undergraduate General Practice Teaching Course', *Medical Education* xvii (1983), pp. 112–19.

[78] See G. Johnson and J. Reynard, 'Assessment of an Objective Structured Clinical Examination', *Journal of Accident Emergence Medicine* xi (1994), pp. 223–6.

existing assessment methods as being unfair and inconsistent.[79] OSCEs were seen as an alternative to problems of subjectivity posed by other examination methods. In 1987 it was suggested that there should be an OSCE at the end of the general surgery firm to 'standardise the marking system'. Staff observed practice in Liverpool and at other centres where OSCEs appeared to work efficiently.[80] An OSCE for first-year students was inaugurated in 1990. The hope was that this could be extended to finals.[81] The CELC curriculum encouraged the adoption of new assessment methods, but no formal structure existed for OSCEs, which were organised on an *ad hoc* basis. Initially, students had problems accepting the validity of the OSCE grade, especially as they often diverged from firm grades. This undermined the value of the examination. Departments also tended to conduct examinations in an idiosyncratic fashion: students were given conflicting advice and examinations were marked in different ways, while some heads of department could not contemplate any alternative to long essays or *vivas*. When OSCEs were introduced, they were initially limited to first-year assessments, where the aim was to identify 'the very small number of students having difficulty with clinical work'.[82] However, the apparent success of the examination suggested that it 'could point the way to changes in the pattern of teaching' and discussions about it merged with debates on the delivery of new teaching methods.[83]

Although the possibility of using OSCEs was gradually accepted, the utility of a joint OSCE to test surgical and medical skills met with resistance. It was not until 1994 that a decision was made to run a joint OSCE to replace short cases in surgery, medicine, obstetrics, gynaecology and therapeutics, with the examination linked to long cases as part of finals.[84] This was part of an overhaul of the assessment procedure which, although not as radical as initially intended, did see a number of changes. The CELC became the first medical school to include OSCEs as part of a finals assessment. Physicians and surgeons were expected to assess a single long case together, treating the case as a clinical whole rather than as specifically a medical or surgical problem.[85] Ironically, although St Bartholomew's was perceived as one of the leading centres in England for the development of OSCEs, in the College doubts and problems about reliability remained, and resistance was encountered.

By the mid-1990s, a mixture of assessment criteria was being used. Project reports and OSCEs in the third and fifth year provided hurdles which

---

[79] David Newble, Brian Jolly and Richard Wakeford, eds, *Certification and Recertification in Medicine* (Cambridge, 1994).
[80] Board of Studies in surgery, 9 April 1987, 2 February 1989, DF.
[81] 1990 annual report, p. 26.
[82] Board of Studies in surgery, 17 January 1992, DF.
[83] College committee, 5 June 1991, MS 28/4.
[84] Board of Studies in surgery, 18 January 1994, DF.
[85] 1993 annual report, p. 41.

students were required to pass to proceed. In-course assessment contributed to the final mark. A number of basic assessment tools were employed: a variety of short-answer questions, MCQs, visual assessments (such as 'spotter' or 'steeplechase' examinations), critical analysis papers and modified essay questions. *Vivas* remained but only for borderline and distinction cases. Not everyone was convinced that this was an improvement.

Medical education and clinical skills

Efforts to reform the curriculum and introduce new methods of assessment stimulated interest in medical education at St Bartholomew's. The need for the creation of departments of medical education had first been voiced in the 1960s.[86] Cull's interest provided a foundation, and in 1984, using funds from the region, JMERG was formed in collaboration with The London. The group under Brian Jolly, assistant director of the audio-visual department, aimed to evaluate the curriculum and shape a new one. It was felt that JMERG 'acted as a stimulus to bring the very real problems of medical education in the future to the centre of the stage'.[87] Although the group had a small staff, it was seen as a unique venture that supplied 'a vital educational input into the development of the new curriculum'.[88] With the creation of CELC, the group was expanded. 'Extreme financial stringency' saw medical illustration combined with the research group to create a new Department of Education and Medical Illustration Services (EMIS). The aim was not driven by academic or service needs, but by a need to improve efficiency and make financial savings, which might allow expansion and reinvestment.

In 1989, EMIS split with the creation of a joint academic unit of medical and dental education. From the start, it was seen as a department of CELC.[89] Given the interest in the University in the need to develop medical education as a discipline, the unit sought to address the 'practical problems associated with the implementation of the new curriculum, provide effective staff development programmes, undertake educational consultations and promote effective teaching and medical educational research'. The anticipation was that it would become a centre of excellence in medical education, and Angela Towle, funded partly by the King's Fund, was appointed in 1989 to investigate teaching practices. She produced a number of groundbreaking studies.[90] The unit tried to tackle the reluctance of some departments to alter how medicine was taught and assessed. It also played an important part in introducing and

---

86 Anderson and Roberts, *A New Look at Medical Education*, p. 24.
87 1985 annual report, p. 9.
88 *Bart's Journal*, summer 1990, p. 3.
89 College committee, 7 June 1989, MS 29/8.
90 Ibid., 5 July 1989, 6 December 1989, MS 29/8.

devising OSCEs. The unit was expanded when Enterprise money enabled the appointment of two half-time staff development officers in 1991. Studies of factual loads were made, along with efforts to increase SDL and improve compatibility between the clinical course at St Bartholomew's and The London. By 1993, it was felt that progress had been made in improving the quality of teaching.[91]

Rising interest in general practice in the 1980s also stimulated new ways of learning through the use of simulated patients, computer-assisted learning and video. The JMERG and its successors were interested in these developments, and in how students were taught clinical skills. The curriculum changes introduced by the CELC provided a focus for debate. Studies based on self-reported evidence revealed that students felt they had received inadequate training in certain clinical skills and had considerable gaps in their practical experience.[92] With patients spending less time in hospital, medical and nursing students were finding it harder to learn by the traditional apprenticeship style of training. It was found that students were not being sufficiently prepared. This concern combined with a growing insistence that students should not practise some clinical skills for the first time on patients. A different way of teaching was needed. The idea that patients were primarily 'teaching aids' had broken down as a new philosophy of medical education emerged in the postwar period. Educational theory had also shifted. Greater emphasis was placed on PBL, small-group and interactive teaching, with the GMC encouraging a move away from rote learning. The introduction of OSCEs encouraged students to spend more time learning clinical skills, and provision for SDL required new facilities and educational techniques.[93] At St Bartholomew's and The London a clinical skills course was designed to meet these needs and to integrate SDL and resource-based learning into the curriculum.

To secure resources for the new clinical skills course, work started on a clinical skills centre in 1991, adding an additional floor to the Robin Brook Centre. During the planning process, learning resources were evaluated and developed. From the start, an inter-professional model was adopted. Aware that healthcare was being increasingly organised into multidisciplinary teams, it was thought important to teach across professional boundaries. Cooperation was therefore secured from the College of Nursing and Midwifery using experience from the joint academic unit in medical education and the EMIS along with work in the College on medical informatics. Good relations between Lesley Rees and Sue Study at the College of Nursing led to the two bodies working together to create the centre as a facility. Here the College was ahead of the Department of Health, and at the time the move to

[91] J. S. Briggs et al., 'Training for Medical Teachers', Medical Education xxviii (1994), pp. 99–106.
[92] Jolly and Macdonald, 'Education for Practice', p. 194.
[93] Medical Education xxii (1988), pp. 200–4.

build a multi-professional training centre at St Bartholomew's was seen as revolutionary. Although tensions surfaced, work on the centre was one of the few programmes that sought to facilitate the 'joint education and training' being attempted at the time.[94] The new centre was modelled on the clinical skills laboratory at the University of Limburg in Maastricht, which had opened in 1975 as part of a new medical school based around a problem-based approach. After twelve years, the methods adopted at Maastricht were seen to work well and to raise skills performance. The centre at St Bartholomew's also borrowed from developments in the teaching of general practice, which had helped pioneer the use of simulated patients, teaching of communications skills and the use of video. It was the first of its kind in England and was trumpeted as pioneering, applying ideas as it did from Maastricht on how clinical and communications skills were taught at a practical level.

In the new centre, students could practice their clinical skills drawing on opportunities for creating simulated clinical encounters implied by the computer-assisted learning packages developed in the College. Students could use manikins (which were initially not of a high standard) in a 'safe environment' to gain confidence and experience before performing procedures on patients. In the communication elements, a combination of real patients with stable signs and actors were used to re-create clinical settings without overwhelming students or exposing patients to distress. Although an accepted procedure for teaching, the use of simulated patients had only gradually caught on in England. As studies argued that such an approach left students better equipped to face patients, greater use was made of these methods.[95] It was also believed that the use of simulated patients would provide an element of consistency suitable for use in an examination setting. With this in mind, the centre also provided a platform for OSCEs.[96] It was divided into a number of skills laboratories: one was set up as a mock ward environment; while another was designed for medical students to learn and practise clinical skills. An information technology training laboratory and communication skills suite formed integral parts of the new centre, reflecting the belief that communication was an essential component of every skill. The skills centre was felt to produce an environment in which a structured approach could be adopted in an interdisciplinary context.[97] Other teaching hospitals soon followed suit.

[94] *In the Patient's Interests, Multi-professional Working across Organisational Boundaries* (London, 1996); Hugh Barr and Ian Shaw, *Shared Learning* (London, 1995).

[95] J. Van Dalen, J. Zuidweg and J. Collett, 'The Curriculum of Communication Skills Teaching at Maastricht Medical School', *Medical Education* xxiii (1989), pp. 55–61; B. McAvoy, 'Teaching Clinical Skills to Medical Students', *Medical Education* xx (1988), p. 193.

[96] 1993 annual report, p. 12.

[97] Rees and Jolly, 'Medical Education', p. 247; Jane Dacre and M. Nicol, *Clinical Skills: The Learning Matrix for Students of Medicine and Nursing* (Oxford, 1996).

Not every department in the College was impressed with the centre but data were gradually collected which demonstrated that it had an impact on clinical competence.[98] Individual general practices were teamed with hospital firms to share the teaching of clinical skills. The move was driven by the problems associated with finding enough patients who stayed in hospitals long enough for students to examine, and by a desire to improve the relationship between general practitioners and hospital consultants. However, hopes that the centre would lead to a greater understanding and respect between medical and nursing students though an identification of common values were slower to emerge. Nor did students always make full use of the centre and, like others elsewhere, it was often underutilised.

Although the new curriculum had pre-empted and influenced *Tomorrow's Doctors*, the GMC's document went further than the CELC curriculum. Improvement was needed to achieve the level of integration, clinical exposure and choice offered. New arrangements were introduced for postgraduate and pre-registration training. In 1996, three years after the publication of the report, four-week clinical SSMs were adopted for fifth-year students to allow them to extend their experience and offer a guide for later careers. However, the College was aware that deficiencies remained. Not everyone was convinced of the value of the new CELC curriculum. Some departments worried about how little input staff from St Bartholomew's had had, while moves to assess departments on research encouraged some to neglect teaching. There were doubts about the utility of vertical integration, which was felt to reduce students' learning time, and about the relative reduction in the science content. Concerns were also expressed that a decrease in general teaching would force students to specialise too early.[99] Gaps emerged, and students voiced complaints about Phase 2. Further changes were made, committing the College to an ongoing process of adaptation. Planning was towards an erosion of the pre-clinical/clinical divisions with an increase in teaching in primary care.[100] However, by 1995 the Committee of Vice-chancellors and Principles acknowledged that St Bartholomew's and The London had 'one of the most modern curricula', with the College confident that it could provide 'academic leadership in curriculum development and in assessment and evaluation of courses'.[101]

---

[98] *BMJ* cccvii (1993), p. 1142.
[99] Joint Board of Studies of obstetrics and gynaecology, 25 June 1993, 10 April 1990, DF; Board of Studies in surgery, 17 November 1988, DF.
[100] College committee, 8 November 1994, MS 29/7.
[101] *Universities and the Health of the Nation* (London, 1995).

Epilogue

Tomlinson and merger

When Ian Kelsey Fry resigned as dean in 1987, it was felt that his successor would have to guide the College through a difficult period.[1] However, at first the situation looked positive. Sweeping reforms to how the University of London was managed promised to end the Byzantine and secretive structure, and delegate greater authority to the constituent colleges. Reforms in the National Health Service (NHS) saw more money directed into teaching hospitals as research and development was emphasised. The threat of a judicial review had given the College a strong hand and a determination to forge ahead with development. For Kelsey Fry, the move to set up the City and East London Confederation (CELC), which came into force in 1990, provided a period of peace and the means to build up the College as a way of protecting it. Under his leadership, and then under Lesley Rees, an opportunity was taken to reverse the planning blight that had affected the College during the protracted discussions in the 1970s and 1980s surrounding the possible merger of St Bartholomew's, The London and Queen Mary College (QMC). Able to develop her interest in medical education as sub-dean, Rees saw in the CELC 'an exciting opportunity to review and refine the philosophy, aims, structure and content of medical education'. She was less constrained by University politics. Rees encouraged a revision of the curriculum (see Chapter 12) and was keen to develop student facilities to maintain the College's corporate identity.[2]

First under Kelsey Fry, and then under Rees, 'much energy' went into 'planning for the development of the Faculty of Basic Medical Sciences . . . and for the design of the New Curriculum for the three . . . schools'.[3] Attention also turned to developing academic space at the Homerton Hospital, and to enlarging research and evidence-based medicine, a move that led to an explosion of research at Charterhouse. To publicise work in the College, William Harvey Day was established in 1990 to promote cross-fertilisation. New departments and research centres were formed, mainly on the initiative of the College after The London and QMC failed to express official interest in using Charterhouse.[4] Several interacting research groups were created and an Institute of Preventive Medicine, known as the Wolfson

---

[1] Report on the procedure for appointment of a new dean, 21 December 1987, DF.
[2] *Barts Journal*, December 1989, p. 3.
[3] Research selectivity exercise, 1989, DF.
[4] College committee, 4 May 1988, MS 29/8.

after the major benefactor, was established. However, plans for an 'innovation centre' (or science park) to 'facilitate the transfer of medical academic achievement to commercial reality', and for a centre for gastroenterology with St Mark's Hospital, had to be abandoned.[5]

Despite the number of projects realised, 1989/90 was a difficult period for the College as it entered the CELC, moved into new buildings, and introduced a new curriculum. The College had decided to join with The London and QMC in the CELC at the last moment at a time when The London and QMC were already pushing ahead with closer collaboration. This placed St Bartholomew's at a disadvantage. The London had undertaken much of the planning for the new faculty of medicine and for the basic medical science (BMS) building, which was included as an integral part of the CELC. It adopted principles that reflected its teaching practices and not necessarily those at St Bartholomew's. Tension between the pre-clinical and clinical staff, the latter welcoming the CELC as a means to redevelop the teaching and laboratory accommodation at Charterhouse, created additional problems for the College. In addition, the suggested level of funding was insufficient to support the new faculty. The unwillingness of the College to reduce student numbers ensured that vacancies went unfilled, so that BMS had one of the worst staff/student ratios in London. Although funding remained problematic, the pre-clinical staff finally moved from Charterhouse Square to the new BMS building at Mile End in July 1990.[6]

The move was greeted with mixed emotions. Over the next few years applications fell, reflecting the end of pre-clinical teaching in the College. Early impressions of BMS were good but were marred by power cuts. Only gradually were facilities for students added. It took longer to adjust to the 'us and them' mentality. The College and the Students' Union (SU) tried to minimise the loss of corporate identity but staff and students in BMS felt a sense of isolation from the rest of the College.[7] However, the CELC had no apparent detrimental effect on examination results: the College continued to rank at the top of the unofficial league table of London's medical schools.[8] A current of reform in the NHS and a growing desire to solve the problems facing the health service in London threatened this position.

NHS reforms and the weakening of medical education

NHS reforms in the 1970s and 1980s had given successive governments greater scope for action. More radical solutions to the perceived problems

---

[5] Ibid., 1 June 1988, 6 December 1989, MS 29/8.
[6] Ibid., 3 October 1990, 4 July 1990, MS 29/8.
[7] *Barts Journal*, spring 1991, p. 8; ibid., summer 1993, p. 7.
[8] College committee, 6 November 1991, MS 28/4.

in the NHS were suggested in the late 1980s, fuelled by rising public expectations about quality and access to treatment, and by scarce resources.[9] Although the continued popularity of the NHS prevented any attempt at privatisation, it could not escape from the Thatcherite doctrine of managed efficiency through competition, devolved budgets and the opportunity to opt out. The 1989 White Paper *Working for Patients* recommended the creation of fund-holding general practices and the introduction of an internal market. This new artificial market was to be divided between purchasers and providers of healthcare. Based on ideas borrowed from American health economists, purchasers and providers were to be linked by contracts and service agreements. The ideal was for money to follow the patient. Emphasis was placed on district services and community care, areas that had attracted increasing interest in the health service in the 1980s as a way of cutting expenditure and meeting local population needs. Hospitals were permitted to opt out of local authority control and apply for trust status, which would permit them to become independent 'service providers'. The hope was that trusts would become major sources of innovation.[10] The devolutionary approach favoured by *Working for Patients* was based on the desire for greater local authority but promised a return to the fragmentation of services that had characterised healthcare before 1939. These changes were embodied in the 1990 NHS and Community Care Act and were the most radical since the service was created in 1948.[11]

Reform provoked fierce opposition. Doctors moved to defend the NHS where they had previously been critical, only to find themselves excluded. Many feared that *Working for Patients* proposed placing financial considerations at the heart of clinical decisions.[12] However, the impact on medical education was initially uncertain. The University of London and the Joint Conference of Metropolitan and Provincial Deans supported the need for reform. They were aware that health authorities, given their size, disparate objectives and tendency to be swayed by politics, had been major obstacles to teaching. Yet they worried that resources for education and research would be starved to the detriment of the health service. At St Bartholomew's anxieties ran high.[13] The College predicted problems, especially over the internal market, and felt that *Working for Patients* would damage teaching and research. Although opinion was divided over the merits of a self-governing trust, those running the hospital felt that the strongest position was to

[9] Charles Webster, *Caring for Health* (Milton Keynes, 1993), p. 134.

[10] *Working for Patients. The Health Service Caring for the 1990s* (London, 1989).

[11] See Judith Allsop, 'Health: From Seamless Service to Patchwork Quilt', in *British Social Welfare*, ed. David Gladstone (London, 1995), pp. 98–123.

[12] Kathleen Jones, *The Making of Social Policy in Britain, 1830–1990* (London, 1991), p. 195.

[13] College committee, 3 May 1989, MS 29/8.

seek trust status. For the College, a trust was perceived as the best way of maintaining undergraduate and postgraduate teaching.[14]

Change was rapid. There was little opportunity for preparation, or for clear objectives to be devised. Teaching hospitals clamoured for trust status in a bid to return to the independence they had lost in 1974. The result was a 'mimic market', which it was anticipated would make the NHS more efficient. More managers were appointed, carrying forward the managerial tendencies present in NHS reorganisations since the 1970s. Without clear guidelines, health authorities and hospitals struggled to devise policies and implement change amidst public fears that the health service was not safe in the Conservative government's hands.[15]

NHS reform and further rationalisation weakened medical education in London. The creation of fund-holding general practitioners made hospital consultants more responsive to their interests, but London's teaching hospitals suffered under the internal market. More money for teaching and research was expected to allow teaching hospitals to compete with other general hospitals as the existing 'knock for knock' (informal cost sharing) arrangements were replaced by contracts. This did not always happen, however. Patient numbers rose, but funding remained static, leading to concerns about resource starvation as beds were closed. This had an immediate impact on teaching. The number of patients students were able to see fell to critical levels, forcing new strategies in an attempt to minimise the effect and greater use of district general hospitals for teaching. As the University Funding Council (UFC) recognised: 'the situation of the main teaching hospitals associated with some of the medical schools in inner London is sufficiently serious as to raise doubts about their future ability to deliver a viable educational programme, unless corrective action is taken.'[16] Fears grew that one or more of London's medical schools would face extinction as the internal market made the existing pattern of hospital services in London unsustainable. Extra cash was pumped into the capital's ailing health service and surveys were commissioned to investigate how the situation might be improved.

A 'savage shake-up of London's hospitals'

The King's Fund was the first to report in 1992. The support it expressed for a reduction in acute services was immediately attacked.[17] An inquiry appointed

---

[14] Joint conference of metropolitan and provincial deans, memorandum, April 1989, DF; College committee, 7 June 1989, 7 February 1990, MS 29/8.

[15] Rudolf Klein, *The New Politics of the NHS* (London, 1995), p. 184; Christopher Ham, Frank Honigsbaum and David Thompson, 'Priority Setting for Health Gain', in *Politics of the Welfare State*, ed. Ann Oakley and A. Susan Williams (London, 1994), p. 99.

[16] Cited in Angela Towle, *Undergraduate Medical Education: London and the Future* (London, 1992), p. 25.

[17] *London Health 2010 – The Report of the King's Fund London Initiative* (London, 1992).

by John Major's Conservative government into the structure of the NHS, research and education under Bernard Tomlinson, former chair of the Northern Regional Health Authority, also appeared in 1992. The decision to hold an inquiry had been made once it had become clear that at least one London teaching hospital might have to close. Major's government was trying to minimise the cost of reform, and the inquiry marked a volte-face to prevent the market from rationalising hospital services.[18] In the run-up to the report, teaching hospitals defended their position but reluctantly admitted the need for further rationalisation. Health specialists feared that in fighting a losing battle to save prized institutions, attention was being diverted from the real problems facing the health service in London.[19]

When the report was published in 1992, it was clear that Tomlinson had been impressed by the ideas expressed in the King's Fund report and returned to recommendations contained in the 1968 Todd report.[20] In arguing for managed rationalisation, the inquiry emphasised the need to improve primary and community care alongside a need to reduce the number of acute beds in central London. The Tomlinson' report anticipated that this would create a more equitable service. St Bartholomew's Hospital became Tomlinson's 'most spectacular' victim. Using arguments that central London had a low resident population and hence little need of a large hospital, the report recommended that St Bartholomew's, The London and the London Chest Hospital should merge 'with the orderly run-down and disposal of the Smithfield site' and the closure of the accident and emergency department in favour of developing services in Whitechapel. The Homerton was to be separated: a move that was interpreted as part of a deliberate attempt to close St Bartholomew's. Other hospitals in London were threatened, but the decision over St Bartholomew's came as a shock.[21]

While the hospital faced closure, the College was pushed towards a merger. Although the Tomlinson inquiry was not overly concerned with medical education, it did call for a reduction in student numbers and the amalgamation of the remaining free-standing medical schools with multi-faculty colleges. It was a policy supported by the Secretary of State of the Department of Education. The inquiry suggested that the College should be merged with The London and become a combined medical school at Queen Mary and Westfield College (QMW).[22] QMW had itself been created by the

---

[18] John Mohan, *A National Health Service? The Restructuring of Health Care in Britain since 1979* (London, 1995), p. 96.
[19] *Financial Times*, 8 October 1992, p. 13.
[20] *Report of the Inquiry into London's Health Service, Medical Education and Research* (London, 1992).
[21] *Guardian*, 18 November 1992, p. 15.
[22] *Inquiry into London's Health Service*.

merger of QMC and Westfield College in 1989.[23] Staff at the College and at
The London were at first in agreement that where a joint clinical school was
to be welcomed, a merger with QMW was not. Merger was felt to offer no
advantage over the CELC and it was strongly believed that separating
St Bartholomew's from the Homerton would be detrimental. QMW stated
that it did not to want to force the issue and agreed that the CELC was
working effectively.[24] The University also declined to support the findings of
the Tomlinson inquiry. It opposed ending the CELC and defended the
plurality of medical education in London.[25] However, Major's government,
without waiting to make decisions on hospital closures, accepted that
medical education should be concentrated at Imperial College, University
College, King's College and QMW.

The 'savage shake-up of London's hospitals' outlined in the Tomlinson
report generated furious condemnation.[26] At St Bartholomew's, the report
and the government's subsequent policy statements were attacked and
undermined. The local community and medical practitioners allied
themselves to the hospital. A local MP was clear: 'we know that, in losing
Bart's, we are losing access to a world-class facility'.[27] Although the hospital
had enemies, the Tomlinson report and Virginia Bottomley, the Minister of
Health responsible for implementing it, were widely attacked in 'the most
ferocious media war ever waged against health service managers and NHS
policy'.[28] A 'Save Bart's' campaign was organised, mobilising sections of the
press through a network of personal and professional contacts. The College
and students fought strenuously for the hospital, and for links with the
Homerton. Lesley Rees played a leading role in helping Michael Besser to
'save' St Bartholomew's, working with him to prepare counter-proposals that
outlined the hospital's future as a specialist unit. While debate raged, the
Department of Health prepared a policy review document. The future of
the College became enmeshed in these debates.

Tomlinson and the events surrounding it did much to damage St
Bartholomew's and its *esprit de corps*. Uncertainties about the future of the
hospital saw funding to the College from external bodies restricted. Research
students and staff were also discouraged from joining the College. Threats

---

[23] Westfield College had been founded in 1882 to provide residence and instruction in 'a
Christian context' for women prepared for University of London examinations. It was
admitted as a school of the University in 1902. In 1964, the Charter was amended to
admit men. In 1983 and 1984, a substantial part of the faculty of science was transferred
to QMC, and in 1989 the two colleges merged.

[24] College committee, 4 November 1992, MS 29/8; *Financial Times*, 24 October 1992,
p. 4.

[25] College committee, 4 November 1992, MS 29/8.

[26] *Daily Mirror*, 30 November 1992, p. 20.

[27] *Hansard*, 5 April 1995, p. 1742.

[28] Geoffrey Rivett, *From Cradle to Grave: Fifty Years of the NHS* (London, 1998), p. 441.

were made in an increasingly acrimonious and emotionally charged atmosphere. However, the power of the campaign to save St Bartholomew's presented Major's government with a dilemma. *Working for Patients* was designed to produce a rational decision-making structure not based on short-term political priorities. A decision to reprieve St Bartholomew's would look like capitulation. Amidst confusion and a sense of crisis, Bottomley partially backed down, a move the press attributed to public pressure and government fears of further embarrassments. When the policy review, *Making London Better*, was published in 1993, it granted the hospital a stay of execution. Three options were outlined: closure, a new trust with The London and the London Chest Hospital, or a move to create a small specialist hospital.[29] Bottomley remained committed to closing the accident and emergency department, however. She continued to argue that the decision about St Bartholomew's was not about finance, even though it was estimated to save £30 million annually, but about 'better specialist services' and meeting Londoners' needs.[30] Although *Making London Better* endorsed Tomlinson's findings in a modified form, it left a number of unresolved issues to the London Implementation Group. The decision was seen as an act of 'political cowardice', devolving responsibility for hospital closures from the Department of Health in an attempt to defuse an already 'acrimonious political debate'.[31] Consultation over the future of the hospital continued and the 'Save Bart's' campaign carried on fighting what it interpreted as a predetermined political agenda to close the hospital.

Whereas the Tomlinson report had only touched on medical education, *Making London Better* presented more detailed proposals. Although it recognised that the academic and research strengths of Charterhouse should be maintained, it stressed the need for 'further and sustained progress' on a merger. Plans were therefore put forward to amalgamate the College and The London with QMW, and University College Hospital with the Royal Free. Northeast Thames Regional Health Authority, of which the College and The London were a part, as well as Rees and Roy Duckworth, dean of The London, argued against *Making London Better*. They felt the CELC should be allowed to continue, 'particularly as one cycle of the new curriculum had not yet been completed'. However, the College's prospects were damaged by a decision by staff at The London to merge with QMW against Duckworth's wishes. Although he pointed to the potential of a 'closer relationship', some departments, especially on the pre-clinical side, saw the merger as a form of salvation to overcome the difficulties they were encountering. At a wider level, staff at The London felt that there was no certain 'future, even in the relatively short-term, for freestanding medical schools in the University . . .

[29] *Making London Better* (Manchester, 1993).
[30] *Hansard*, 5 April 1995, p. 1736.
[31] *Daily Mirror*, 17 January 1992, p. 2.

and there was a risk in trying to maintain such status'. They hoped that the College would join discussions.[32] It was a view shared by QMW. Although the Higher Education Funding Council for England (HEFCE) and the University of London claimed they would not force the College into a merger, they were clear that progress should be made.[33] In 1989, the University had supported the creation of academic clusters and links with multi-faculty institutions to limit the damage created by NHS cuts and rationalisation.[34] *Making London Better* made this vital. However, The London did not favour a union of the clinical schools. It argued that this would only delay a merger with QMW.

The College adopted a different approach. While it agreed to explore amalgamation with The London, it was hostile to QMW. Debates over amalgamation in the 1970s and 1980s, and the troubled relationship between the College and QMC, had left a legacy of ill-feeling on both sides. In addition, the College saw QMW as a weak institution, a poor relation in the University. The College felt that the CELC had produced an innovative curriculum and that a merger with QMW would not be advantageous to teaching or research. The College also worried that if QMW made a bid to become a separate university it would also lose the ability to confer University of London degrees.[35] A working party under Sir Michael Palliser, chairman of the CELC, was formed with The London to discuss these ideas.

Merger

However, there was little room for manoeuvre. Managers of the hospital, in a bid to prevent closure, had decided to join with The London and the London Chest Hospital in a trust as recommended in *Making London Better*. The *Guardian* interpreted this as surrender; others as a plausible survival plan.[36] By embracing the proposal, clinical services could be continued at West Smithfield, a move that delighted the College. With closer links being forged between the three hospitals as trust status was pursued, and with outside pressure to merge with The London and QMW, the College was left in a poor position. Staff morale was low. The future of the West Smithfield site remained precarious, and plans to replace the casualty department with a minor injuries unit created significant problems for senior house officer and pre-registration posts. Funding cuts and cancelled operations were also damaging clinical teaching.

---

[32] College committee, 3 March 1993, 3 June 1993, MS 29/8.
[33] HEFCE was successor to the UFC and had been created in 1992.
[34] University of London, *The Best Medicine for London* (London, 1989).
[35] College committee, 3 June 1993, MS 29/8.
[36] *Guardian*, 18. February 1993, p.2.

The College felt bullied. Although initially the HEFCE was not prepared to force through the Tomlinson report and *Making London Better*, it did press for a joint development plan. Other forces were at work. Many of the grant-awarding bodies increasingly preferred to fund research in a multi-faculty environment, while QMW and The London were anxious for the merger to go ahead. QMW felt that neither the College nor The London would be able to compete in an environment where 'enormously powerful amalgamations and unions are taking shape'. QMW did admit that it would derive considerable benefit, but argued that a merger was the natural outcome of the 1968 Todd report and the creation of the CELC in 1990. The College was adamant that there had been 'no suggestion whatsoever that the new Confederation was the first stage of a process leading to merger'.[37] It continued to press for a federal structure but agreed to enter discussions to explore the practical implications of a merger. A hard-fought and controversial compromise was reached that committed the College to a merger with QMW largely because The London, fearful of the College, had refused to contemplate uniting the two clinical schools ahead of an amalgamation with QMW. In agreeing to a merger, the College noted that it had been 'mindful of its duty to honour the inheritance of the . . . past, its duty to . . . present staff and students and its duty to ensure that the College handed over to the [school] sound strategies for the future'.[38] Negotiations were begun to include the Eastman Dental Institute as part of the new school, and regular meetings were organised in the College to discuss developments. Implementation was aided by the prospect of additional funding from the HEFCE, which had set aside £50 million to help meet the aims of *Making London Better*.[39] Three faculties were created in basic medical sciences, clinical medicine and clinical dentistry ahead of the merger, and renewed interest was expressed in the need for joint departments to help bring teaching into line.[40]

During discussions relations between QMW and St Bartholomew's deteriorated further. Staff in the College felt that QMW showed little sensitivity and that the merger was being push through to match a political agenda in the health service. Many became despondent. They feared a takeover by The London and suspected that staff there wanted to see St Bartholomew's closed so that a new hospital could be built at Whitechapel. It was a policy favoured by the shadow NHS trust, and ill-advised statements in the press appeared to confirm these fears. Suspicion grew in all three institutions, with staff at QMW expressing reservation and anxiety about the role the College would seek to play in the new school. Difficulties were encountered between the schools over the name of the new institution,

---

[37] Rees to Rutherford, 11 April 1995, Merger Bill, DF.
[38] Special meeting of the governors, 9 November 1994, MS 27/5.
[39] College committee, 5 October 1994, MS 29/8.
[40] Ibid., 4 May 1994, MS 29/8.

which was eventually fixed at 'St Bartholomew's and the Royal London Hospital School of Medicine and Dentistry'. The selection of a new warden to run the institution soured relations further. The appointment of Colin Berry, dean of The London, as warden over Rees did not find favour at St Bartholomew's and polarised the institutions. Rees had worked hard to provide the best possible base for the new school and expressed confidence that it could be a success. Staff in the College became disenchanted, and voiced anxiety about the level of consultation and what they considered to be a 'lack of vision'. The Eastman was equally troubled, pulling out of discussions at the last minute. Rumours that Charterhouse had a limited future were denied and assurances were sought that 'academically successful departments' would not be transferred until corresponding facilities existed at QMW. The retention and attraction of staff became difficult. The continuing uncertainties about the future of the hospital and rumours of rationalisation and redundancies only increased anxiety. Rees was aware that the College was in an 'unstable position'.[41]

Opposition to the merger persisted: the SU looked for assurances but recognised that the result by 1994 was a foregone conclusion. Those most opposed to the merger, or worried about the implications of the Tomlinson report, started to resign. All were felt to be a 'significant loss to the new School' and produced anxiety at QMW and St Bartholomew's.[42] While the College continued to express reservations and worried about the future of hospital services in West Smithfield, it was recognised by QMW and The London that in hindsight 'many mistakes had been made'.[43]

To secure the merger of the three institutions legislation was required: a merger bill was drawn up under which the College's 1921 Charter of incorporation was revoked and Charterhouse transferred to an independent trust managed by the College. The bill quickly ran into difficulties. The College was accused of not being committed 'in the way the rest of us are', and of 'using the Bill as an opportunity to decided whether or not' to proceed.[44] A degree of bullying was suspected and anxieties existed on both sides. In the House of Commons, the bill became caught up in the fight to save St Bartholomew's. Attacks became personal and accusations were made about the 'well intentioned but uninspiring' management at QMW.[45] Efforts were made to dispel the notion that a merger and what was happening in the newly formed Royal Hospitals' NHS Trust constituted a takeover by The London. Despite reassurances from the Secretary of State for health that the

[41] Ibid., 8 November 1994, 5 April 1995, MS 29/8.
[42] Ibid., 5 April 1995, MS 29/8.
[43] Ibid., 7 December 1994, 4 October 1995, MS 29/8.
[44] Merger implementation committee correspondence, DF; College Council, 1 November 1994.
[45] *Hansard*, 19 April 1995, p. 290; ibid., 5 April 1995, pp. 1736–46.

'Barts ethos' and culture would 'be preserved', the support that continued to be expressed for concentrating acute and specialist services at Whitechapel increased tension.[46] BMS also faced uncertainty as rumours circulated of restructuring in the faculty. By January 1995, the potential exodus of 'able people from Bart's' was 'widening and deepening' and the SU was expressing fears of dilution.[47] Even when difficulties had been smoothed over and the bill was allowed to proceed, delays occurred. It was not until November 1995 that the bill finally received the Royal ascent.

St Bartholomew's Medical College was formally dissolved on 7 November 1995 and the new school came into being the following day. Doubts continued over the nature of the hospital's future. A reception was organised in December to mark the end of the College. Personal tributes were paid to Rees, and it was felt that the new school had 'an optimistic and bright future'.[48] However, the merger had come at a high cost that left a legacy of ill-feeling and resentment.

Retrospect

The merger of the College with The London and QMW in 1995 was felt to mark the end of an era, and of an institution. During debates over the merger, the College was seen as a traditional, conservative institution, one which had a very different ethos from that of The London or QMW. Both feared that the College would try to dominate the new school and impose its perceived values.

Part of the problem arose from a confusion of hospital and college: the two were often seen as synonymous. Although relations were at times strained, and disputes emerged over who should control teaching, from the early nineteenth century the College had regularly appealed to the hospital's governors in its attempt to extend teaching accommodation. Consequently, the College had come to play an important role in shaping clinical services at St Bartholomew's, in particular through the introduction of new specialties and the development of laboratory accommodation. At the same time, the hospital's governors acquired a stake in how the College was run and resourced. The creation of the NHS in 1948, and the privileged position of St Bartholomew's as a teaching hospital in the new service, blurred the boundaries yet further. Clinical services and teaching needs often became inseparable, especially in relation to the district and region. There was a considerable overlap of staff, with the College playing an active role in the hospital's management. However, although the College became immersed in

---

[46] College committee, 5 April 1995, MS 29/8.
[47] Merger implementation committee correspondence, DF.
[48] College committee, 1 November 1995, MS 29/8.

some of the traditions and ethos of the hospital, it had a different history, one intimately connected with the nature of medical education in London, with the development of academic medicine in the University, and with the state, leading to tensions that were not easily resolved. It was this history, the personalities involved and the notions of academic medicine adopted that influenced the development of a corporate identity and gave the College its character.

Although the presence of medical students was first noted in the seventeenth century, it was in the eighteenth century that formal teaching and a medical school began to emerge at St Bartholomew's. A product of a transition from book-learning to bedside instruction, of the growing market for medicine and medical knowledge, and of individual initiatives, St Bartholomew's under the influence of John Abernethy became an important part of the metropolitan educational community. As such, it reflected an institutional style of training that was adopted across London's medical schools but one that was relative slow to emerge in the hospital. The College became part of the London lecturing empire, a bastion of the medical establishment. However, it was shaped by fears of competition and the need to deliver lecturers and courses that matched student demand and the requirements of the examining boards. These two external forces were to continue to play a central role in the College's history. This ensured that the instruction underwent regular adaptation as the College modified its teaching to reflect the demands of the examining bodies, and to take account of changing ideas and constructions of medicine and treatment.

Concerns about competition with other medical schools intensified in the period following Abernethy's death in 1830. Abernethy had not only given the College its institutional form, but his difficult and domineering personality had also led to tensions. Without Abernethy, the College declined at a time when medical education was experiencing a period of rationalisation. Fears of competition, an awareness in the mid-1840s that the College had reached a low point, and changes to ideas about learning, forced reform. Although the style of teaching did not dramatically change, new subjects were added and the College sought to impose a system of discipline and academic standards that had much in common with the style of education associated with Oxbridge.

Reform and rebuilding ensured that by the 1880s the College had become the largest school in London, adopting a model of training that was to ally it closely with the academic ethos of the University of London. It was an alliance that had benefits for the College, as it increasingly matched its teaching and administration to reflect the University's MB BS examination. The College became a staunch advocate of university medicine and in the twentieth century repeatedly reaffirmed the need for medical education to be conducted in a university atmosphere. The College conceived itself as an important institution in the University, although for contemporaries and reformers it was University College Hospital that was intimately associated with the university ideal. However, in the late nineteenth century few could doubt that the College had become a central institution in the development of London medicine and medical education; a position which was to earn it a degree of enmity a hundred years later.

Although the College moved closer to the University, its position also encouraged complacency, pointing to continuities in the structure of teaching and mentalities in the College that were only gradually eroded in the late nineteenth and early twentieth centuries. A series of attacks in the early nineteenth century had labelled St Bartholomew's as conservative, a defender of the status quo, accusations that were to be repeated in the 1970s, 1980s and 1990s. In the late nineteenth century, there was some truth to these accusations. Staff in the College defended the medical establishment and retained a traditional style of bedside instruction that found favour with the patrician medical class. They were resistant to adopting an experimental and laboratory approach, advocating a clinical art that reacted slowly to the shift in attitudes on the content of training. A strong individualistic and empirical outlook ensured that old practices continued at the bedside and in the lecture theatre, pointing to continuities in experience and training. Although the paradigm of bedside instruction found apparent favour with students, staff in the College were forced to adapt by the licensing bodies. Change was prompted by a growing interest in pathology (and bacteriology) as an aid to diagnosis. When linked to external pressure from the licensing bodies, this promoted a more scientific approach to medicine and training. Initially, this was limited to pre-clinical teaching, setting up divisions with the clinical staff that later were to frustrate the development of pre-clinical teaching. The College, like many other schools in London, was initially caught somewhere between a traditional, empirical approach and one characterised by the laboratory.

Although divisions between an empirical approach and one associated with the laboratory remained in the first half of the twentieth century, debates over the structure of the University of London and the nature of medical education saw the College move closer to the academic, scientific model favoured by reformers. Reworking debates on academic medicine to reflect the realities of London medical education, the clinical teaching and the intellectual organisation of the College were rethought. The value of research was emphasised and moves made to adopt a clinical, academic model that attempted to integrate laboratory medicine with the clinic. Using money from the recently formed University Grants Committee (UGC), in 1919 the College established the first two clinical units headed by full-time professors in London, marking a modern approach that was widely applauded. By the 1920s, academic clinical units were seen as the desired goal in medical education and a number of units had been established by London's teaching hospitals. The units at St Bartholomew's sought to embody values of scientific, academic medicine and research that had emerged in the College and in debates on medical education from the 1890s onwards.

In the interwar period, the units at St Bartholomew's (or elsewhere) did not bring about the immediate fusion of medicine with science that had been foreseen by the College, UGC or by reformers. An academic style of medicine had been accepted, but financial problems in the early 1920s ensured that the optimistic schemes for reconstruction in the College were never fully implemented. Problems first encountered in the late nineteenth century of how to include new specialties in an already overburdened curriculum, hospital and school re-emerged. However, in the interwar period the outpatient clinic was seen as one part of the solution, with the College developing links with other institutions to provide the facilities it could not. It was a model that was to be extended under the NHS. Tension also existed between those who saw the College as a teaching institution and those who wanted to encourage research. Traditional patterns of clinical training and a clinical, gentlemanly ethos were fitfully merged with the academic and laboratory ideal represented by the units. Staff defended their own fields and a focus on academic and clinical medicine restricted the pre-clinical departments. It was not until 1930 that agreement was reached over the need to rethink pre-clinical teaching. In moving the pre-clinical departments to Charterhouse Square, teaching was revitalised, but the result proved a mixed blessing, heralding tensions that were to resurface after 1945.

Although a fragile consensus on the desired nature of medical education had emerged by the late 1930s, change was cut short by war in 1939. War proved a harrowing experience for the College. Staff and students adapted to being dispersed, but severe bomb damage threatened the future of the College. Planning for reconstruction became entangled in debates about a national health service and the postwar shape of medical education. Once more, a university model of training was defended. Outside the College, an academic model of medicine was endorsed by the 1944 Goodenough report on medical education, returning to ideas expressed before 1914.

War created a new mood of social expectation, seemingly embodied in the creation of the NHS and the renewed expansion of universities. However, the immediate postwar years were not 'golden years' for the College. As teaching hospitals adapted (financially and culturally) to the NHS, debate focused on achieving an integrated curriculum in an academic framework to fulfil the ideas outlined in the Goodenough report. How integration was to be reconciled with the existing curriculum and the nature of healthcare in London was less certain.

The College adapted to the NHS and tried to match reconstruction to efforts to implement those aspects of the Goodenough report that had not already been adopted. It underwent a troubled renaissance and worked to re-establish services and create new departments. Although efforts were made to develop a research culture and revise teaching, rebuilding throughout the 1950s and 1960s disturbed teaching, delayed expansion and strained resources. Ambitious schemes adopted by other teaching hospitals were not attempted in favour of returning the college to its prewar level. In comparison to other London teaching hospitals, facilities in the College remained overstretched, while the extension of educational links with non-teaching hospitals was not enough to solve problems in clinical teaching. Some of the dynamism of the first half of the twentieth century was lost and it was only in the 1960s that the College reclaimed some of the ground lost through the war.

By 1966, a feeling existed in the College that it needed to be reorganised to reflect changing patient, doctor and student needs. This was coupled with efforts to rethink the curriculum as the nature of university education was revised. However, while the college's submission to the Todd Commission echoed wider debates in medical education, the report's recommendations that the College merge with The London and become part of the multi-faculty environment at QMC raised questions about its future. The circular and difficult discussions about a possible merger were to dominate the College's history for the next twenty-five years, resulting in a planning blight and a defence of the College's position that many saw as confirmation that it was a traditional, conservative institution.

The Todd report split the College. At one level, it continued to adapt teaching and promote reform to reflect ideas on medical education pioneered elsewhere. Curriculum reform led to new modes of assessment, the development of general practice teaching, and research into medical education and the technology of learning. Efforts were also made to develop the College's research culture and it became highly successful in attracting outside funding. These ideas clashed with the more traditional approaches in the College, but the curriculum and teaching methods introduced with the CELC were by 1995 considered to be one of the most modern.

However, the implications of the Todd report also threatened the College, which was pressed increasingly into accepting a merger with The London and QMC. In the process, the College suffered from a blight that frustrated development. The divide between the pre-clinical and clinical departments, already present in the interwar period, became more pronounced as each had a slightly different conception of how the College should develop. Although the College continued to accept the importance of an academic model of medicine, relations with the University and UGC deteriorated, prompting the threat of a judicial review that sent 'shivers through the academic medical world' and challenged the authority of the UGC.[49] The College could accept a university model and the need for cooperation with The London, provided it retained its independence, protected Charterhouse, and did not mean working with QMC. The forced compromise in the CELC proved short-lived, but represented a period of innovation and growing cooperation (in some areas) with The London. The Tomlinson report and the 'savage shake-up of London's hospitals' upset this balance. Together, they forced the pace of change and deepened the sense of crisis, a process that led to a merger which left all sides with concerns.

[49] *Hansard*, 19 April 1995, p. 286.

The College's history therefore represents not only internal forces and traditions, but also the nature of medical education in London and the pressures exerted on it. It is one where the College's identity and way of doing things was shaped by competition, curriculum demands, and the growing intervention of the state in healthcare and medical education. Tradition was represented in a series of continuities and set of values associated with the College's position in the medical establishment and the defence of its independence within the University of London. However, for much of its history, the College remained a number of institutions. At one level, it was conservative and defended an approach that applauded bedside medicine and the teaching of clinical skills through apprenticeship. It was an approach that upheld the art of medicine and reflected the opposition of London's teaching hospitals to too much academic direction, their self-confidence, and their independence. At another, the College adopted an academic model and sought to reform the curriculum to reflect (if sometimes belatedly) changing ideas on medical education. In doing so, the College became an important part of university medical education in London, but one all too often misrepresented and labelled as conservative.

Select bibliography

Unpublished primary sources

St Bartholomew's Hospital archives, West Smithfield, London
Records of St Bartholomew's Medical School (MS)
Records of St Bartholomew's Medical School: Deans' Files (DF)
Records of St Bartholomew's Hospital
Records of the Abernethian Society (SA)
Records of the Cambridge Graduate Club (SC)
Records of the Students' Union (SU)
Diary of George Saunders, 1841–78 (X5/17)
George Dance's plans for lecture theatre, 1791 (X5/12)
G. W. Mackenzie lecture notes, 1845–6 (X48)
James Matthews Duncan, miscellaneous letters
Journal of Ludford Harvey, 1804–26 (X54/1)
Journal of William Meacher, 1887 (X55)
Julia Smith, 'A glimpse of my life at St. Bartholomew's' (X5/25)
Notebook of Edward Stanley, 1837–48 (X/16)
Medical students at St Bartholomew's, 1839–59 (X5/18–20)
Memoirs of William Henry Cross, 1866–1905 (X5/26)
Papers of Sir Dyce Duckworth (X45)
Press-cuttings (X19)
Queen Victoria' visit, 1869 (X5/21)
Resignation speech of Luther Holden, 1871 (X5/22)
Shuter to Graham (X64)
W. Thomas lecture notes, 1817–18 (X50)
St Bartholomew's Hospital Journal
St Bartholomew's Hospital Reports
College Calendar
Holmes Coote, MS *Notes on Anatomy and Physiology* (1847)
William Girling Ball, 'The History of the Medical College of St Bartholomew's Hospital' (1941)
—— 'Autobiography' (typescript)
—— Scrapbook
Herbert Williamson, MS *Lectures on Midwifery and Gynaecology* (1904)

Archives and Manuscripts (Wellcome), Wellcome Library for the Understanding of Medicine, 18 Euston Road, London
London student notebook (MS 6922)

'Notes of Andrew Thynne's lectures on midwifery', 1804–7 (MS 4788)
'Notes of Mr Abernethy's lectures', 1808–9 (MS 5600)
'Notes of Lectures delivered by Mr Abernethy', 1814 (MS 5606)
Papers of Anthony Alfred Bowlby (GC/181)
Papers of George Newman (MS 6201–6)
Papers of George Pickering (PP/GWP)
Papers of James Paget (MS 5702–5)
Papers of Thomas Lewis (PP/LEW)
Percival Pott, 'Lectures on surgery', c.1770 (MS 3957)
Records of the Medical Women's Federation (SA/MWF)
Records of the Royal College of Physicians 'Younger Fellows Club', 1940–43
    (GC/186/3)
Records of the Society for Social Medicine (SA/SSM)
Sir Lauder Brunton notes, 5 vols (MS 5966–70)
Royal Commission on Medical Education (SA/CME)

Guildhall Library (Guildhall), Aldermanbury Road, London
Merchant Taylors' Company court minutes, 1922–33

Royal London Hospital archive and museum, St Augustine with St Philip's
    Church, Newark Street, London
Records of the Royal London School of Medicine

**London Metropolitan Archive (LMA), Northampton Road, Clerkenwell,
    London**
Records of Friern Hospital (H12/CH)
Records of the King's Fund (KE)
Records of the LCC (LCC)

Imperial College, London
Papers of Henry Armstrong (B/Armstrong)

Public Record Office (PRO), Kew
Records of the Board of Education (ED)
Records of the Medical Research Council (FD)
Records of the Ministry of Health (MH)
Records of the University Grants Committee (UGC)

Royal College of Physicians, St Andrew's Place, Regent's Park, London
Casebook of Peter Mere Latham (MSS 393–94, 396)
Dyce Duckworth, 'Some Requirements for Modern Clinical Teaching' (MS
    695)
Papers of Samuel Gee (MS 32–43)

Royal College of Surgeons, Lincoln's Inn Fields, London
Papers of Geoffrey Keynes: National blood transfusion service
Papers of William Lawrence

University of London Library (ULL), Senate House, Malet Street, London
Records of the University of London

Official documents and publications (in date order)

SC on Anatomy, PP (1828) viii
SC on Medical Education, PP (1834) xiii
RC on Oxford, PP (1852) xxii
Report of the RC on the Practice of Subjecting Live Animals to Experiments for Scientific Purposes, PP (1876) xli
RC on Grant of Medical Degrees, PP (1882) xxix
RC on a University for London, PP (1889) xxxix
SC of the House of Lords on Metropolitan Hospitals, etc., First Report, PP (1890) xvi
RC to Consider the Draft Charter for the Proposed Gresham University in London, PP (1894) xxxiv
RC on Medical Education in London; Third Report, PP (1911) xx; *Fifth Report*, PP (1912) xxii; *Final Report*, PP (1913) xl
Report of the Inter-Departmental Committee on Medical Schools (London, 1944)
Report of the Committee of Enquiry into the Cost of the National Health Service (London, 1956)
Report of the Committee to Consider the Future Numbers of Medical Practitioners and the Appropriate Intake of Medical Students (London, 1957)
Report of the RC on Medical Education (London, 1968)
Patients First. Consultative Paper on the Structure and Management of the National Health Service in England and Wales (London, 1979)
Towards a Balance (London, 1980)
Promoting Better Health. The Government's Programme for Improving Primary Health Care (London, 1987)
Working for Patients. The Health Service caring for the 1990s (London, 1989)
Report of the Inquiry into London's Health Service, Medical Education and Research (London, 1992)
Making London Better (Manchester, 1993)

Newspapers and periodicals

Archives of the Roetengen Ray
Association Medical Journal

Blackwood
British Journal of Medical Education
British Journal of Nursing
British Journal of Radiology
British Medical Journal
Changes in Medical Education
Charity Organisation Review
Citizen
City Press
Contemporary Review
Daily Mirror
Daily Sketch
Daily Telegraph
Dial
Edinburgh Medical Journal
Evening Standard
Financial Times
Gentleman's Magazine
Guardian
Hospital
Independent
Journal of Mental Science
Journal of the Sanitary Institute
Lancet
London Medical and Physical Journal
London Medical Gazette
London University Gazette
Medical Education
Medical Times and Gazette
Medical Press and Circular
Medico-Chirurgical Review
Morning Post
Pall Mall Gazette
Proceedings of the Abernethian Society
Proceedings of the Society of Medicine
Provincial Medical and Surgical Journal
Punch
Saturday Review
Sunday Times
Surgery
Telegraph
The Times
Times Education Supplement
Times Higher Education Supplement

Pre-1948 printed publications

The Amalgamated Clubs of St Bartholomew's Hospital, 1893–4 (London, 1893)

Annual Report of the Medical Officer of the Local Government Board (London, 1896)

Annual Report of the Ministry of Health (London, 1934–5)

Committee Reports of the Royal College of Physicians (London, 1942–7)

Interim Report of the Departmental Committee on Maternal Mortality and Morbidity (London, 1930)

Maternal Mortality Report (London, 1934)

Medical Education in London: Being a Guide to the Schools of the University of London in the Faculty of Medicine (London, 1908)

A Memoir of Howard Marsh (London, 1921)

Memorandum on the Training of Medical Students in Midwifery and Gynaecology (London, 1932)

Methods and Problems of Medical Education, 7th series (New York, 1930)

Proposed New Medical College Buildings (London, 1942)

Report of the Department of Pathological Chemistry of University College London, New Series, 1896–1902

UGC Report. Academic Year 1928–29 (London, 1930)

Abernethy, John, *Surgical and Physiological Essays* (London, 1793)

—— *Reflections on Gall and Spruzheim's System of Physiognomy and Phrenology* (London, 1821)

Armstrong, Henry, *The Teaching of Scientific Method and Other Papers on Education* (London, 1925)

Atlay, J. B., *Sir Henry Wentworth Acland* (London, 1903)

Blackwell, Elizabeth, *Pioneer Work in Opening the Medical Profession to Women: Autobiographic Sketches* (London, 1895)

Bowlby, Anthony A., *Surgical Pathology and Morbid Anatomy* (London, 1887)

Brockbank, Edward Mansfield, *The Foundation of Provincial Medical Education in England and of the Manchester School in Particular* (Manchester, 1936)

Burrows, George, *Introductory Lecture to a Course on Forensic Medicine, delivered in the Anatomical Theatre of St Bartholomew's Hospital* (London, 1831)

Butlin, Henry, *Diseases of the Joints* (London, 1886)

—— *On the Operative Surgery of Malignant Disease* (London, 1887)

Campbell Thomson, H., *The Story of the Middlesex Medical School* (London, 1935)

Christison, Robert, *Life of Robert Christison*, 3 vols (London, 1885/6)

Cobb, Frances Power, 'Medicine and Morality', *Modern Review* xi (1881), p. 323

Coote, Holmes, *On Joint Diseases; Their Pathology, Diagnosis and Treatment Including the Nature and Treatment of Deformities, and Curvatures of the Spine* (London, 1867)

Davies, Richard, *General State of Education in the Universities* (Bath, 1759)

Duckworth, Dyce, *Knowledge and Wisdom in Medicine* (London, 1902)

—— *The Chirurgical Works of Percival Pott* (London, 1790)

Earle, James, ed., *The Chirurgical Works of Percival Pott. To which are added, a short account of the life of the author* (London, 1775)

—— ed., *The Chirurgical Works of Percival Pott* (London, 1790 edn)

Farre, Frederick, *On Self-Culture and the Principles to be Observed in the Study of Medicine* (London, 1849)

Feltoe, Charles Lett, *Memoirs of John Flint South* (London, 1884)

Flexner, Abraham, *Medical Education in the United States and Canada* (New York, 1910)

—— *Medical Education in Europe: A Report to the Carnegie Foundation for the Advancement of Teaching* (New York, 1912)

—— *I Remember: The Autobiography of Abraham Flexner* (New York, 1940)

Foster, Michael, *On Medical Education at Cambridge* (London, 1878)

Gairdner, William T., *On Medicine and Medical Education* (Edinburgh, 1858)

Gee, Samuel, *Medical Lectures and Aphorisms* (London, 1902)

Girling Ball, William, *St Bartholomew's Hospital in the 'Blitz'* (London, 1943)

Grey Glover, James, *The Gaps in Medical Education: Considered in the Light of the Reports of the Inspectors and Examinations of the Medical Council* (London, 1889)

Halliburton, W. D., ed., *Physiology and National Needs* (London, 1919)

Harris, Vincent Dormer and D'Arcy Power, *Manual for the Physiological Laboratory* (London, 1880)

Herringham, Wilmot Parker, Archibald Garrod and W. J. Gow, *A Handbook of Medical Pathology, for the Use of Students in the Museum of St Bartholomew's Hospital* (London, 1894)

Holden, Luther, *Landmarks, Medical and Surgical* (London, 1876)

Horder, Mervyn, *The Little Genius: A Memoir of the First Lord Horder* (London, 1966)

Horder, Thomas, *Clinical Pathology in Practice: With a Short Account of Vaccine-therapy* (London, 1910)

Jex-Blake, Sophia, *Medical Women: A Thesis and a History* (Edinburgh, 1886)

Kanthack, Alfredo A. and John H. Drysdale, *A Course of Elementary Practical Bacteriology: Including Bacteriological Analysis and Chemistry* (London, 1895)

Keetley, Charles Bell, *The Student's and Junior Practitioner's Guide to the Medical Profession* (London, 1885)

Kershaw, Richard, *Special Hospitals: Their Origin, Development and Relationship to Medical Education; Their Economic Aspects and Relative Freedom from Abuse* (London, 1909)

Keynes, George, *Blood Transfusion* (London, 1922)

Klein, Edward Emanuel *Micro-organisms and Disease: An Introduction to the Study of Specific Micro-organisms* (London, 1896)

Latham, Peter Mere, *Lectures on Subjects Connected with Clinical Medicine* (London, 1836)

—— *Lectures on Subjects Connected with Clinical Medicine, comprising Diseases of the Heart* (London, 1846)

Lauder Brunton, Thomas, *Textbook of Pharmacology, Therapeutics and Materia Medica* (London, 1885)

Lawrence, William, *Lectures on Surgery, Medical and Operative* (London, 1832)

—— *A Treatise on the Diseases of the Eye* (London, 1844)

—— *Hunterian Oration* (London, 1846)

Lockwood, Charles B., *Aseptic Surgery* (London, 1896)

Lucas, James, *A Candid Inquiry into the Education, Qualifications and Offices of a Surgeon-Apothecary* (Bath, 1800)

MacAlister, Edith F., *Sir Donald Macalister of Tarbert* (London, 1935)

Macilwain, George, *The Memoirs of John Abernethy* (London, 1856)

McWhinnie, Andrew M., *Introductory Address Delivered at St Bartholomew's Hospital on the Opening of the Medical Session, October 1st, 1856* (London, 1856)

Marsh, Howard, *Diseases of the Joints* (London, 1886)

Marshall, William Barrett, *An Essay on Medical Education* (London, 1827)

Martindale, Louisa, *The Woman Doctor and her Future* (London, 1922)

Miles, Alexander, *A Guide to the Study of Medicine* (London, 1925)

Moore, Norman, *Pathological Anatomy of Disease: Arranged According to the Nomenclature of Diseases of the Royal College of Physicians of London* (London, 1889)

—— *Principles and Practice of Medicine* (London, 1893)

—— *The History of the Study of Medicine in the British Isles* (Oxford, 1908)

Newman, George, *Bacteria, Especially as they are Related to the Economy of Nature, to Industrial Processes, and to the Public Health* (London, 1900)

—— *Infant Mortality: A Social Problem* (London, 1906)

—— *Some Notes on Medical Education in England: A Memorandum Addressed to the President of the Board* (London, 1918)

—— *Recent Advances in Medical Education in England* (London, 1923)

—— *An Outline of the Practice of Preventive Medicine: A Memorandum Addressed to the Minister of Health* (London, 1926)

—— *The Foundations of National Health* (London, 1928)

—— and Harold Swithinbank, *Bacteriology of Milk* (London, 1903)

Oppenheimer, Jane M., *New Aspects of John and William Hunter* (London, 1946)

Paget, Stephen, ed., *Memoirs and Letters of Sir James Paget* (London, 1901)

Parkinson, James, *The Hospital Pupil; or, an Essay Intended to Facilitate the Study of Medicine and Surgery* (London, 1800)

Pettigrew, Thomas Joseph, *Medical Portrait Gallery*, 2 vols (London, 1838–40)

Power, D'Arcy, *British Masters of Medicine* (London, 1936)

Pye, Walter and Thomas Lauder Brunton, 'Action of *Erythrophleum guinense*', *Philosophical Transactions* clxvii (1877), p. 627

Rigby, Edward, *On the Constitutional Treatment of Female Diseases* (London, 1857)

Rivington, Walter, *The Medical Profession* (Dublin, 1888)

Rosen, George, *The Specialisation of Medicine with Particular Reference to Ophthalmology* (New York, 1944)

Ross, Ronald, *Memoirs: With a Full Account of the Great Malaria Problem and its Solution* (London, 1923)

Royal College of Physicians Planning Committee, *Report on Medical Education* (London, 1944)

Sharpey-Schafer, Edward, *History of the Physiological Society During its First Fifty Years, 1876–1926* (London, 1927)

Skey, Frederick Carpenter, *The Principles and Practice of Operative Surgery* (London, 1858)

—— *Hysteria: Remote Causes of Disease in General Treatment of Disease by Tonic Agency Local or Surgical Forms of Hysteria*, 2nd edn (London, 1867)

Sprigge, Samuel Squire, *Life and Times of Thomas Wakley* (London, 1897)

—— *Some Considerations of Medical Education* (London, 1910)

—— *Physics and Fiction* (London, 1921)

Stanley, Edward, *A Manual of Practical Anatomy, For the Use of Students Engaged in Dissections* (London, 1822)

Strangeways, T. S. P. and F. L. Hopwood, 'Effects of X-rays upon Mitotic Cell Division', *Proceedings of the Royal Society* c (1926), p. 283

Thorne Thorne, Richard, 'Aetiology, Spread and Prevention of Diphtheria', *Journal of the Sanitary Institute* xv (1894), pp. 7–20

University of London, *Report of the Academic Council on Medical Education of Women in London*, Part i (London, 1916)

—— *Report of the Committee on the Medical Education of Women Undergraduates* (London, 1929)

—— *Report of the Committee on the Medical Education of Women Undergraduates* (London, 1942)

—— *Report of the Special Committee of the University of London to Consider the Medical Education of Women in London* (London, 1944)

—— *Minority Report of the Special Committee of the University of London to Consider the Medical Education of Women in London* (London, 1944)

—— *The Best Medicine for London* (London, 1989)

Wrottesley, John and Samuel Smith, 'St Bartholomew's Hospital', *32nd Report of the Charity Commissions*, Part vi (London, 1840)

Post-1948 printed books and articles

Dr Anthony Dawson: 21 Years at Bart's (London, 1986)

Edinburgh Declaration, World Conference on Medical Education (s.n., 1988)

Fifty Years of Medicine (London, 1950)

The Hospital Building Programme: A Revision of the Hospital Plan for England and Wales (London, 1966)

In the Patient's Interests, Multi-professional Working across Organisational Boundaries (London, 1996)

London Medical Education – A New Framework (London, 1980)

'Physicians for the Twenty First Century', *Report of the Panel on the General Professional Education of the Physician and College Preparation for Medicine*, (s.n., 1984)

Proceedings of the Twenty-fifth Annual Conference on Research in Medical Education (Washington, 1986)

Review of Medical Services in Great Britain (London, 1963)

Undergraduate Medical Education in General Practice (Exeter, 1984)

The University and Health Care in London (London, 1976)

Abel-Smith, Brian, *The Hospitals, 1800–1948: A Study in Social Administration in England and Wales* (London, 1964)

Ackerknecht, Erwin H., *Medicine at the Paris Hospital, 1794–1848* (Baltimore, 1967)

Aldcroft, Derek H., *From Versailles to Wall Street, 1919–1929* (London, 1977)

Allsop, Judith, 'Health: From Seamless Service to Patchwork Quilt', *British Social Welfare*, ed. David Gladstone (London, 1995), pp. 98–123.

Anderson, John and Frederick John Roberts, *A New Look at Medical Education* (London, 1965)

Anderson, R. D., *The Student Community at Aberdeen, 1860–1939* (Aberdeen, 1988)

——*Universities and Elites in Britain since 1800* (Cambridge, 1992)

Ashby, Eric and Mary Anderson, *The Rise of the Student Estate in Britain* (Basingstoke, 1970)

Austoker, Joan, 'The Politics of Cancer Research', *Bulletin of the Society for the Social History of Medicine* xxxvii (1985), pp. 63–7

—— *A History of the Imperial Cancer Research Fund, 1902–1986* (Oxford, 1988)

—— 'Walter Morley Fletcher and the Origins of a Basic Biomedical Research Policy', in *Historical Perspectives on the Role of the Medical Research Council: Essays in the History of the Medical Research Council*, ed. Joan Austoker and Linda Bryder (Oxford, 1989), pp. 23–35

Babaei-Mahani, L., 'Evaluation of a Health Advocate's Training Course', *Medical Education* xxvi (1992), pp. 71–2

Barr, Hugh and Ian Shaw, *Shared Learning* (London, 1995)

Bashford, Alison, *Purity and Pollution: Gender, Embodiment and Victorian Medicine* (Basingstoke, 1998)

Bearn, Alexander G. and Elizabeth D. Miller, 'Archibald Garrod and the Development of the Concept of Inborn Errors of Metabolism', *BHM* liii (1979), 315–28

Becker, Howard S, Blanche Geer, Everett C. Hughes and Anselm L. Strauss, *Boys in White. Student Culture in Medical School* (Chicago, 1961)

Bell, E. Moberly, *Storming the Citadel: The Rise of the Woman Doctor* (London, 1953)

Berridge, Virginia, *Health and Society in Britain Since 1939* (Cambridge, 1999)

Blake, Catriona, *The Charge of the Parasols: Women's Entry to the Medical Profession* (London, 1990)

Bliss, Michael, *William Osler: A Life in Medicine* (Oxford, 1999)

Blume, Stuart S., *Insight and Industry: On the Dynamic of Technological Change in Medicine* (Cambridge, Mass., 1992)

Bonner, Thomas N., 'Abraham Flexner as Critic of British and Continental Medical Education', *Medical History* xxxiii (1989), pp. 472–9

—— *To the Ends of the Earth: Women's Search for Education in Medicine* (Cambridge, Mass., 1992)

—— *Becoming a Physician: Medical Education in Britain, France, Germany, and the United States, 1750–1945* (New York, 1995)

Booth, Christopher C., 'Clinical Research', in *Historical Perspectives on the Role of the Medical Research Council: Essays in the History of the Medical Research Council*, ed. Joan Austoker and Linda Bryder (Oxford, 1989), pp. 205–41

—— 'Clinical Research', in *Companion Encyclopaedia of the History of Medicine*, ed. W. F. Bynum and Roy Porter, 2 vols (London, 1997), Vol. 1, pp. 205–29

Bosanquet, Nick, 'The Ailing State of the National Health', in *British Social Attitudes*, ed. R. Jowell, S. Witherspoon and L. Brook (Aldershot, 1988), pp. 93–108

Bourne, Geoffrey, *We Met at Bart's: The Autobiography of a Physician* (London, 1963)

Bradley, James, Anne Crowther and Margaret Dupree, 'Mobility and Selection in Scottish University Medical Education, 1858–1886', *Medical History* xl (1996), pp. 1–24

Brieger, Gert H., '"Fit to Study Medicine"', *BHM* lvii (1983), pp. 1–21

British Medical Association, *Recruitment to the Medical Profession* (London, 1962)

Brock, W. H., 'Science Education', *Companion to the History of Modern Science*, R. C. Olby, G. N. Canto, J. R. R. Christie and M. J. S. Hodge (London, 1990), pp. 946–9

Brooke, Christopher N., *A History of the University of Cambridge* (Cambridge, 1993)

Burgess, Robert G., 'Aspects of Education in Post-war Britain', in *Understanding Postwar Britain*, ed. James Obelkevich and Peter Catteral (London, 1994), pp. 45–64

Burnby, Juanita, 'An Examined and Free Apothecary', in *The History of Medical Education in Britain*, ed. Vivian Nutton and Roy Porter (Amsterdam, 1995), pp. 16–36

Burnett, John, *Plenty and Want: A Social History of Diet in England from 1815 to the Present Day* (London, 1979)

Burstyn, Joan, *Victorian Education and the Ideal of Womanhood* (London, 1980)

—— 'Educators' Response to Scientific and Medical Studies of Women in England, 1860–1900', in *Is Higher Education Fair to Women?*, ed. Sandra Acker and David Warren Piper (Guildford, 1984), pp. 65–80

Butler, Stella V. F., 'A Transformation in Training: The Formation of University Medical Faculties in Manchester, Leeds and Liverpool, 1870–84', *Medical History* xxx (1986), pp. 115–32

—— 'Centres and Peripheries: The Development of British Physiology, 1870–1914', *Journal of the History of Biology* xxi (1988), pp. 473–500

Bynum, W. F., *Science and the Practice of Medicine in the Nineteenth Century* (Cambridge, 1994)

—— 'Sir George Newman and the American Way', in *The History of Medical Education in Britain*, ed. Vivian Nutton and Roy Porter (Amsterdam, 1995), pp. 37–50

Bynum, W. F. and Roy Porter, eds, *William Hunter and the Eighteenth-Century Medical World* (Cambridge, 1985)

Calder, Angus, *The People's War: Britain, 1939–45* (London, 1992)

Cameron, H. C., *Mr Guy's Hospital, 1726–1948* (London, 1954)

Cantor, David, 'MRC's Support for Experimental Radiology during the Inter-war Years', in *Historical Perspectives on the Role of the Medical Research Council: Essays in the History of the Medical Research Council*, ed. Joan Austoker and Linda Bryder (Oxford, 1989), pp. 181–204

—— 'Cancer', in *Companion Encyclopaedia of the History of Medicine*, ed. W. F. Bynum and Roy Porter, 2 vols (London, 1997), Vol. 1, pp. 537–61

Carswell, John, *Government and Universities in Britain: Programme and Performance, 1960–1980* (Cambridge, 1985)

Chambers, Peggy, *A Doctor Alone: A Biography of Elizabeth Blackwell, the First Woman Doctor, 1821–1910* (London, 1956)

Chapple, J. A. V., *Science and Literature in the Nineteenth Century* (London, 1986)

Christie, Ronald, *Medical Education and the State* (London, 1969)

Clarke, Peter, *Hope and Glory: Britain, 1900–1990* (London, 1997)

Committee of Vice-chancellors and Principals, *Universities and the Health of the Nation* (London, 1995)

Conrad, Lawrence, Michael Neve, Vivian Nutton, Roy Porter and Andrew Wear, *Western Medical Tradition, 800 BC to AD 1800* (Cambridge, 1996)

Cook, Harold, 'The New Philosophy and Medicine in Seventeenth Century England', in *Reappraisals of the Scientific Revolution*, ed. David Lindberg and Robert Westman (Cambridge, 1990), pp. 397–436

Cooter, Roger, *Cultural Meaning of Popular Science: Phrenology and the Organisation of Consent in Nineteenth-Century Britain* (Cambridge, 1984)

—— *Surgery and Society in Peace and War: Orthopaedics and the Organisation of Modern Medicine, 1880–1948* (Basingstoke, 1993)

—— and Steve Sturdy, 'Science, Scientific Management, and the

Transformation of Medicine in Britain, c.1870–1950', *History of Science* xxxvi (1998), pp. 421–66

Cope, Zachary, 'Surgical Lectures of 150 Years Ago', in *Sidelights on the History of Medicine*, ed. Zachary Cope (London, 1957), pp. 151–60

—— *Royal College of Surgeons of England* (London, 1959)

—— 'Private Medical Schools of London (1746–1914)', in *The Evolution of Medical Education in Britain*, ed. F. N. L. Poynter (London, 1966), pp. 89–109

Crawford, Catherine, 'A Scientific Profession: Medical Reform and Forensic Medicine in British Periodicals of the Early Nineteenth Century', in *British Medicine in an Age of Reform*, ed. Roger French and Andrew Wear (London, 1991), pp. 203–30

Cunningham, Andrew, *The Anatomical Renaissance: The Resurrection of the Anatomical Projects of the Ancients* (Aldershot, 1997)

Cunningham, Andrew and Perry Williams, eds, *The Laboratory Revolution in Medicine* (Cambridge, 1992)

Curthoys, M. C., 'The "Unreformed" Colleges', in *The History of the University of Oxford: Nineteenth Century Oxford*, ed. M. G. Brock and M. C. Curthoys (Oxford, 1997), Vol. 6, pp. 146–73

—— 'The Examination System', in *The History of the University of Oxford: Nineteenth Century Oxford*, ed. M. G. Brock and M. C. Curthoys (Oxford, 1997), Vol. 6, pp. 339–74

Dacre, Jane and M. Nicol, *Clinical Skills: The Learning Matrix for Students of Medicine and Nursing* (Oxford, 1996)

Dainton, Frederick, *Reflections on the Universities and the National Health Service* (London, 1983)

Davidson, Luke, '"Identities Ascertained": British Ophthalmology in the First Half of the Nineteenth Century', *SHM* ix (1996), pp. 313–33

Delamont, Sara, *Knowledgeable Women: Structuralism and the Reproduction of Elites* (London, 1989)

Dewhurst, K., *Dr Thomas Sydenham (1624–1689): His Life and Original Writings* (London, 1966)

Dickens, Charles, *The Pickwick Papers* (Oxford, 1988)

Digby, Anne and Nick Bosanquet, 'Doctors and Patients in an Era of National Health Insurance and Private Practice, 1913–1938', *EcHR* xli (1988), pp. 74–94

—— *Making a Medical Living: Doctors and Patients in the English Market of Medicine, 1720–1911* (Cambridge, 1994)

—— *The Evolution of British General Practice, 1850–1948* (Oxford, 1999)

Donnison, Jean, *Midwives and Medical Men: A History of the Struggle for the Control of Childbirth* (London, 1988)

Draper, F. W., *Four Centuries of Merchant Taylors' School, 1561–1961* (London, 1962)

Dunn, C. L., *The Emergency Medical Services*, 2 vols (London, 1952–3)

Durey, M. J., 'Bodysnatchers and Benthamites: The Implications of the Dead

Body Bill for the London Schools of Anatomy, 1820–42', *London Journal* ii (1976), pp. 200–25

Dwork, Deborah, *War is good for babies and other young children: A History of the Infant and Child Welfare Movement in England, 1898–1918* (London, 1987)

Dyhouse, Carol, *Girls Growing up in Late-Victorian and Edwardian England* (London 1981)

—— 'Storming the Citadel or Storm in a Tea Cup? The Entry of Women into Higher Education, 1860–1920', in *Is Higher Education Fair to Women?*, ed. Sandra Acker and David Warren Piper (Guildford, 1984), pp. 51–64

—— *No Distinction of Sex? Women in British Universities, 1870–1939* (London, 1995)

—— 'Women Students and the London Medical Schools, 1914–39: The Anatomy of a Masculine Culture', *Gender and History* x (1998), pp. 110–32

Eckstein, Harry, *The English Health Service: Its Origins, Structure and Achievements* (Cambridge, Mass., 1958)

Ellis, John, *LHMC, 1785–1985* (London, 1986)

Elston, Mary Ann, 'Women Doctors in a Changing Profession: The Case of Britain', in *Gender, Work and Medicine: Women and the Medical Division of Labour*, ed. Elaine Riska and Katarina Wegar (London, 1993)

Engel, Arthur J., '"Immoral Intentions": The University of Oxford and the Problem of Prostitution, 1827–1914', *Victorian Studies* xxiii (1979–80), pp. 79–107

Feldberg, W. S., 'Henry Hallet Dale', *Biographical Memoirs of the Fellows of the Royal Society* xvi (1970), pp. 77–174

Fisher, Donald, 'The Rockefeller Foundation and the Development of Scientific Medicine in Great Britain', *Minerva* xvi (1978), pp. 20–41

Fissell, M. E., *Patients, Power and the Poor in Eighteenth Century Bristol* (Cambridge, 1991)

Ford, John M. T., ed., *A Medical Student at St Thomas's Hospital, 1801–2: The Weekes Family Letters*, *Medical History* Supplement No. 7 (1987)

Foster, W. D., 'The Early History of Clinical Pathology in Great Britain', *Medical History* iii (1959), pp. 173–87

Foucault, Michel, *The Birth of the Clinic: An Archaeology of Medical Perceptions*, trans. A. M. Sheridan (London, 1972)

Fox, Daniel M., *Health Policies, Health Politics: The Experience of Britain and America, 1911–1965* (Princeton, 1986)

—— 'The National Health Service and the Second World War: The Elaboration of Consensus', in *War and Social Change: British Society in the Second World War*, ed. Harold L. Smith (Manchester, 1986), pp. 32–57

Fraser, Derek, *The Evolution of the British Welfare State: A History of Social Policy Since the Industrial Revolution* (London, 1984)

French, Roger, 'The Anatomical Tradition', in *Companion Encyclopaedia of the History of Medicine*, ed. W. F. Bynum and Roy Porter, 2 vols (London, 1994), Vol. 1, pp. 81–101

French, Roger and Andrew Wear, eds, *The Medical Revolution of the Seventeenth Century* (Cambridge, 1989)

Garner, James Stuart, 'The Great Experiment: The Admission of Women Students to St Mary's Hospital Medical School, 1916–25', *Medical History* xlii (1998), pp. 68–88

Geison, Gerald L., 'Social and Institutional Factors in the Stagnancy of English Physiology, 1840–1870', *BHM* xlvi (1972), pp. 30–58

—— *Michael Foster and the Cambridge School of Physiology: The Scientific Enterprise in Late Victorian Society* (Princeton, 1978)

—— 'Scientific Change, Emerging Specialties, and Research Schools', *History of Science* ix (1981), pp. 20–40

Gelfand, Toby, 'The "Paris Manner" of Dissection: Student Anatomical Dissection in Early Eighteenth-century Paris', *BHM* xlvi (1972), pp. 99–130

—— *Professionalising Modern Medicine: Paris Surgeons and Medicine Science and Institutions in the Eighteenth Century* (Westport, Conn., 1980)

—— '"Invite the Philosopher, as well as the Charitable": Hospital Teaching as Private Enterprise in Hunterian London', in *William Hunter and the Eighteenth-Century Medical World*, ed. W. F. Bynum and Roy Porter (Cambridge, 1985), pp. 129–51

Getz, Faye, 'John Mirfield and the *Breviarium Bartholomei*: The Medical Writings of a Clerk at St Bartholomew's Hospital in the Later Fourteenth Century', *Bulletin (Society for the Social History of Medicine)* xxxvii (1985), pp. 24–6

—— 'Charity, Translation and the Language of Medical Learning in Medieval England', *BHM* lxiv (1990), pp. 1–17

GMC, *Recommendations as to the Medical Curriculum* (London, 1957)

—— *Recommendations as to Basic Medical Education* (London, 1967)

—— *Recommendations on Basic Medical Education* (London, 1980)

—— *The Teaching of Behavioural Sciences, Community Medicine and General Practice in Basic Medical Education* (London, 1987)

—— *Tomorrow's Doctors: Recommendations on Undergraduate Medical Education* (London, 1993)

Gow, A. S. F., *Letters from Cambridge, 1939–1944* (London, 1945)

Granshaw, Lindsay, '"Fame and fortune by means of bricks and mortar": The Medical Profession and Specialist Hospitals in Britain, 1800–1948', in *The Hospital in History*, ed. Lindsay Granshaw and Roy Porter (London, 1989), pp. 199–220

—— '"Upon this principle I have based a practice": The Development and Reception of Antisepsis in Britain, 1867–90', in *Medical Innovation in Historical Perspective*, ed. John V. Pickstone (Basingstoke, 1992), pp. 17–46

—— 'The Rise of the Modern Hospital in Britain', in *Medicine in Society: Historical Essays*, ed. Andrew Wear (Cambridge, 1994), pp. 197–218

Glynn, Sean, 'The Establishment of Higher Education in London', in *London Higher*, ed. Roderick Floud and Sean Glynn (London, 1998), pp. 1–35

Graham, George, 'The Formation of the Medical and Surgical Professorial Units in the London Teaching Hospitals', *Annals of Science* xxvi (1970), pp. 1–22

Haigh, Elizabeth, 'William Brande and the Chemical Education of Medical Students', in *British Medicine in an Age of Reform*, ed. Roger French and Andrew Wear (London, 1991), pp. 186–202

Haldane, Richard B., *Education and Empire: Addresses on Certain Topics of the Day* (London, 1902)

—— *An Autobiography* (London, 1929)

Hall-Turner, W., 'An Experimental Assessment Carried out in an Undergraduate General Practice Teaching Course', *Medical Education* xvii (1983), pp. 112–19

Halsey, A. H., *Decline of Donnish Dominion: The British Academic Professions in the Twentieth Century* (Oxford, 1992)

Ham, Christopher, *Policy-Making in the National Health Service: A Case Study of the Leeds Regional Hospital Board* (London, 1981)

——, Frank Honigsbaum and David Thompson, 'Priority Setting for Health Gain', in *Politics of the Welfare State*, ed. Ann Oakley and A. Susan Williams (London, 1994), pp. 98–126

Hamad, B., 'Community-oriented Medical Education: What is it?', *Medical Education* xxv (1991), pp. 16–22

Hammerstein, Notker, 'The Modern World, Sciences, Medicine and Universities', *History of Universities* viii (1989), pp. 151–78

Hannaway, Caroline and Ann La Berge, eds, *Constructing Paris Medicine* (Amsterdam, 1998)

Hannay, David, 'University Medical Education and General Practice', in *General Practice under the National Health Service, 1848–1997*, ed. Irvine Loudon, John Horder and Charles Webster (Oxford, 1998), pp. 165–81

Hannay, David and P. D. Campion, 'University Departments of General Practice', *British Journal of General Practice* xlvi (1996), pp. 35–6

Harden, R. M. and F. A. Glesson, 'Assessment of Clinical Competence Using an Objective Structured Clinical Examination', *Medical Education* xiii (1979), pp. 41–54

——, Susette Sowden and W. R. Dunn, 'Some Educational Strategies in Curriculum Development', *Medical Education* xviii (1984), pp. 284–97

Hardy, Anne, 'On the Cusp: Epidemiology and Bacteriology at the Local Government Board, 1890–1905', *Medical History* xlii (1998), pp. 328–46

Harris, José, *Private Lives, Public Spirit: Britain, 1870–1914* (London, 1994)

Harrison, Barbara, 'Women and Health', in *Women's History: Britain, 1850–1945: An Introduction*, ed. June Purvis (London, 1995), pp. 157–92

Harrison, Brian, *Drink and the Victorians: The Temperance Question in England, 1815–1872* (Pittsburgh, 1971)

Harte, Negley, *The University of London, 1836–1986* (London, 1986)

Hays, J. N., 'The London Lecturing Empire, 1800–50', in *Metropolis and*

Provinces: Science in British Culture, 1780–1850, ed. Ian Inkster and Jack Morrell (Philadelphia, 1983), pp. 91–119

Heyck, T. W., *Transformation of Intellectual Life in Victorian England* (London, 1982)

Holloway, S. W. F., 'The Apothecaries Act, 1815: A Reinterpretation', *Medical History* x (1966), pp. 107–29, 221–36

Holt, R. J., *Sport and the British: A Modern History* (Oxford, 1989)

Honigsbaum, Frank, *Health, Happiness and Security: The Creation of the National Health Service* (London, 1989)

Howarth, Janet, 'Science Education in late-Victorian Oxford: A Curious Case of Failure?', *EHR* cii (1987), pp. 334–71

Humphries, Stephen, *Hooligans or Rebels? An Oral History of Working-class Childhood and Youth, 1889–1939* (Oxford, 1995)

Iliffe, S., 'All That is Solid Melts in Air – The Implications of Community Based Undergraduate Medical Education', *British Journal of General Practice* xlii (1992), pp. 390–3

Inkster, Ian, 'Marginal Men: Aspects of the Social Role of Medical Community in Sheffield, 1780–1850', in *Health Care and Popular Medicine in Nineteenth Century England: Essays in the Social History of Medicine*, ed. John Woodward and David Richards (New York, 1977), pp. 128–63

Jacyna, L. S., 'Principles of General Physiology: The Comparative Dimension to British Neuroscience in the 1830s and 1840s', *Studies in the History of Biology* vii (1984), pp. 47–92

—— 'The Laboratory and the Clinic: The Impact of Pathology on Surgical Diagnosis in the Glasgow Western Infirmary, 1875–1910', *BHM* lxii (1988), pp. 384–406

Johnson G. and J. Reynard, 'Assessment of an Objective Structured Clinical Examination', *Journal of Accident Emergence Medicine* xi (1994), pp. 223–6

Jolly, Brian and Lesley Rees, *Room for Improvement* (London, 1984)

Jolly, Brian and Margaret Macdonald, 'Education for Practice', *Medical Education* xxiii (1989), pp. 189–95

Jones, Colin, 'Montpellier Medical Students and the Medicalisation of Eighteenth- Century France', in *Problems and Methods in the History of Medicine*, ed. Roy Porter and Andrew Wear (London, 1987), pp. 57–80

Jones, David R., *The Origins of Civic Universities: Manchester, Liverpool and Leeds* (London, 1988)

Jones, H. S., 'Student Life and Sociability 1860–1930', *History of Universities* xiv (1995/6), pp. 225–46

Jones, Kathleen, *The Making of Social Policy in Britain, 1830–1990* (London, 1991)

Jones, Noel and Parry Jones, *The Rise of the Medical Profession: A Study of Collective Social Mobility* (London, 1976)

Jones, Peter Murray, 'Reading Medicine in Tudor Cambridge', in *The History of Medical Education in Britain*, ed. Vivian Nutton and Roy Porter (Amsterdam, 1995), pp. 153–83

Kelly, Thomas, *Early Public Libraries: A History of Public Libraries in Britain before 1850* (London, 1966)

Kent, Susan Kingsley, *Making Peace: The Reconstruction of Gender in Interwar Britain* (Princeton, 1993)

Kershen, Anne J., 'Higher Education in the London Community', in *London Higher*, ed. Roderick Floud and Sean Glynn (London, 1998), pp. 77–95

Keynes, George, *The Life of William Harvey* (Oxford, 1966)

—— *The Gates of Memory* (Oxford, 1981)

Kidd, Alan J., 'Philanthropy and the "Social History Paradigm"', *Social History* xxi (1996), pp. 180–92

King's Fund, *London Health 2010 – The Report of the King's Fund London Initiative* (London, 1992)

Klein, Rudolf, *The New Politics of the NHS* (London, 1995)

Kohler, Robert E., 'Walter Fletcher, F. G. Hopkins and the Dunn Institute of Biochemistry: A Case Study in the Patronage of Science', *Isis* lxix (1978), pp. 331–55

Land, Andrew, Rodney Lowe and Noel Whiteside, *The Development of the Welfare State, 1939–1951* (London, 1992)

Lane, Joan, 'The Role of Apprenticeship in Eighteenth-Century Medical Education in England', in *William Hunter and the Eighteenth Century Medical World*, ed. W. F. Bynum and Roy Porter (Cambridge, 1985), pp. 57–103

Lawrence, Christopher, 'Incommunicable Knowledge: Science, Technology and Clinical Art in Britain, 1850–1914', *Journal of Contemporary History* xx (1985), pp. 503–20

—— 'Alexander Monro *Primus* and the Edinburgh Manner of Anatomy', *BHM* lxii (1988), pp. 193–214

—— *Medicine in the Making of Modern Britain, 1700–1920* (London, 1994)

—— 'Still Incommunicable: Clinical Holists and Medical Knowledge in Interwar Britain', in *Greater than the Parts: Holism in Biomedicine, 1920–1950*, ed. Christopher Lawrence and George Weisz (Oxford, 1998), pp. 94–112

——'A Tale of Two Sciences: Bedside and Bench in Twentieth Century Britain', *Medical History* xliii (1999), pp. 421–49

—— and R. Dixley, 'Practising on Principle: Joseph Lister and the Germ Theories of Diseases', in *Medical Theory; Surgical Practice: Studies in the History of Surgery*, ed. Christopher Lawrence (London, 1992), pp. 153–215

Lawrence, Susan C., '"Desirous of Improvement in Medicine": Pupils and Practitioners in the Medical Societies at Guy's and St Bartholomew's Hospitals, 1795–1815', *BHM* lix (1985), pp. 89–104

—— 'Entrepreneurs and Private Enterprise: The Development of Medical Lecturing in London, 1775–1820', *BHM* lxii (1988), pp. 171–92

—— 'Private Enterprise and Public Interest: Medical Education and the Apothecaries' Act, 1780–1825', in *British Medicine in an Age of Reform*, ed. Roger French and Andrew Wear (London, 1991), pp. 45–73

—— 'Educating the Senses: Students, Teachers and Medical Rhetoric in Eighteenth Century London', in *Medicine and the Five Senses*, ed. W. F. Bynum and Roy Porter (Cambridge, 1993), pp. 154–78

—— 'Medical Education', in *Companion Encyclopaedia of the History of Medicine*, ed. W. F. Bynum and Roy Porter, 2 vols (London, 1994) Vol 2, pp. 1151–79

—— 'Anatomy and Address: Creating Medical Gentlemen in Eighteenth Century London', in *The History of Medical Education in Britain*, ed. Vivian Nutton and Roy Porter (Amsterdam, 1995), pp. 199–228

—— *Charitable Knowledge: Hospital Pupils and Practitioners in Eighteenth-Century London* (Cambridge, 1996)

Leader, Damian, *A History of the University of Cambridge* (Cambridge, 1988)

L'Esperance, Jean, 'Doctors and Women in Nineteenth-Century Society: Sexuality and Role', in *Health Care and Popular Medicine in Nineteenth Century England: Essays in the Social History of Medicine*, ed. John Woodward and David Richards (New York, 1977), pp. 105–27

Le Grand, Julian, David Winter and Francis Woolley, 'The National Health Service: Safe in Whose Hands?', in *The State of Welfare: The Welfare State in Britain Since 1974*, ed. John Hills (Oxford, 1990), pp. 88–134

Le Quesne, L. P., 'Medicine', in *The University and the World of Learning*, ed. F. M. L. Thompson (London, 1990), pp. 125–45

Levine, Philippa, *Feminist Lives in Victorian England: Private Roles and Public Commitment* (Oxford, 1990)

Lewis, Jane, *Politics of Motherhood: Child and maternal welfare in England, 1900–1939* (London, 1980)

—— 'The Public's Health: Philosophy and Practice in Britain in the Twentieth Century', in *A History of Education in Public Health*, ed. Elizabeth Fee and R. Acheson (Oxford, 1991), pp. 195–229

Loudon, Irvine, *Medical Care and the General Practitioner, 1750–1850* (Oxford, 1986)

—— *Death in Childbirth: An International Study of Maternal Care and Maternal Mortality, 1800–1950* (Oxford, 1992)

—— 'Medical Practitioners and Medical Reform in Britain 1750–1850', in *Medicine in Society: Historical Essays*, ed. Andrew Wear (Cambridge, 1994), pp. 219–37

—— and Jean Loudon, 'Medicine, Politics and the Medical Periodicals 1800–50', in *Medical Journals and Medical Knowledge: Historical Essays*, ed. W. F. Bynum, Stephen Lock and Roy Porter (London, 1992), pp. 49–69

Lowerson, John, *Sport and the English Middle Classes, 1870–1914* (Manchester, 1993)

Lowry, Stella, *Medical Education* (London, 1993)

Ludmerer, Kenneth, *Learning to Heal: The Development of American Medical Education* (New York, 1985)

McAvoy, B., 'Teaching Clinical Skills to Medical Students', *Medical Education* xxii (1988), p. 193

McClellan, James E., *Science Reorganised: Scientific Societies in the Eighteenth Century* (New York, 1985)

McCrorie, Peter, F. Lefford and F. Perrin, *Medical Undergraduate Community-Based Teaching* (Dundee, 1991)

McInnes, E M., *St Thomas's Hospital* (London, 1963)

McMenemey, W. H., 'Education and the Medical Reform Movement', in *The Evolution of Medical Education in Britain*, ed. F. N. L. Poynter (London, 1966), pp. 135–54

MacLeod, Roy, 'Support for Victorian Science: The Endowment of Science Movement in Great Britain', *Minerva* iv (1971), pp. 197–230

—— 'Science and Examinations in Victorian England', in *Days of Judgement: Science, Examinations and the Organisation of Knowledge in Late Victorian England*, ed. Roy MacLeod (North Humberside, 1982), pp. 2–23

Mangan, J. A., *Athleticism in the Victorian and Edwardian Public School: The Emergence and Consolidation of an Educational Ideology* (Cambridge, 1981)

Mansell, A. L., 'Examinations and Medical Education: The Preliminary Sciences in the Examinations of London University and the English Conjoint Board, 1861–1911', in *Days of Judgement: Science, Examinations and the Organisation of Knowledge in Late Victorian England*, ed. Roy MacLeod (North Humberside, 1982), pp. 87–107

Manton, J., *Elizabeth Garrett Anderson* (New York, 1965)

Marks, Lara, 'Mothers, Babies and Hospitals: "The London" and the Provision of Maternity Care in East London, 1870–1939', in *Women and Children First: International Maternal and Infant Welfare, 1870–1945*, ed. Valerie Fildes, Lara Marks and Hilary Marland (London, 1992), pp. 48–73

—— *Metropolitan Maternity: Maternal and Infant Welfare Services in Early-Twentieth Century London* (Amsterdam, 1996)

Marland, Hilary, *Medicine and Society in Wakefield and Huddersfield, 1780–1870* (Cambridge, 1987)

Maulitz, Russell, '"Physician versus Bacteriologist": The Ideology of Science in Clinical Medicine', in *The Therapeutic Revolution*, ed. Morris J. Vogel and Charles E. Rosenberg (Philadelphia, 1979), pp. 91–107

—— *Morbid Appearances: The Anatomy of Pathology in the Early Nineteenth Century* (Cambridge, 1987)

Medvei, Victor and John Thornton, *The Royal Hospital of Saint Bartholomew's, 1123–1973* (London, 1974)

Merrington, W. R., *University College Hospital and its Medical School: A History* (London, 1976)

Merton, R. K., George C. Reader and Patricia L. Kendall, *The Student-Physician. Introductory Studies in the Sociology of Medical Education* (Cambridge: Mass., 1957)

Mitchell, David, *Women on the Warpath: The Story of the Women of the First World War* (London, 1966)

Mohan, John, *A National Health Service? The Restructuring of Health Care in Britain since 1979* (London, 1995)

Morrell, Jack, 'The Chemist Breeders: The Research Schools of Liebig and Thomson', *Ambix* xix (1972), pp. 1–46

—— *Science at Oxford, 1914–1939: Transforming an Arts University* (Oxford, 1997)

Moscucci, Ornella, *The Science of Woman: Gynaecology and Gender in England, 1800–1929* (Cambridge, 1990)

Moss, G. P. and M. V. Saville, *From Palace to College: An Illustrated Account of Queen Mary College* (London, 1985)

Murley, Reginald, 'Breast Cancer: Keynes and Conservatism', *British Journal of Clinical Practice* xl (1986), pp. 49–58

Nead, Lynda, *Myths of Sexuality: Representations of Women in Victorian Britain* (Oxford, 1988)

Newble, David, Brian Jolly and Richard Wakeford, eds, *Certification and Recertification in Medicine* (Cambridge, 1994)

Newman, Charles, *Evolution of Medical Education in the Nineteenth Century* (London, 1957)

Noack, Horst, ed., *Medical Education and Primary Health Care* (London, 1980)

Nutton, Vivian, ed., *Medicine at the Courts of Europe, 1500–1837* (London, 1989)

Ormerod, Henry A., *Early History of the Liverpool Medical School from 1834 to 1877* (Liverpool, 1953)

Oswald, Nigel, 'Long-Term Community-Based Attachments', *Medical Education* xxix (1995), pp. 72–6

—— 'Training Doctors for the National Health Service: Social Medicine, Medical Education and the GMC, 1936–48', in *Social Medicine and Medical Sociology in the Twentieth Century*, ed. Dorothy Porter (Amsterdam, 1997), pp. 59–80

Pater, John E., *The Making of the National Health Service* (London, 1981)

Peachey, George C., *Memoir of William and John Hunter* (Plymouth, 1924)

Pederson, Joyce Senders, *The Reform of Girls' Secondary and Higher Education in Victorian England. A Study of Elites and Educational Change* (New York, 1987)

Pelling, Margaret and Charles Webster, 'Medical Practitioners', in *Health, Medicine and Mortality in the Sixteenth Century*, ed. Charles Webster (Cambridge, 1979), pp. 165–235

—— 'Medical Practice in Early Modern England: Trade or Profession?', in *The Professions in Early Modern England*, ed. Wilfred Prest (London, 1987), pp. 90–128

—— 'Knowledge Common and Acquired: The Education of Unlicensed Medical Practitioners in Early-Modern London', in *The History of Medical Education in Britain*, ed. Vivian Nutton and Roy Porter (Amsterdam, 1995), pp. 250–79

Pennington, T. H., 'Listerism, its Decline and its Persistence: The Introduction of Aseptic Surgical Techniques in three British Teaching Hospitals, 1890–99', *Medical History* xxxix (1995), pp. 35–60

Pereira Gray, D., 'The Emergence of the Disciplines of General Practice', *Journal of the Royal College of General Practitioners* xxxix (1989), pp. 228–33

Perkin, Harold, *The Rise of Professional Society: England Since 1880* (London, 1989)

Perry, Mark, 'Academic General Practice in Manchester Under the Early NHS: A Failed Experiment in Social Medicine', *SHM* xiii (2000), pp. 111–29

Peterson, M. Jeanne, *The Medical Profession in Mid-Victorian London* (Berkeley, 1978)

—— 'Sir George Paget and Cambridge Medical Education, 1851–1892', in *History of Medical Education*, ed. Teizo Ogawa (Osaka, 1983), pp. 27–54

—— 'Gentlemen and Medical Men: The Problem of Professional Recruitment', *BHM* lviii (1984), pp. 457–73

Phillips, Catherine, *Robert Bridges: A Biography* (Oxford, 1992)

Pickstone, John V., 'Ways of Knowing: Towards a Historical Sociology of Science, Technology and Medicine', *British Journal for the History of Science* xxvi (1993), pp. 433–58

Porter, Dorothy, 'Changing Disciplines: John Ryle and the Making of Social Medicine in Britain in the 1940s', *History of Science* xxx (1992), pp. 137–64

Porter, Roy, 'William Hunter: A Surgeon and a Gentleman', in *William Hunter and the Eighteenth-Century Medical World*, ed. W. F. Bynum and Roy Porter (Cambridge, 1985), pp. 7–34

—— *London: A Social History* (London, 1994)

—— 'Medical Lecturing in Georgian London', *British Journal of the History of Science* xxviii (1995), pp. 91–9

—— *The Greatest Benefit of Mankind* (London, 1997)

Preston-Whyte, F., 'Training for Medical Teachers: A UK Survey (Briggs et al.)', *Medical Education* xxviii (1994), pp. 99–106

Prochaska, Frank K., *Philanthropy and the Hospitals of London: The King's Fund, 1897–1990* (Oxford, 1992)

Rather, Lelland, *The Genesis of Cancer: A Study in the History of Ideas* (Baltimore, 1978)

Rawcliffe, Carole, 'The Hospitals of Later Medieval London', *Medical History* xxviii (1984), pp. 1–21

Rees, Lesley and Brian Jolly, 'Medical Education into the Next Century', in *Medical Education in the Millennium*, ed. Lesley Rees and Brian Jolly (Oxford, 1998), pp. 245–59

Reiser, Stanley J., *Medicine and the Reign of Technology* (Cambridge, 1990)

Richardson, Ruth, *Death, Dissection and the Destitute* (London, 1989)

—— '"Trading Assassins" and the Licensing of Anatomy', in *British Medicine in an Age of Reform*, ed. Roger French and Andrew Wear (Cambridge, 1991), pp. 74–91

—— and Brian Hurwitz, 'Celebrating New Year in Bart's Dissecting Room', *Clinical Anatomy* ix (1996), pp. 408–13

Rivett, Geoffrey, *The Development of the London Hospital System, 1823–1982* (London, 1986)

—— *From Cradle to Grave: Fifty Years of the NHS* (London, 1998)

Roach, J. P. C., *Public Examinations in England, 1850–1900* (Cambridge, 1971)

Rose, Craig, 'Politics and the Royal London Hospitals, 1683–92', in *The Hospital in History*, ed. Lindsay Granshaw and Roy Porter (London, 1990), pp. 123–48

Rosner, Lisa, *Medical Education in the Age of Improvement: Edinburgh Students and Apprentices, 1760–1826* (Edinburgh, 1991)

—— 'Student Culture at the Turn of the Century: Edinburgh and Philadelphia', *Caduceus* x (1994), pp. 65–86

Rothblatt, Sheldon, *The Revolution of the Dons: Cambridge and Society in Victorian England* (London, 1968)

—— 'London: A Metropolitan University?', in *The University and the City*, ed. T. Bender (New York, 1988), pp. 119–49

Rothstein, William, *American Medical Schools and the Practice of Medicine* (New York, 1987)

Rupke, Nicholaas A., 'Pro-Vivisection in England in the early 1880s', in *Vivisection in Historical Perspective*, ed. Nicolaas A. Rupke (London, 1987), pp. 188–208

—— *Richard Owen: Victorian Naturalist* (New Haven, 1994)

Rushton, W. A., 'Hamilton Hartridge', *Biographical Memoirs of Fellows of the Royal Society* xxii (1977), pp. 193–211

Sanderson, Michael, ed., *The Universities in the Nineteenth Century* (London, 1975)

Schaffer, Simon, 'Natural Philosophy and Public Spectacle in the Eighteenth Century', *History of Science* xxi (1983), pp. 1–43

Searby, Peter, *A History of the University of Cambridge*, 3 vols (Cambridge, 1997)

Shattock, Michael, *The UGC and the Management of British Universities* (Bristol, 1994)

Sheppard, Francis, *London 1808–1870: The Infernal Wen* (London, 1971)

Shortt, S. E. D., 'Physicians, Science and Status: Issues in the Professionalisation of Anglo-American Medicine in the Nineteenth Century', *Medical History* xxvii (1983), pp. 51–68

Simon, Brian, *Studies in the History of Education, 1780–1870* (London, 1960)

Siraisi, Nancy G., *Medieval and Early Renaissance Medicine: An Introduction to Knowledge and Practice* (Chicago, 1990)

Smith, R. G., 'The Development of Ethical Guidance for Medical Practitioners by the General Medical Council', *Medical History* xxxvii (1993), pp. 56–67

Snow, C. P., *Two Cultures and the Scientific Revolution* (Cambridge, 1959)

Stevens, Rosemary, *Medical Practice in Modern England: The Impact of Specialisation and State Medicine* (Harvard, 1966)

Stow, John, *A Survey of London Written in the Year 1598*, Introduction by Antonia Fraser (Stroud, 1997)

Sturdy, Steve, 'The Political Economy of Scientific Medicine: Science, Education and the Transformation of Medical Practice in Sheffield, 1890–1922', *Medical History* xxxiv (1992), pp. 125–99

—— 'From the Trenches to the Hospitals at Home: Physiologists, Clinicians and Oxygen Therapy, 1914–1930', in *Medical Innovations in Historical Perspective*, ed. John V. Pickstone (Basingstoke, 1992), pp. 104–23

—— 'Medical Chemistry and Clinical Medicine: Academics and the Scientisation of Medical Practice in Britain, 1900–25', in *Medicine and Change: Historical and Social Studies of Medical Innovation*, ed. Ilana Löwy (Montrouge, 1993), pp. 352–74

—— 'Hippocrates and State Medicine: George Newman outlines the Foundling Policy of the Ministry of Health', in *Greater than the Parts: Holism in Biomedicine, 1920–1950*, ed. Christopher Lawrence and George Weisz (Oxford, 1998), pp. 112–34

Sutherland, Gillian, 'The Plainest Principles of Justice: The University of London and the Higher Education of Women', in *University of London and the World of Learning, 1836–1986*, ed. F. M. L. Thompson (London, 1990), pp. 35–56

Sykes, A. H., 'A. D. Walker and the University of London Physiological Laboratory', *Medical History* xxxiii (1989), pp. 217–34

Taylor, David, 'Policing the Community', in *Social Conditions, Status and Community, 1860-c.1920*, ed. Keith Laybourne (Stroud, 1997), pp. 104–22

Thompson, E. P. and E. Yeo, eds, *The Unknown Mayhew: Selections from the Morning Chronicle, 1849–50* (London, 1973)

Thornton, John, *John Abernethy: A Biography* (London, 1953)

Timmins, Nicholas, *The Five Giants: A Biography of the Welfare State* (London, 1995)

Towle, Angela, *Undergraduate Medical Education: London and the Future* (London, 1992)

—— *Community-Based Teaching* (London, 1992)

Tranter, N., *Sport, Economy and Society in Britain, 1750–1914* (Cambridge, 1998)

Twigg, John, 'The Limits of "Reform"', *History of Universities* iv (1984), pp. 99–114

—— *A History of Queens' College, Cambridge, 1448–1986* (Woodbridge, 1987)

Van Dalen, J., J. Zuidweg and J. Collett, 'The Curriculum of Communication Skills Teaching at Maastricht Medical School', *Medical Education* xxiii (1989), pp. 55–61

Van Zwanenberg, David, 'The Training and Careers of those Apprenticed to Apothecaries in Suffolk, 1815–1858', *Medical History* xxvii (1983), pp. 139–50

Vernon, Keith, 'Pus, Sewage, Beer and Milk: Microbiology in Britain, 1870–1940', *History of Science* xxviii (1990), pp. 289–325

Waddington, Ivan, 'General Practitioners and Consultants in Early Nineteenth Century England: The Sociology of an Intra-Professional Conflict', in *Health Care and Popular Medicine in Nineteenth Century England: Essays in the Social History of Medicine*, ed. John Woodward and David Richards (New York, 1977), pp. 164–88

—— *The Medical Profession in the Industrial Revolution* (Dublin, 1984)

Waddington, Keir, 'The Nursing Dispute at Guy's Hospital', *Social History of Medicine*, viii (1995), pp. 211–30

—— 'Mayhem and Medical Students: Image, Conduct and Control in the Victorian and Edwardian London Teaching Hospital', *Social History of Medicine* xv (2002), pp. 45–64

Walvin, James, *Leisure and Society, 1839–1950* (London, 1978)

Warner, John Harley, 'Science in Medicine', *Osiris* 2nd ser. 1 (1985), pp. 37–58

—— 'Idea of Science in English Medicine: The "Decline of Science" and the Rhetoric of Reform, 1815–45', in *British Medicine in an Age of Reform*, ed. Roger French and Andrew Wear (Cambridge, 1991), pp. 136–64

—— 'American Doctors in London during the Age of Paris Medicine', in *The History of Medical Education in Britain*, ed. Vivian Nutton and Roy Porter (Amsterdam, 1995), pp. 341–65

Weatherall, Mark W., 'Making Medicine Scientific: Empiricism, Rationality, and Quackery in mid-Victorian Britain', *SHM* ix (1996), pp. 175–94

—— *Gentlemen, Scientists, and Doctors: Medicine at Cambridge, 1800–1940* (Woodbridge, 2000)

Webb-Peploe, M. M., *Challenge of Medical Education* (London, 1976)

Webster, Charles, 'The Medical Profession and its Radical Critics', in *Change and Continuity in Seventeenth Century England*, ed. John E. Hill (London, 1974), pp. 157–78

—— *From Paracelsus to Newton: Magic and the Making of Modern Science* (Cambridge, 1982)

—— *The Health Service since the War*, Vol. 1. *Problems of Health Care. The National Health Service before 1957* (London, 1988)

—— 'Conflict and Consensus: Explaining the British Health Service', *Twentieth Century British History* i (1990), pp. 115–51

—— ed., *Aneurin Bevan on the National Health Service* (Oxford, 1991)

—— *Caring for Health* (Milton Keynes, 1993)

—— *The Health Service Since the War*, Vol. 2. *Government and Health Care: The British National Health Service 1958–1979* (London, 1996)

—— *The National Health Service: A Political History* (Oxford, 1998)

Whitteridge, Gweneth, *William Harvey and the Circulation of the Blood* (London, 1971)

Williams, P. O. and Mary J. Rowe, eds, *Undergraduate Medical Curricula Changes in Britain* (London, 1963)

Witz, Anne, *Professions and Patriarchy* (London, 1992)

Woodward, John, *To do the sick no harm: A Study of the British Voluntary Hospital System to 1875* (London, 1974)

Worboys, Michael, 'Vaccine Therapy and Laboratory Medicine in Edwardian Britain', in *Medical Innovation in Historical Perspective*, ed. John V. Pickstone (Basingstoke, 1992), pp. 84–103

—— *Spreading Germs: Disease Theories and Medical Practice in Britain, 1865–1900* (Cambridge, 2000)

World Health Organisation, *Community-based Education of Health Personnel* (s.n., 1987)

Wormald, Francis and C. Wright, eds, *The English Library before 1700* (London, 1958)

Zuckerman, S. and H. P. Gilding, eds, *Proceedings of the First World Conference on Medical Education* (London, 1954)

Unpublished theses, books and papers

Bates, Donald, 'Thomas Sydenham: The Development of his Thought, 1666–1676' (MD, Baltimore, 1975)

Butler, Stella V. F., 'Science and the Education of Doctors during the Nineteenth Century: A Study of British Medical Schools with Particular Reference to the Development and Uses of Physiology' (Ph.D. diss., UMIST, 1981)

Cassar, Claire L. J., '"Of Mary's and Men": Admissions to the St. Mary's Hospital Medical School "Experience", 1883–1916' (B.Sc. diss., University College London, 1999)

Cunningham, Andrew, 'Aspects of Medical Education in the Seventeenth and Early Eighteenth Centuries' (Ph.D. diss., London, 1974)

Hammer, Margaret A. E., 'The Building of a National's Health: The Life and Work of George Newman to 1921' (Ph.D. diss., Cambridge, 1995)

Kirkpatrick, Robert, 'Nature's Schools: The Hunterian Revolution in London Hospital Medicine, 1780–1825' (Ph.D. diss., Cambridge, 1988)

Lawrence, Susan C., 'Science and Medicine at the London Hospitals: The Development of Teaching and Research, 1750–1815' (Ph.D. diss., Toronto, 1985)

Marks, Lara, 'Irish and Jewish Women's Experience of Childbirth and Infant Care in East London, 1870–1939' (D.Phil. diss., Oxford, 1990)

Richardson, Ruth, 'On the Anatomy Act of 1832' (Ph.D. diss, Sussex, 1982)

Watkin, Dorothy E., 'The English Revolution in Social Medicine, 1889–1911' (Ph.D. diss., London, 1984)

Index

445

report, 408; in wartime, 263, 268, 276, 277–8, 279
University of London Union (ULU), 257
urology, teaching in, 381

vaccine therapy, 154, 155
venereal disease, 103, 186, 205
venereology, 156, 381
Venn, John, 278–9
Vermont, university of, 396
vernacular, medical literature, 14, 19, 43
'Vicarage', 272–3
Vick, Reginald, 145
Vincent, John, 51
Virchow, Rudolf, 99, 106, 135, 137, 138, 149
viva voces, see examinations
vivisection, 123, 127
voluntary hospitals, *see* hospitals, *individual hospitals*
Voluntary Hospitals Committee for London, 192, 290–1

Wakefield, 224
Wakley, Thomas: attitude to St Bartholomew's, 50, 53, 59, 70, 72, 82; dispute with Abernethy, 50, 53; and medical reform, 43, 70–1; student life, 244
Wald, Nicholas, 370
Waller, Augustus, 165
Walsham, William, 97
war, 172; damage, 273–6; First World, 172–3, 176, 183, 222, 248, 256, 262, 296, 303, 306; impact of, 176, 222, 256, 261–87; 296, 303, 306; Second World, 183, 217, 261–87; students and, 222, 256, 269–73, 303; teaching during, 263, 264–9
War Damage Commission, 277, 279
warden, 81, 82–3, 89, 241, 242. *See also* College Hall, James Paget
Waring, Holburt Jacob, 150, 181; and University of London, 150, 163, 164, 165–6, 176
Wass, John, 386
Waterhouse, Alfred, 108
Waterlow, Sydney, 108, 239

Webb, Sidney, 160
Well Street clinic, 396
Wellcome Research Laboratory, 319
Wellcome Trust, 334, 375
West, Charles, 298
West, Samuel Hatch, 90
West Smithfield: conditions in, 190, 213, 236–7; public houses in, 235–6, 271
Westfield College, 303, 408
Westminster Dispensary, 71
Westminster Hospital, 49, 51, 129, 165, 255, 307, 365
Wheeler, Charles, 59
Whitechapel, 235, 361, 407, 411, 413
Wickham Legg, John, 138, 300
Wilkinson, George, 214
Willet, Alfred, 133
William Harvey Research Institute, 375
Willink, Henry, 285
Willink report, 338, 345
Wills, Eric, 396
Winchmore Hill, 246, 255, 257
Witts, Leslie, 198, 199
Wix, Samuel, 85
Wolfson Institute, *see* Institute of Preventive Medicine
Womack, Frederick, 129
women: admissions of to medical schools, 296–312; doctors, attitudes to, 299–302, 304, 305; Goodenough commission and, 307–10; and University Grants Commission (UGC), 307, 309–10, 312; and University of London, 302, 304–10
Women's Guild, 214
Woollard, Herbert, 210, 213, 215, 216–17
World Health Organisation, 391, 395
Wormald, Thomas, 42, 59, 80, 90, 103
Wormall, Arthur, 217, 264; and research, 331, 333
Wright, Almroth, 154, 248
Wykeham Balme, Harold, 311

X-ray, 202; therapy, 203–4, 332–3

Zachray Merton Convalescent Home, 294
zoology, department of, 316, 375; lectures on, 127